FIFTH EDITION

CASE FILES®
Internal Medicine

Eugene C. Toy, MD
Assistant Dean for Educational Programs
Director of Doctoring Courses
Director of Scholarly Concentrations in
    Women's Health
Professor and Vice Chair of Medical Education
Department of Obstetrics and Gynecology
McGovern Medical School at The University
    of Texas Health Science Center at Houston
    (UTHealth)
Houston, Texas

John T. Patlan Jr., MD
Associate Professor of Medicine
Department of General Internal Medicine
MD Anderson Cancer Center
Houston, Texas

Mark T. Warner, MD
Assistant Professor
Division of Critical Care Medicine
Department of Internal Medicine
McGovern Medical School at The University
    of Texas Health Science Center at Houston
    (UTHealth)
Houston, Texas

Mc
Graw
Hill
Education

New York   Chicago   San Francisco   Athens   London   Madrid   Mexico City
Milan   New Delhi   Singapore   Sydney   Toronto

Notice

Medicine is an ever-changing science. As new research and clinical experience broaden our knowledge, changes in treatment and drug therapy are required. The authors and the publisher of this work have checked with sources believed to be reliable in their efforts to provide information that is complete and generally in accord with the standard accepted at the time of publication. However, in view of the possibility of human error or changes in medical sciences, neither the editors nor the publisher nor any other party who has been involved in the preparation or publication of this work warrants that the information contained herein is in every respect accurate or complete, and they disclaim all responsibility for any errors or omissions or for the results obtained from use of the information contained in this work. Readers are encouraged to confirm the information contained herein with other sources. For example and in particular, readers are advised to check the product information sheet included in the package of each drug they plan to administer to be certain that the information contained in this work is accurate and that changes have not been made in the recommended dose or in the contraindications for administration. This recommendation is of particular importance in connection with new or infrequently used drugs.

This book was set in Adobe Jenson Pro by Cenveo® Publisher Services.
The editors were Catherine A. Johnson and Cindy Yoo.
The production supervisor was Catherine H. Saggese.
Project management was provided by Raghavi Khullar, Cenveo Publisher Services.
RR Donnelley was printer and binder.

Library of Congress Cataloging-in-Publication Data

Names: Toy, Eugene C., author. | Patlan, John T., Jr., author. | Warner, Mark (Mark T.), author.
Title: Case files. Internal medicine / Eugene C. Toy, John T. Patlan Jr., Mark Warner.
Other titles: Internal medicine
Description: Fifth edition. | New York : McGraw-Hill Education, [2017] |
   Includes bibliographical references and index.
   Identifiers: LCCN 2016022294| ISBN 9780071843355 (pbk.) | ISBN 0071843353
Subjects: | MESH: Internal Medicine | Diagnosis, Differential | Physical
   Examination | Problems and Exercises | Case Reports
Classification: LCC RC66 | NLM WB 18.2 | DDC 616—dc23 LC record available at
   https://lccn.loc.gov/2016022294

*To our coach Victor, and our father-son teammates Bob & Jackson,
Steve & Weston, Ron & Wesley, and Dan & Joel. At the inspirational JH Ranch
Father-Son Retreat, all of us, including my loving son Andy, arrived as strangers,
but in 6 days, we left as lifelong friends.*

– ECT

*To my parents who instilled an early love of learning and of the written word,
and who continue to serve as role models for life.*

*To my beautiful wife Elsa and children Sarah and Sean,
for their patience and understanding, as precious family time was
devoted to the completion of "the book."*

*To all my teachers, particularly Drs. Carlos Pestaña, Robert Nolan,
Herbert Fred, and Cheves Smythe, who make the complex understandable,
and who have dedicated their lives to the education of physicians,
and served as role models of healers.*

*To the medical students and residents at the
McGovern Medical School at The University of Texas
Health Science Center at Houston (UTHealth) whose enthusiasm, curiosity,
and pursuit of excellent and compassionate care provide
a constant source of stimulation, joy, and pride.*

*To all readers of this book everywhere in the hopes that it might help them
to grow in wisdom and understanding,
and to provide better care for their patients
who look to them for comfort and relief of suffering.*

*And to the Creator of all things, Who is the source of all knowledge
and healing power, may this book serve as an instrument of His will.*

– JTP

*To my beloved wife, Dean-na, and my lovely daughter, Kayley,
forever gratitude for your undying love and support in this journey.
You two have provided me the necessary margin and energy
to complete this task and furthered my ability
to continue on in the pursuit of Medicine.*

– MTW

CONTENTS

Javier Barreda-Garcia, MD
Assistant Professor of Medicine
Divisions of Critical Care, Pulmonary and Sleep Medicine
McGovern Medical School at the University of Texas Health Science Center at
Houston (UTHealth)
Houston, Texas
Tuberculosis (Pulmonary), Cavitary Lung Lesions

Sujith Cherian, MD
Assistant Professor of Medicine
Divisions of Critical Care, Pulmonary and Sleep Medicine
McGovern Medical School at the University of Texas Health Science Center at
Houston (UTHealth)
Houston, Texas
Pleural Effusion, Parapneumonic Effusions

Rosa M. Estrada-Y-Martin, MD, MSc, CMQ, FCCP
Associate Professor of Medicine
Divisions of Critical Care, Pulmonary and Sleep Medicine
McGovern Medical School at the University of Texas Health Science Center at
Houston (UTHealth)
Houston, Texas
HIV and Pneumocystis Pneumonia

Reeba Mathew, MD
Assistant Professor of Medicine
Divisions of Critical Care, Pulmonary and Sleep Medicine
McGovern Medical School at the University of Texas Health Science Center at
Houston (UTHealth)
Houston, Texas
Chronic Cough/Asthma

Sandeep Sahay, MD
Assistant Professor of Medicine
Divisions of Critical Care, Pulmonary and Sleep Medicine
Baylor College of Medicine
Houston, Texas
Chronic Obstructive Pulmonary Disease

Mary Alice Sallman, MS4
Medical Student, Class of 2017
McGovern Medical School at the University of Texas
Health Science Center at Houston (UTHealth)
Houston, Texas
Review Questions and Answers

Lilit Sargsyan, MD
Clinical Fellow, Pulmonary and Critical Care Medicine
McGovern Medical School at the University of Texas Health Science Center at
    Houston (UTHealth)
Houston, Texas
Community-Acquired Pneumonia

Allison L. Toy
Registered Nurse
Baylor Scott & White Hillcrest Medical Center
Waco, Texas
Manuscript Reviewer

Erik Vakil, MD
Clinical Fellow, Pulmonary and Critical Care Medicine
McGovern Medical School at the University of Texas Health Science Center at
    Houston (UTHealth)
Houston, Texas
Hemoptysis, Lung Cancer

I have been deeply amazed and grateful to see how the *Case Files®* books have been so well received, and have helped students to learn more effectively. In the 12 short years since *Case Files®: Internal Medicine* was first printed, the series has now multiplied to span most of the clinical and the basic science disciplines, and has been translated into over a dozen foreign languages. Numerous students have sent encouraging remarks, suggestions, and recommendations. Four completely new cases have been written. The cases have been reorganized into organ systems for better ability to integrate knowledge. Case correlation references are also used in this edition. This fifth edition has been a collaborative work with my wonderful coauthors and contributors, and with the suggestions from five generations of students. Truly, the enthusiastic encouragement from students throughout not just the United States but worldwide provides me the inspiration and energy to continue to write. It is thus with humility that I offer my sincere thanks to students everywhere … for without students, how can a teacher teach?

Eugene C. Toy

The curriculum that evolved into the ideas for this series was inspired by Philbert Yau and Chuck Rosipal, two talented and forthright students, who have since graduated from medical school. It has been a tremendous joy to work with my excellent coauthors, Dr. John Patlan, who exemplifies the qualities of the ideal physician— caring, empathetic, and avid teacher, and who is intellectually unparalleled, and Dr. Mark Warner who has a magnificent grasp of the breadth of medicine and also is an accomplished and passionate educator. Dr. Warner would like to acknowledge Drs. Javier Barreda-Garcia, Rosa Estrada-Y-Martin and Reeba Mathew, wonderful colleagues and contributors, Drs. Erik Vakil and Lilit Sargsyan, colleagues and fellows that continue to teach him and Drs. Sandeep Sahay and Sujith Cherian, wonderful students who have now, themselves, become teachers.

I am greatly indebted to Catherine Johnson, whose exuberance, experience, and vision helped to shape this series. I appreciate McGraw-Hill's believing in the concept of teaching through clinical cases. I am also grateful to Catherine Saggese for her excellent production expertise, and Cindy Yoo for her wonderful and meticulous role as development editor. I cherish the ever-organized and precise project manager, Raghavi Khullar. It has been a privilege and honor to work with one of the brightest medical students I have encountered, Alice Sallman, who directed the review questions and answers, and gave input on the explanations for all the comprehension questions. Most of all, I appreciate my ever-loving wife Terri, and our four wonderful children, Andy and his wife Anna, Michael, Allison, and Christina, for their patience and understanding.

Eugene C. Toy

Mastering the cognitive knowledge within a field such as internal medicine is a formidable task. It is even more difficult to draw on that knowledge, procure and filter through the clinical and laboratory data, develop a differential diagnosis, and, finally, to make a rational treatment plan. To gain these skills, the student learns best at the bedside, guided and instructed by experienced teachers, and inspired toward self-directed, diligent reading. Clearly, there is no replacement for education at the bedside. Unfortunately, clinical situations usually do not encompass the breadth of the specialty. Perhaps the best alternative is a carefully crafted patient case designed to stimulate the clinical approach and the decision-making process. In an attempt to achieve that goal, we have constructed a collection of clinical vignettes to teach diagnostic or therapeutic approaches relevant to internal medicine.

Most importantly, the explanations for the cases emphasize the mechanisms and underlying principles, rather than merely rote questions and answers. This book is organized for versatility: it allows the student "in a rush" to go quickly through the scenarios and check the corresponding answers, and it allows the student who wants thought-provoking explanations to obtain them. The answers are arranged from simple to complex: the bare answers, an analysis of the case, an approach to the pertinent topic, a comprehension test at the end, clinical pearls for emphasis, and a list of references for further reading. The clinical vignettes are purposely placed in random order to simulate the way that real patients present to the practitioner. A listing of cases is included in Section III to aid the student who desires to test his/her knowledge of a certain area, or to review a topic, including basic definitions. Finally, we intentionally did not use a multiple choice question format in the case scenarios, because clues (or distractions) are not available in the real world.

HOW TO GET THE MOST OUT OF THIS BOOK

Each case is designed to simulate a patient encounter with open-ended questions. At times, the patient's complaint is different from the most concerning issue, and sometimes extraneous information is given. The answers are organized into four different parts:

CLINICAL CASE FORMAT: PART I

1. **Summary:** The salient aspects of the case are identified, filtering out the extraneous information. Students should formulate their summary from the case before looking at the answers. A comparison to the summation in the answer will help to improve their ability to focus on the important data, while appropriately discarding the irrelevant information—a fundamental skill in clinical problem solving.
2. **A Straightforward Answer** is given to each open-ended question.

3. The **Analysis of the Case** is comprised of two parts:
   a. **Objectives of the Case:** A listing of the two or three main principles that are crucial for a practitioner to manage the patient. Again, the students are challenged to make educated "guesses" about the objectives of the case upon initial review of the case scenario, which helps to sharpen their clinical and analytical skills.
   b. **Considerations:** A discussion of the relevant points and brief approach to the specific patient.

PART II

Approach to the Disease Process: It consists of two distinct parts:
a. **Definitions:** Terminology pertinent to the disease process.
b. **Clinical Approach:** A discussion of the approach to the clinical problem in general, including tables, figures, and algorithms.

PART III

Comprehension Questions: Each case contains several multiple-choice questions, which reinforce the material, or which introduce new and related concepts. Questions about material not found in the text will have explanations in the answers.

PART IV

Clinical Pearls: Several clinically important points are reiterated as a summation of the text. This allows for easy review, such as before an examination.

LISTING BY CASE NUMBER

LISTING BY DISORDER (ALPHABETICAL)

How to Approach Clinical Problems

Part 1. Approach to the Patient

The transition from the textbook or journal article to the clinical situation is one of the most challenging tasks in medicine. Retention of information is difficult; organization of the facts and recall of a myriad of data in precise application to the patient is crucial. The purpose of this text is to facilitate in this process. The first step is gathering information, also known as establishing the database. This includes taking the history (asking questions), performing the physical examination, and obtaining selective laboratory and/or imaging tests. Of these, the historical examination is the most important and useful. Sensitivity and respect should always be exercised during the interview of patients.

CLINICAL PEARL

▶ The history is the single most important tool in obtaining a diagnosis. All physical findings and laboratory and imaging studies are first obtained and then interpreted in the light of the pertinent history.

HISTORY

1. **Basic information:** Age, gender, and ethnicity must be recorded because some conditions are more common at certain ages; for instance, pain on defecation and rectal bleeding in a 20-year-old may indicate inflammatory bowel disease, whereas the same symptoms in a 60-year-old would more likely suggest colon cancer.

2. **Chief complaint:** What is it that brought the patient into the hospital or clinic? Is it a scheduled appointment, or an unexpected symptom? The patient's own words should be used if possible, such as, "I feel like a ton of bricks are on my chest." The chief complaint, or real reason for seeking medical attention, may not be the first subject the patient talks about (in fact, it may be the last thing), particularly if the subject is embarrassing, such as a sexually transmitted disease, or highly emotional, such as depression. It is often useful to clarify exactly what the patient's concern is, for example, they may fear their headaches represent an underlying brain tumor.

3. **History of present illness:** This is the most crucial part of the entire database. The questions one asks are guided by the differential diagnosis one begins to consider the moment the patient identifies the chief complaint, as well as the clinician's knowledge of typical disease patterns and their natural history. The duration and character of the primary complaint, associated symptoms, and exacerbating/relieving factors should be recorded. Sometimes, the history will be convoluted and lengthy, with multiple diagnostic or therapeutic interventions at different locations. For patients with chronic illnesses, obtaining prior medical records is invaluable. For example, when extensive evaluation of a complicated medical problem has been done elsewhere, it is usually better to

first obtain those results than to repeat a "million-dollar workup." When reviewing prior records, it is often useful to review the primary data (eg, biopsy reports, echocardiograms, serologic evaluations) rather than to rely upon a diagnostic label applied by someone else, which then gets replicated in medical records and by repetition, acquires the aura of truth, when it may not be fully supported by data. Some patients will be poor historians because of dementia, confusion, or language barriers; recognition of these situations and querying of family members is useful. When little or no history is available to guide a focused investigation, more extensive objective studies are often necessary to exclude potentially -serious diagnoses.

4. **Past history:**

   a. **Illness:** Any illnesses such as hypertension, hepatitis, diabetes mellitus, cancer, heart disease, pulmonary disease, and thyroid disease should be elicited. If an existing or prior diagnosis is not obvious, it is useful to ask exactly how it was diagnosed; that is, what investigations were performed. Duration, severity, and therapies should be included.

   b. **Hospitalization:** Any hospitalizations and emergency room (ER) visits should be listed with the reason(s) for admission, the intervention, and the location of the hospital.

   c. **Blood transfusion:** Transfusions with any blood products should be listed, including any adverse reactions.

   d. **Surgeries:** The year and type of surgery should be elucidated and any complications documented. The type of incision and any untoward effects of the anesthesia or the surgery should be noted.

5. **Allergies:** Reactions to medications should be recorded, including severity and temporal relationship to the medication. An adverse effect (such as nausea) should be differentiated from a true allergic reaction.

6. **Medications:** Current and previous medications should be listed, including dosage, route, frequency, and duration of use. Prescription, over-the-counter, and herbal medications are all relevant. Patients often forget their complete medication list; thus, asking each patient to bring in all their medications—both prescribed and nonprescribed—allows for a complete inventory.

7. **Family history:** Many conditions are inherited, or are predisposed in family members. The age and health of siblings, parents, grandparents, and others can provide diagnostic clues. For instance, an individual with first-degree family members with early onset coronary heart disease is at risk for cardiovascular disease.

8. **Social history:** This is one of the most important parts of the history in that the patient's functional status at home, social and economic circumstances, and goals and aspirations for the future are often the critical determinant in what the best way to manage a patient's medical problem is. Living arrangements, economic situations, and religious affiliations may provide important clues for puzzling diagnostic cases, or suggest the acceptability of various diagnostic

or therapeutic options. Marital status and habits such as alcohol, tobacco, or illicit drug use may be relevant as risk factors for disease.

9. **Review of systems:** A few questions about each major body system ensure that problems will not be overlooked. The clinician should avoid the mechanical "rapid-fire" questioning technique that discourages patients from answering truthfully because of fear of "annoying the doctor."

PHYSICAL EXAMINATION

The physical examination begins as one is taking the history, by observing the patient and beginning to consider a differential diagnosis. When performing the physical examination, one focuses on body systems suggested by the differential diagnosis, and performs tests or maneuvers with specific questions in mind; for example, does the patient with jaundice have ascites? When the physical examination is performed with potential diagnoses and expected physical findings in mind ("one sees what one looks for"), the utility of the examination in adding to diagnostic yield is greatly increased, as opposed to an unfocused "head-to-toe" physical.

1. **General appearance:** A great deal of information is gathered by observation, as one notes the patient's body habitus, state of grooming, nutritional status, level of anxiety (or perhaps inappropriate indifference), degree of pain or comfort, mental status, speech patterns, and use of language. This forms your impression of "who this patient is."

2. **Vital signs:** Vital signs like temperature, blood pressure, heart rate, respiratory rate, height, and weight are often placed here. Blood pressure can sometimes be different in the two arms; initially, it should be measured in both arms. In patients with suspected hypovolemia, pulse and blood pressure should be taken in lying and standing positions to look for orthostatic hypotension. It is quite useful to take the vital signs oneself, rather than relying upon numbers gathered by ancillary personnel using automated equipment, because important decisions regarding patient care are often made using the vital signs as an important determining factor.

3. **Head and neck examination:** Facial or periorbital edema and pupillary responses should be noted. Funduscopic examination provides a way to visualize the effects of diseases such as diabetes on the microvasculature; papilledema can signify increased intracranial pressure. Estimation of jugular venous pressure is very useful to estimate volume status. The thyroid should be palpated for a goiter or nodule, and carotid arteries auscultated for bruits. Cervical (common) and supraclavicular (pathologic) nodes should be palpated.

4. **Breast examination:** Inspect for symmetry and for, skin or nipple retraction with the patient's hands on her hips (to accentuate the pectoral muscles) and also with arms raised. With the patient sitting and supine, the breasts should then be palpated systematically to assess for masses. The nipple should be assessed for discharge, and the axillary and supraclavicular regions should be examined for adenopathy.

5. **Cardiac examination:** The point of maximal impulse (PMI) should be ascertained for size and location, and the heart auscultated at the apex of the heart as well as at the base. Heart sounds, murmurs, and clicks should be characterized. Murmurs should be classified according to intensity, duration, timing in the cardiac cycle, and changes with various maneuvers. Systolic murmurs are very common and often physiologic; diastolic murmurs are uncommon and usually pathologic.

6. **Pulmonary examination:** The lung fields should be examined systematically and thoroughly. Wheezes, rales, rhonchi, and bronchial breath sounds should be recorded. Percussion of the lung fields may be helpful in identifying the hyperresonance of tension pneumothorax, or the dullness of consolidated pneumonia or a pleural effusion.

7. **Abdominal examination:** The abdomen should be inspected for scars, distension, or discoloration (such as the Grey Turner sign of discoloration at the flank areas indicating intraabdominal or retroperitoneal hemorrhage). Auscultation of bowel sounds to identify normal versus high-pitched and hyperactive -versus hypoactive. Percussion of the abdomen can be utilized to assess the size of the liver and spleen, and to detect ascites by noting shifting dullness. Careful palpation should begin initially away from the area of pain, involving one hand on top of the other, to assess for masses, tenderness, and peritoneal signs. Tenderness should be recorded on a scale (eg, 1-4 where 4 is the most severe pain). Guarding, and whether it is voluntary or involuntary, should be noted.

8. **Back and spine examination:** The back should be assessed for symmetry, tenderness, and masses. The flank regions are particularly important to assess for pain on percussion, which might indicate renal disease.

9. **Genitalia:**
   a. **Females:** The pelvic examination should include an inspection of the external genitalia, and with the speculum, evaluation of the vagina and cervix. A pap smear and/or cervical cultures may be obtained. A bimanual examination to assess the size, shape, and tenderness of the uterus and adnexa is important.
   b. **Males:** An inspection of the penis and testes is performed. Evaluation for masses, tenderness, and lesions is important. Palpation for hernias in the inguinal region with the patient coughing to increase intraabdominal pressure is useful.

10. **Rectal examination:** A digital rectal examination is generally performed for those individuals with possible colorectal disease, or gastrointestinal bleeding. Masses should be assessed, and stool for occult blood should be tested. In men, the prostate gland can be assessed for enlargement and for nodules.

11. **Extremities:** An examination for joint effusions, tenderness, edema, and cyanosis may be helpful. Clubbing of the nails might indicate pulmonary diseases such as lung cancer or chronic cyanotic heart disease.

12. **Neurologic examination:** Patients who present with neurologic complaints usually require a thorough assessment, including the mental status, cranial nerves, motor strength, sensation, and reflexes.

13. **Skin examination:** The skin should be carefully examined for evidence of pigmented lesions (melanoma), cyanosis, or rashes that may indicate systemic disease (malar rash of systemic lupus erythematosus).

LABORATORY AND IMAGING ASSESSMENT

1. **Laboratory:**

    a. **Complete blood count** (CBC): To assess for anemia and thrombocytopenia.

    b. **Serum chemistry:** Chemistry panel is most commonly used to evaluate renal and liver function.

    c. **Lipid panel:** Lipid panel is particularly relevant in cardiovascular diseases.

    d. **Urinalysis:** Urinalysis is often referred to as a "liquid renal biopsy," because the presence of cells, casts, protein, or bacteria provides clues about underlying glomerular or tubular diseases.

    e. **Infection:** Gram stain and culture of urine, sputum, and cerebrospinal fluid, as well as blood cultures, are frequently useful to isolate the cause of infection.

2. **Imaging procedures:**

    a. **Chest radiography:** Chest radiography is extremely useful in assessing cardiac size and contour, chamber enlargement, pulmonary vasculature and infiltrates, and the presence of pleural effusions.

    b. **Ultrasonographic examination:** Ultrasonographic examination is useful for identifying fluid-solid interfaces, and for characterizing masses as cystic, solid, or complex. It is also very helpful in evaluating the biliary tree, kidney size, and evidence of ureteral obstruction, and can be combined with Doppler flow to identify deep venous thrombosis. Ultrasonography is noninvasive and has no radiation risk, but cannot be used to penetrate through bone or air, and is less useful in obese patients.

CLINICAL PEARL

▶ Ultrasonography is helpful in evaluating the biliary tree, looking for ureteral obstruction, and evaluating vascular structures, but has limited utility in obese patients.

    c. **Computed tomography:** Computed tomography (CT) is helpful in possible intracranial bleeding, abdominal and/or pelvic masses, and pulmonary processes, and may help to delineate the lymph nodes and retroperitoneal -disorders. CT exposes the patient to radiation and requires the patient to be immobilized during the procedure. Generally, CT requires administration of a radiocontrast dye, which can be nephrotoxic.

d. **Magnetic resonance imaging:** Magnetic resonance imaging (MRI) identifies soft-tissue planes very well and provides the best imaging of the brain parenchyma. When used with gadolinium contrast (which is not nephrotoxic), MR angiography (MRA) is useful for delineating vascular structures. MRI does not use radiation, but the powerful magnetic field prohibits its use in patients with ferromagnetic metal in their bodies, for example, many prosthetic devices.

e. **Cardiac procedures:**
   i **Echocardiography:** Uses ultrasonography to delineate the cardiac size, function, ejection fraction, and presence of valvular dysfunction.
   ii **Angiography:** Radiopaque dye is injected into various vessels, and radiographs or fluoroscopic images are used to determine the vascular occlusion, cardiac function, or valvular integrity.
   iii **Stress treadmill tests:** Individuals at risk for coronary heart disease are monitored for blood pressure, heart rate, chest pain, and electrocardiogram (ECG) while increasing oxygen demands on the heart, such as running on a treadmill. Nuclear medicine imaging of the heart can be added to increase the sensitivity and specificity of the test. Individuals who cannot run on the treadmill (such as those with severe arthritis) may be given medications such as adenosine or dobutamine to "stress" the heart.

INTERPRETATION OF TEST RESULTS: USING PRETEST PROBABILITY AND LIKELIHOOD RATIO

Because no test is 100% accurate, it is essential when ordering a test to have some knowledge of the test's characteristics, as well as how to apply the test results to an **individual patient's clinical** situation. Let us use the example of a patient with chest pain. The first diagnostic concern of most patients and physicians regarding chest pain is **angina pectoris**, that is, the pain of myocardial ischemia caused by coronary insufficiency. Distinguishing angina pectoris from other causes of chest pain relies upon two important factors: the clinical history, and an understanding of how to use objective testing. In making the diagnosis of angina pectoris, the clinician must establish whether the pain satisfies the **three criteria for typical anginal pain:** (1) retrosternal in location, (2) precipitated by exertion, and (3) relieved within minutes by rest or nitroglycerin. Then, the clinician considers other factors, such as patient age and other risk factors, to determine a **pretest probability** for angina pectoris.

After a pretest probability is estimated by applying some combination of statistical data, epidemiology of the disease, and clinical experience, the next decision is whether and how to use an objective test. **A test should only be ordered if the results would change the posttest probability high enough or low enough in either direction that it will affect the decision-making process.** For example, a 21-year-old woman with chest pain that is not exertional and not relieved by rest or nitroglycerin has a very low pretest probability of coronary artery disease, and any positive results on a cardiac stress test are very likely to be false positive. Any test result is unlikely to change her management; thus, the test should not be obtained.

Similarly, a 69-year-old diabetic smoker with a recent coronary angioplasty who now has recurrent episodes of typical angina has a very high pretest probability that the pain is a result of myocardial ischemia. One could argue that a negative cardiac stress test is likely to be falsely negative, and that the clinician should proceed directly to a coronary angiography to assess for a repeat angioplasty. **Diagnostic tests, therefore, are usually most useful for those patients** in the midranges of pretest probabilities in whom a positive or negative test will move the clinician past some decision threshold.

In the case of diagnosing a patient with atherosclerotic coronary artery disease (CAD), one test that is frequently used is the exercise treadmill test. Patients are monitored on an electrocardiogram, while they perform graded exercise on a treadmill. A positive test is the development of ST-segment depression during the test; the greater the degree of ST depression, the more useful the test becomes in raising the posttest probability of CAD. In the example illustrated by Figure I–1, if a

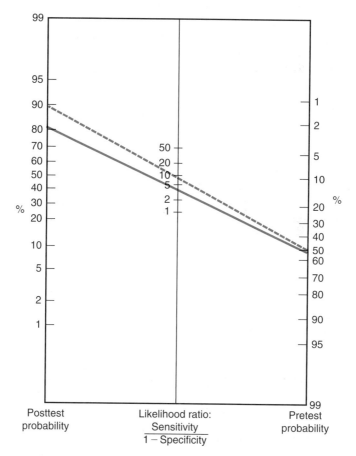

Figure I–1. Nomogram illustrating the relationship between pretest probability, posttest probability, and likelihood ratio. (Reproduced with permission from Braunwald E, Fauci AS, Kasper KL, et al. *Harrison's Principles of Internal Medicine.* 16th ed. New York, NY: McGraw-Hill; 2005:10.)

patient has a pretest probability of CAD of 50%, then the test result of 2 mm of ST-segment depression raises the posttest probability to 90%.

If one knows the sensitivity and specificity of the test used, one can calculate the **likelihood ratio** of the positive test as **sensitivity/(1 – specificity)**. Posttest probability is calculated by multiplying the positive likelihood ratio by the pretest probability, or plotting the probabilities using a nomogram (see Figure I–1).

Thus, knowing something about the characteristics of the test you are employing, and how to apply them to the patient at hand is essential in reaching a correct diagnosis and to avoid falling into the common trap of "positive test = disease" and "negative test = no disease." Stated another way, **tests do not make diagnoses; doctors do, considering test results quantitatively in the context of their clinical assessment.**

> ## CLINICAL PEARL
>
> ▶ If test result is positive,
> Posttest Probability = Pretest Probability × Likelihood Ratio
> Likelihood Ratio = Sensitivity/(1 – Specificity)

Part 2. Approach to Clinical Problem Solving

There are typically four distinct steps to the systematic solving of clinical problems:

1. Making the diagnosis

2. Assessing the severity of the disease (stage)

3. Rendering a treatment based on the stage of the disease

4. Following the patient's response to the treatment

MAKING THE DIAGNOSIS

There are two ways to make a diagnosis. Experienced clinicians often make a diagnosis very quickly using **pattern recognition**, that is, the features of the patient's illness match a scenario the physician has seen before. If it does not fit a readily recognized pattern, then one has to undertake several steps in diagnostic reasoning:

1. The first step is to **gather information with a differential diagnosis in mind.** The clinician should start considering diagnostic possibilities with initial contact with the patient, which are continually refined as information is gathered. Historical questions and physical examination tests and findings are all tailored to the potential diagnoses one is considering. This is the principle that "you find what you are looking for." When one is trying to perform a thorough head-to-toe examination, for instance, without looking for anything in particular, one is much more likely to miss findings.

2. The next step is to try to move from subjective complaints or nonspecific symptoms to focus on objective abnormalities in an effort to **conceptualize**

the patient's objective problem with the greatest specificity one can achieve. For example, a patient may come to the physician complaining of pedal edema, a relatively common and nonspecific finding. Laboratory testing may reveal that the patient has renal failure, a more specific cause of the many causes of edema. Examination of the urine may then reveal red blood cell casts, indicating glomerulonephritis, which is even more specific as the cause of the renal failure. The patient's problem, then, described with the greatest degree of specificity, is glomerulonephritis. The clinician's task at this point is to consider the differential diagnosis of glomerulonephritis rather than that of pedal edema.

3. The last step is to **look for discriminating features** of the patient's illness. This means the features of the illness, which by their presence or their absence narrow the differential diagnosis. This is often difficult for junior learners because it requires a well-developed knowledge base of the typical features of disease, so the diagnostician can judge how much weight to assign to the various clinical clues present. For example, in the diagnosis of a patient with a fever and productive cough, the finding by chest x-ray of bilateral apical infiltrates with cavitation is highly discriminatory. There are few illnesses besides tuberculosis that are likely to produce that radiographic pattern. A negatively predictive example is a patient with exudative pharyngitis who also has rhinorrhea and cough. The presence of these features makes the diagnosis of streptococcal infection unlikely as the cause of the pharyngitis. Once the differential diagnosis has been constructed, the clinician uses the presence of discriminating features, knowledge of patient risk factors, and the epidemiology of diseases to decide which potential diagnoses are most likely.

CLINICAL PEARL

► There are three steps in diagnostic reasoning:
   1. Gathering information with a differential diagnosis in mind
   2. Identifying the objective abnormalities with the greatest specificity
   3. Looking for discriminating features to narrow the differential diagnosis

Once the most specific problem has been identified, and a differential diagnosis of that problem is considered using discriminating features to order the possibilities, the next step is to consider using diagnostic testing, such as laboratory, radiologic, or pathologic data, to confirm the diagnosis. Quantitative reasoning in the use and interpretation of tests was discussed in Part 1. Clinically, the timing and effort with which one pursues a definitive diagnosis using objective data depend on several factors: the potential gravity of the diagnosis in question, the clinical state of the patient, the potential risks of diagnostic testing, and the potential benefits or harms of empiric treatment. For example, if a young man is admitted to the hospital with bilateral pulmonary nodules on chest x-ray, there are many possibilities including metastatic malignancy, and aggressive pursuit of a diagnosis is necessary, perhaps -including a thoracotomy with an open-lung biopsy. The same radiographic findings in an elderly bed-bound woman with advanced Alzheimer dementia who would not be a good candidate for chemotherapy might be best left alone without any diagnostic testing. Decisions like this are difficult, require solid medical knowledge, as well as a thorough understanding of one's patient and the patient's background and inclinations, and constitute the art of medicine.

ASSESSING THE SEVERITY OF THE DISEASE

After ascertaining the diagnosis, the next step is to characterize the severity of the disease process; in other words, it is describing "how bad" a disease is. There is usually prognostic or treatment significance based on the stage. With malignancy, this is done formally by cancer staging. Most cancers are categorized from stage I (localized) to stage IV (widely metastatic). Some diseases, such as congestive heart failure, may be designated as mild, moderate, or severe based on the patient's functional status, that is, their ability to exercise before becoming dyspneic. With some infections, such as syphilis, the staging depends on the duration and extent of the infection, and follows along the natural history of the infection (ie, primary syphilis, secondary, latent period, and tertiary/neurosyphilis).

RENDERING A TREATMENT BASED ON THE STAGE OF THE DISEASE

Many illnesses are stratified according to severity because prognosis and treatment often vary based on the severity. If neither the prognosis nor the treatment was affected by the stage of the disease process, there would not be a reason to subcategorize as mild or severe. As an example, a man with mild chronic obstructive pulmonary disease (COPD) may be treated with inhaled bronchodilators as needed and advice for smoking cessation. However, an individual with severe COPD may need round-the-clock oxygen supplementation, scheduled bronchodilators, and possibly oral corticosteroid therapy.

The treatment should be tailored to the extent or **"stage" of the disease**. In making decisions regarding treatment, it is also essential that the clinician identify the therapeutic objectives. When patients seek medical attention, it is generally because they are bothered by a symptom and want it to go away. When physicians institute therapy, they often have several other goals besides symptom relief, such as prevention of short- or long-term complications or a reduction in mortality. For example, patients with congestive heart failure are bothered by the symptoms of edema and dyspnea. Salt restriction, loop diuretics, and bed rest are effective at reducing these symptoms. However, heart failure is a progressive disease with a high mortality, so other treatments such as angiotensin-converting enzyme (ACE) inhibitors and some beta-blockers are also used to reduce mortality in this condition. It is essential that the clinician know what the therapeutic objective is, so that one can monitor and guide therapy.

CLINICAL PEARL

▶ The clinician needs to identify the objectives of therapy: symptom relief, prevention of complications, or reduction in mortality.

FOLLOWING THE PATIENT'S RESPONSE TO THE TREATMENT

The final step in the approach to disease is to follow the patient's response to the therapy. The "measure" of response should be recorded and monitored. Some responses are clinical, such as the patient's abdominal pain, or temperature, or pulmonary examination. Obviously, the student must work on being more skilled in eliciting the data in an unbiased and standardized manner. Other responses may be followed by imaging tests, such as CT scan of a retroperitoneal node size in a patient receiving chemotherapy, or a tumor marker such as the prostate-specific antigen (PSA) level in a man receiving chemotherapy for prostatic cancer. For syphilis, it may be the nonspecific treponemal antibody test rapid plasma reagent (RPR) titer over time. The student must be prepared to know what to do if the measured marker does not respond according to what is expected. Is the next step to retreat, or to repeat the metastatic workup, or to follow up with another more specific test?

Part 3. Approach to Reading

The clinical problem–oriented approach to reading is different from the classic "systematic" research of a disease. Patients rarely present with a clear diagnosis; hence, the student must become skilled in applying the textbook information to the clinical setting. Furthermore, one retains more information when one reads with a purpose. In other words, the student should read with the goal of answering specific questions. There are several fundamental questions that facilitate **clinical thinking**. These questions are:

1. What is the most likely diagnosis?
2. What should be the next step?
3. What is the most likely mechanism for this process?
4. What are the risk factors for this condition?
5. What are the complications associated with the disease process?
6. What is the best therapy?
7. How would you confirm the diagnosis?

CLINICAL PEARL

▶ Reading with the purpose of answering the seven fundamental clinical questions improves retention of information and facilitates the application of "book knowledge" to "clinical knowledge."

WHAT IS THE MOST LIKELY DIAGNOSIS?

The method of establishing the diagnosis was discussed in the previous part. One way of attacking this problem is to develop standard "approaches" to common -clinical problems. It is helpful to understand the most common causes of various presentations, such as "the most common causes of pancreatitis are gallstones and alcohol." (See the **Clinical Pearls** at end of each case.)

The clinical scenario would entail something such as:

A 28-year-old pregnant woman complains of severe epigastric pain radiating to the back, nausea and vomiting, and an elevated serum amylase level. What is the most likely diagnosis?

With no other information to go on, the student would note that this woman has a clinical diagnosis of pancreatitis. Using the "most common cause" information, the student would make an educated guess that the patient has gallstones, because being female and pregnant are risk factors. If, instead, cholelithiasis is removed from the equation of this scenario, a phrase may be added such as:

"The ultrasonogram of the gallbladder shows no stones."

CLINICAL PEARL

▶ The two most common causes of pancreatitis are gallstones and alcohol abuse.

Now, the student would use the phrase "patients without gallstones who have pancreatitis most likely abuse alcohol." Aside from these two causes, there are many other etiologies of pancreatitis.

WHAT SHOULD BE THE NEXT STEP?

This question is difficult because the next step may be more diagnostic information, or staging, or therapy. It may be more challenging than "the most likely diagnosis," because there may be insufficient information to make a diagnosis and the next step may be to pursue more diagnostic information. Another possibility is that there is enough information for a probable diagnosis, and the next step is to stage the disease. Finally, the most appropriate action may be to treat. Hence, from clinical data, a judgment needs to be rendered regarding how far along one is on the road of:

Make a diagnosis → Stage the disease → Treatment based on stage → Follow response

Frequently, the student is "taught" to regurgitate the same information that someone has written about a particular disease, but is not skilled at giving the next step. This talent is learned optimally at the bedside, in a supportive environment, with freedom to make educated guesses, and with constructive feedback. A sample scenario may describe a student's thought process as follows:

1. **Make the diagnosis:** "Based on the information I have, I believe that Mr. Smith has stable angina because he has retrosternal chest pain when he walks three blocks, but it is relieved within minutes by rest and with sublingual nitroglycerin."

2. **Stage the disease:** "I don't believe that this is severe disease because he does not have pain lasting for more than 5 minutes, angina at rest, or congestive heart failure."

3. **Treatment based on stage:** "Therefore, my next step is to treat with aspirin, beta-blockers, and sublingual nitroglycerin as needed, as well as lifestyle changes."

4. **Follow response:** "I want to follow the treatment by assessing his pain (I will ask him about the degree of exercise he is able to perform without chest pain), performing a cardiac stress test, and reassessing him after the test is done."

In a similar patient, when the clinical presentation is unclear or more severe, perhaps the best "next step" may be diagnostic in nature such as thallium stress test, or even coronary angiography. The **next step** depends upon the **clinical state of the patient** (if unstable, the next step is therapeutic), the **potential severity** of the disease (the next step may be staging), or the **uncertainty of the diagnosis** (the next step is diagnostic).

Usually, the vague question, "What is your next step?" is the most difficult question, because the answer may be diagnostic, staging, or therapeutic.

WHAT IS THE MOST LIKELY MECHANISM FOR THIS PROCESS?

This question goes further than making the diagnosis, but also requires the student to understand the underlying mechanism for the process. For example, a clinical scenario may describe an "18-year-old woman who presents with several months of severe epistaxis, heavy menses, petechiae, and a normal CBC except for a platelet count of 15,000/mm^3." Answers that a student may consider to explain this condition include immune-mediated platelet destruction, drug-induced thrombocytopenia, bone -marrow suppression, and platelet sequestration as a result of hypersplenism.

The student is advised to learn the mechanisms for each disease process, and not merely memorize a constellation of symptoms. In other words, rather than solely committing to memory the classic presentation of idiopathic thrombocytopenic purpura (ITP) (isolated thrombocytopenia without lymphadenopathy or offending drugs), the student should understand that ITP is an autoimmune process whereby the body produces IgG antibodies against the platelets. The platelet-antibody complexes are then taken from the circulation in the spleen. Because the disease process is specific for platelets, the other two cell lines (erythrocytes and leukocytes) are normal. Also, because the thrombocytopenia is caused by excessive platelet peripheral destruction, the bone marrow will show increased megakaryocytes (platelet precursors). Hence, treatment for ITP includes oral corticosteroid agents to decrease the immune process of antiplatelet IgG production, and, if refractory, then splenectomy.

WHAT ARE THE RISK FACTORS FOR THIS PROCESS?

Understanding the risk factors helps the practitioner to establish a diagnosis and to determine how to interpret tests. For example, understanding the risk factor analysis may help to manage a 45-year-old obese woman with sudden onset of dyspnea and pleuritic chest pain following an orthopedic surgery for a femur fracture. This patient has numerous risk factors for deep venous thrombosis and pulmonary embolism. The physician may want to pursue angiography even if the ventilation/perfusion scan result is low probability. Thus, the number of risk factors helps to categorize the likelihood of a disease process.

> **CLINICAL PEARL**
>
> ▶ When the pretest probability of a disease is high based on risk factors, even with a negative initial test, more definitive testing may be indicated.

WHAT ARE THE COMPLICATIONS ASSOCIATED WITH THE DISEASE PROCESS?

A clinician must understand the complications of a disease so that one may monitor the patient. Sometimes the student has to make the diagnosis from clinical clues and then apply his/her knowledge of the sequelae of the pathological process. For example, the student should know that chronic hypertension may affect various end organs, such as the brain (encephalopathy or stroke), the eyes (vascular changes), the kidneys, and the heart. Understanding the types of consequences also helps the clinician to be aware of the dangers to a patient. The clinician is acutely aware of the need to monitor for the end-organ involvement and undertakes the appropriate intervention when involvement is present.

WHAT IS THE BEST THERAPY?

To answer this question, the clinician needs to reach the correct diagnosis, assess the severity of the condition, and weigh the situation to reach the appropriate intervention. For the student, knowing exact dosages is not as important as understanding the best medication, route of delivery, mechanism of action, and possible complications. It is important for the student to be able to verbalize the diagnosis and the rationale for the therapy. A common error is for the student to "jump to a treatment," like a random guess, and therefore be given "right or wrong" feedback. In fact, the student's guess may be correct, but for the wrong reason; conversely, the answer may be a very reasonable one, with only one small error in thinking. Instead, the student should verbalize the steps so that feedback may be given at every reasoning point.

For example, if the question is, "What is the best therapy for a 25-year-old man who complains of a nontender penile ulcer?" the incorrect manner of response is for the student to blurt out "azithromycin." Rather, the student should reason it out in a way similar to this: "The most common cause of a nontender infectious ulcer of the penis is syphilis. Nontender adenopathy is usually associated. Therefore, the best treatment for this man with probable syphilis is intramuscular penicillin (but I would want to confirm the diagnosis). His partner also needs treatment."

> **CLINICAL PEARL**
>
> ▶ Therapy should be logical based on the severity of disease. Antibiotic therapy should be tailored for specific organisms.

HOW WOULD YOU CONFIRM THE DIAGNOSIS?

In the scenario above, the man with a nontender penile ulcer is likely to have syphilis. Confirmation may be achieved by serology (rapid plasma reagent [RPR] or Venereal Disease Research Laboratory [VDRL] test); however, there is a significant possibility that patients with primary syphilis may not have developed antibody response yet, and have negative serology. Thus, confirmation of the diagnosis is attained with dark-field microscopy. Knowing the limitations of diagnostic tests and the manifestations of disease aids in this area.

SUMMARY

1. There is no replacement for a careful history and physical examination.

2. There are four steps to the clinical approach to the patient: making the diagnosis, assessing severity, treatment based on severity, and following response.

3. Assessment of pretest probability and knowledge of test characteristics are essential in the application of test results to the clinical situation.

4. There are seven questions that help to bridge the gap between the textbook and the clinical arena.

REFERENCES

Bordages G. Elaborated knowledge: a key to successful diagnostic thinking. *Acad Med.* 1994;69(11): 883-885.

Bordages G. Why did I miss the diagnosis? Some cognitive explanations and educational implications. *Acad Med.* 1999;74(10):138-143.

Sox HC, HIggins MC, Owens DK. Medical decision making, 2nd ed. Hoboken, NJ: Wiley-Blackwell publishers; 2013:7-76.

Mark DB. Decision-making in clinical medicine. In: Kasper DL, Fauci AS, Longo D, et al., eds. *Harrison's Principles of Internal Medicine.* 19th ed. New York, NY: McGraw-Hill; 2015:16-23.

Cases

A 66-year-old woman comes in for a routine physical examination. She volunteers that her menopause occurred at age 51. The medical history is unremarkable. Her family history includes one maternal cousin with ovarian cancer. On examination, she is found to have blood pressure 120/70 mm Hg, heart rate 70 bpm, and temperature 98°F. Her weight is 140 lb, and her height is 5 ft 4 in. The thyroid is normal to palpation. Breast examination reveals no masses or discharge. Abdominal, cardiac, and lung evaluations are within normal limits. Pelvic examination shows a normal multiparous cervix, a normal-size uterus, and no adnexal masses. She had undergone a mammogram 3 months ago. The patient states that she has regular Papanicolaou (Pap) smears, and that the last one performed 1 year ago was normal.

▶ What is your next step?
▶ What would be the most common cause of mortality for this patient?

ANSWERS TO CASE 1:

Health Maintenance

Summary: A 66-year-old woman presents for health maintenance. A mammogram had been performed 3 months ago.

- **Next step:** Each of the following should be performed: stool for occult blood or colonoscopy or sigmoidoscopy, pneumococcal vaccine, influenza vaccine, tetanus vaccine (if not within 10 years), cholesterol screening, fasting blood glucose.

- **Most common cause of mortality:** Cardiovascular disease.

ANALYSIS

Objectives

1. Understand which health maintenance studies should be performed for a patient older than 65 years.

2. Know the most common cause of mortality in a woman in this age group.

3. Understand that preventive maintenance consists of immunizations, cancer screening, and screening for common diseases.

Considerations

The approach to health maintenance consists of three parts: (1) screening for cancer, cardiovascular disease or other conditions, (2) immunizations, and (3) behavioral counseling regarding healthy behaviors such as regular exercise and tobacco cessation. For a 66-year-old woman, this includes mammography for breast cancer screening, colon cancer screening, tetanus booster every 10 years, pneumococcal vaccine, and yearly influenza immunization. Screening for hypercholesterolemia every 5 years up to age 75 and fasting blood glucose levels every 3 years also are recommended. The most common cause of mortality in men or women over 65 is cardiovascular disease. Cervical cancer screening can be stopped at age 65 if all previous Pap smears have been normal.

APPROACH TO:

Health Maintenance

DEFINITIONS

COST-EFFECTIVENESS: Comparison of resources expended (dollars) in an intervention versus the benefit, which may be measured in life-years or quality-adjusted life-years.

PRIMARY PREVENTION: Identifying and modifying risk factors in subjects who have never had the disease of concern.

SCREENING TEST: Device used to identify asymptomatic disease in the hope that early detection will lead to an improved outcome. An optimal screening test has high sensitivity and specificity, is inexpensive, and is easy to perform.

SECONDARY PREVENTION: Actions taken to reduce the morbidity or mortality once a disease has been diagnosed.

CLINICAL APPROACH

Aside from episodic care to treat acute or chronic illnesses, a major part of medical practice includes preventive care, that is, medical care to prevent disease, or to detect it early enough that interventions are more likely to be effective. There are several types of preventive care:

1. **Immunizations:** Aside from childhood immunizations, routine adult immunizations include influenza, pneumococcal, diphtheria, tetanus, and acellular pertussis (Td/Tdap), zoster, as well as others in certain situations such as hepatitis A or B vaccines.

2. **Behavioral counseling:** Inquiry and counseling regarding regular exercise, avoidance or cessation of tobacco, moderate alcohol use, or screening for depression.

3. **Chemoprevention:** Use of medication to prevent disease, such as use of folate during pregnancy to prevent neural tube defects, or low-dose aspirin to prevent cardiovascular events.

4. **Screening:** Identification of disease or risk factors in an asymptomatic patient.

Of these preventive measures, screening requires firm medical evidence that it may offer benefit, and thoughtful consideration from the practitioner before he or she initiates screening, and recommends to an asymptomatic patient that he/she undergoes a medical intervention with potential harms (such as cost, radiation exposure, anxiety regarding false-positive tests, biopsies, or other follow-up examinations). The World Health Organization outlined the principles of screening:

1. The condition must be an important health problem.

2. There should be an effective treatment for the condition.

3. Facilities for diagnosis and treatment of the condition should be available to the patient.

4. There needs to be a latent or preclinical stage of the disease in which it can be detected.

5. There should be an accurate test to detect the condition.

6. The test should be acceptable to the patient or the population.

7. The natural history of the disease should be understood to guide intervention or treatment.

8. The cost of case-finding should be balanced within the context of overall medical expenditures.

Using these criteria, one may deduce that it would not be useful to screen for Alzheimer dementia since there is no curative treatment and no evidence that early intervention alters the course of the disease, or to perform cancer screening in developing countries where treatment facilities may not be available or accessible to large portions of the population. Regarding cost-effectiveness, health care economists perform sophisticated analysis for screening and other medical care, but one rough measure of cost-effectiveness is quality-adjusted life-year (QALY), combining longevity with quality of life in a single measure. In the United States, medical interventions including cancer screening are often considered cost-effective at a cost of $50,000 to 100,000 per QALY gained.

Among Americans between ages 15 and 45, accidents and homicide are the leading causes of death, so preventive care may include counseling regarding behavioral risk reduction, such as seatbelt use, avoiding alcohol or texting while driving, or substance abuse. After age 45, the leading causes of death are malignancy and cardiovascular disease, so screening is focused on risk factor reduction for those diseases (such as tobacco cessation, or control of blood pressure and hyperlipidemia), or early detection of cancers. Regarding cancer screening tests, the American Cancer Society and various subspecialty organizations publish various recommendations, which are often not in agreement. The US Preventive Services Task Force (USPSTF) is an independent panel of physicians and epidemiologists appointed by the Department of Health and Human Services to systematically review the evidence of effectiveness of clinical preventive services (though they do not consider cost-effectiveness). The USPSTF recommendations for cancer and other health screening are listed in Table 1–1:

For older patients, other preventive care is important. Routine immunizations include annual influenza vaccine (especially important in the geriatric population, since >90% of influenza-related deaths occur in patients over 60 years), pneumococcal vaccines (23-valent polysaccharide vaccine and 13-valent pneumococcal conjugate vaccine should be given sequentially), and Herpes zoster vaccine for patients over age 60. Offering cancer screening to older patients should consider estimated life expectancy (typically at least 10 years), comorbid conditions, and ability or willingness to undergo cancer treatment if a cancer is detected (eg, to tolerate a hemicolectomy if a colon cancer is found). There is little data to support screening for most diseases after age 75.

Table 1–1 • US PREVENTIVE SERVICES TASK FORCE SCREENING RECOMMENDATIONS

Health Problem	Population	Intervention
Cardiovascular disease		
Hypertension	All patients	BP screening
Hyperlipidemia	No risk factors: M >35, F >45	Check lipids
	With risk factors: M >25, F >35	
Diabetes	With hypertension or hyperlipidemia	Screen for diabetes every 3 y
	With BMI >25 kg/m²	Screen
Abdominal aortic aneurysm M age 65-75 with history of smoking		Ultrasound
Cancer		
Breast cancer	Women >40 y	Mammography every 1-2 y
Cervical cancer	Women 21-29 y	Pap smear every 3 y
	Women >30 y	Pap smear every 3 y or
		Pap smear + HPV testing every 5 y
Colorectal cancer	Patients >50 y	Screening: fecal occult blood testing annually, or flexible sigmoidoscopy every 5 y, or colonoscopy every 10 y
Lung cancer	Patients 55-74 y, ≥30 pack-year smoking history (current smoker or quit <15 y)	Low-dose CT chest annually
Prostate cancer	Men ≥50 y or high-risk men ≥40 y	Discuss screening, individual decision
Infectious diseases		
Hepatitis C	All persons born between 1945 and 1965	Anti-HCV Ab assay (one-time screening)
HIV	Pregnant women and all patients age 15-65	Rapid HIV or immunoassay

The US Preventive Services Task Force Guide to Clinical Preventive Services 2007, *American Cancer Society Screening Guidelines,* 2008.

COMPREHENSION QUESTIONS

1.1 A 59-year-old woman is being seen for a health maintenance appointment. She has not seen a doctor for over 10 years. She had undergone a total hysterectomy for uterine fibroids 12 years ago. The patient takes supplemental calcium. The physician orders a fasting glucose level, lipid panel, mammogram, colonoscopy, and a Pap smear of the vaginal cuff. Which of the following statements is most accurate regarding the screening for this patient?

A. The Pap smear of the vaginal cuff is unnecessary.

B. In general, colon cancer screening should be initiated at age 60 but this patient has very sporadic care; therefore colonoscopy is reasonable.

C. Because the patient takes supplemental calcium, a dual-energy x-ray absorptiometry (DEXA) scan is not needed.

D. Pneumococcal vaccination should be recommended.

1.2 A 63-year-old man has had annual health maintenance appointments and has followed all the recommendations offered by his physician. The physician counsels him about varicella zoster vaccine. Which of the following is the most accurate statement about this vaccine?

A. This vaccine is recommended for patients who are aged 65 and older.

B. This vaccine is not recommended if a patient has already developed shingles.

C. This vaccine is a live attenuated immunization.

D. This vaccine has some cross-reactivity with herpes simplex virus (HSV) and offers some protection against HSV.

1.3 An 18-year-old woman is being seen for a health maintenance appointment. She has not had a Pap smear previously. She currently takes oral contraceptive pills. She began sexual intercourse 6 months previously. Which of the following statements is most accurate regarding health maintenance for this individual?

A. A Pap smear should not be performed in this patient at this time.

B. The human papilloma virus (HPV) vaccine should be administered only if she has a history of genital warts.

C. The most common cause of mortality for this patient would be suicide.

D. Hepatitis C vaccination should be offered to this patient.

ANSWERS

1.1 **A.** Cervical cytology of the vaginal cuff is unnecessary when the hysterectomy was for benign indications (not cervical dysplasia or cervical cancer) and when there is no history of abnormal Pap smears. Colon cancer screening is generally started at age 50 and not at age 60. DEXA scan for osteoporosis is recommended for women starting at age 65, or earlier for women with elevated fracture risk. Pneumococcal vaccine is generally given at age 65.

1.2 **C.** The varicella zoster vaccine is a live attenuated vaccine, recommended for individuals aged 60 and above. It has been shown to greatly reduce the incidence of herpes zoster (shingles) and the severity and likelihood of postherpetic neuralgia. It has no efficacy in preventing HSV.

1.3 **A.** Cervical cytology should be deferred until age 21. This is due to the fact that adolescents many times will clear the HPV infection and cause an abnormal Pap smear to normalize. **The Advisory Committee on Immunization Practices (ACIP) recommends that the HPV vaccine should be recommended to both males and females between the age of 9 and 26.** The most common cause of mortality for adolescent females is motor vehicle accidents. No vaccine is currently available for hepatitis C.

CLINICAL PEARLS

▶ The basic approach to health maintenance is age-appropriate immunizations, cancer screening, and screening for common diseases.

▶ The most common cause of mortality in a woman younger than 20 years is motor vehicle accidents.

▶ The top two causes of mortality in men or women age 45 or older are cardiovascular disease and cancer.

▶ Women older than 65 years should be screened for osteoporosis, heart disease, breast cancer, and depression.

▶ Obesity is a major concern and has numerous complications including diabetes, hyperlipidemia, heart disease, sleep apnea, and respiratory difficulties.

▶ Tobacco use should be queried at each visit, and patients should be counseled actively about cessation; pharmacologic therapy is associated with a higher success rate.

REFERENCES

Martin GJ. Screening and prevention of disease. In: Kasper DL, Fauci AS, Hauser SL, et al., eds. *Harrison's Principles of Internal Medicine.* 19th ed. New York, NY: McGraw-Hill Education; 2015: 26-31.

US Preventive Services Task Force. Guide to clinical prevention services 2014. http://www.ahrq. gov/professionals/clinicians-providers/guidelines-recommendations/guide/index.html. Accessed November 1, 2015.

A 35-year-old man presents to your clinic for a general checkup and cholesterol screening. He denies having medical problems and takes no medications on a regular basis. He works as a computer programmer, exercises regularly at a gym, and does not smoke or use illicit drugs. He drinks two to three beers on the weekend. His father suffered his first heart attack at age 42 and eventually died of complications of heart disease at age 49. The patient's older brother recently was diagnosed with "high cholesterol."

The patient's blood pressure is 125/74 mm Hg and heart rate 72 bpm. He is 69 in tall and weighs 165 lb. His physical examination is unremarkable.

Fasting lipid levels are drawn. The next day, you receive the results: total cholesterol 362 mg/dL, triglycerides 200 mg/dL, high-density lipoprotein (HDL) 36 mg/dL, and low-density lipoprotein (LDL) 266 mg/dL.

▶ What is the most likely diagnosis?
▶ What is your next step?
▶ What are the possible complications if left untreated?

ANSWERS TO CASE 2:

Hypercholesterolemia

Summary: A healthy 35-year-old man presents for a physical examination and is found to have markedly elevated total and LDL cholesterol and triglycerides and low HDL cholesterol. He has an unremarkable physical examination. He is normotensive and is a nonsmoker, but he has a strong family history of hypercholesterolemia and premature atherosclerotic coronary artery disease (CAD).

- **Likely diagnosis:** Familial hypercholesterolemia.

- **Next step:** Counsel regarding lifestyle modification with a low-fat diet and exercise, and offer treatment with a β-hydroxy-β-methylglutaryl-coenzyme A (HMG-CoA) reductase inhibitor (also known as a "statin" agent).

- **Complications if untreated:** Development of atherosclerotic vascular disease, including coronary heart disease (CHD).

ANALYSIS

Objectives

1. Know the risk factors for developing coronary artery disease and know how to estimate the risk for coronary events using available risk calculators.

2. Be familiar with the recommendations for cholesterol screening and for the treatment of high-risk patients.

3. Understand how the different classes of lipid-lowering agents affect lipid levels and the potential side effects of those agents.

4. Know the secondary causes of hyperlipidemia.

Considerations

A young man presents to the clinic for a checkup and is found to have markedly elevated total cholesterol (normal <200 mg/dL) and LDL levels (normal <100 mg/dL), and low HDL levels (normal >45 mg/dL). He does not have any apparent secondary causes of dyslipidemia, and has no signs or symptoms of vascular disease. He does have a strong family history of hypercholesterolemia and premature death caused by myocardial infarction (MI). The decisions regarding the method and intensity of lipid-lowering therapy are based on one's **estimation of the patient's 10-year risk of major coronary events.** Because of his very high lipid levels and family history, he is a high-risk patient and, thus, should be counseled about lipid-lowering medical therapy. The very high cholesterol levels at a young age in the absence of secondary causes lead one to suspect familial hypercholesterolemia, a condition caused by defective or absent LDL surface receptors and subsequent inability to metabolize LDL particles. Meanwhile, the importance of lifestyle modification cannot be overemphasized.

APPROACH TO:
Hyperlipidemia

DEFINITIONS

HYPERLIPIDEMIA: An excess of fats or lipids in the blood, principally due to either elevated cholesterol or triglycerides.

ATHEROSCLEROSIS: Deposition of atheromatous plaques containing cholesterol and lipids on the innermost layer of the walls of large- and medium-sized arteries.

STATIN MEDICATIONS: A class of agents that lower total and LDL cholesterol by inhibiting 3-hydroxy-3-methylglutaryl-coenzyme A (HMG-CoA) reductase, a key enzyme in cholesterol synthesis.

CLINICAL APPROACH

Atherosclerotic coronary artery disease is the **leading cause of death of both men and women** in the United States. Because of the association of hypercholesterolemia and development of atherosclerotic heart disease, most authorities recommend routine screening of average-risk individuals at least every 5 years. Clinical laboratories usually measure total cholesterol, HDL, and triglycerides. The LDL cholesterol may be calculated by using the formula:

$$LDL = \text{Total cholesterol} - HDL - (\text{Triglycerides}/5)$$

A fasting sample should be measured, if possible, but the total cholesterol and HDL are still reliable in a nonfasting sample. The triglycerides and the calculated LDL levels are affected by recent dietary intake and should be drawn in the fasting state (Table 2–1).

One should exclude a *secondary* **cause of lipid disorder**, either by clinical or laboratory evaluation. The most common underlying causes of dyslipidemia are **hypothyroidism** and **diabetes mellitus**. Other conditions to consider are obstructive liver disease, chronic renal failure/nephrotic syndrome, and medication side effects (progestins, anabolic steroids, corticosteroids). Very high cholesterol levels in young patients in the absence of secondary causes suggest familial hypercholesterolemia, a condition caused by defective or absent LDL surface receptors and subsequent inability to metabolize LDL particles. Homozygotes for this condition

Table 2–1 • CHD RISK FACTORS

Cigarette smoking
Hypertension (elevated blood pressure when seen, or patient on antihypertensives)
Low HDL cholesterol (<40 mg/dL)
Family history of premature coronary artery disease (in men <55 y or in women <65 y)
Age of the patient (men >45 y, women >55 y)
Diabetes mellitus

may develop atherosclerotic disease in childhood and usually require intensive lipid-lowering drug therapy.

Epidemiologic studies have found a graded relationship between the total cholesterol concentration and risk of cardiovascular events. Lowering serum cholesterol levels decrease the risk of major coronary events and death in hypercholesterolemic patients without a prior history of CHD (**primary prevention**), as well as reducing the overall mortality and coronary disease mortality in patients who have established cardiovascular disease (**secondary prevention**). All patients should first be educated regarding therapeutic lifestyle changes. These changes include a diet low in saturated fat (<7% of total daily calories) and low in cholesterol (<200 mg/d), as well as exercise, which can help to lower cholesterol.

Multiple trials have shown that statin therapy is effective in cardiovascular risk reduction for secondary prevention, as well as for primary prevention, over a wide range of baseline LDL-cholesterol levels and lipid profiles. For patients treated with statins, the risk for a heart attack or stroke drops by about 20% for each 39 mg/dL reduction in LDL cholesterol. The 2013 guidelines from the American College of Cardiology and the American Heart Association recommend statin therapy for the following groups:

1. Patients with known atherosclerotic cardiovascular disease (history of MI, angina, stroke or transient ischemic attack (TIA), peripheral arterial disease, coronary or other revascularization procedure).

2. Diabetic patients age 40 to 75.

3. Patients with LDL cholesterol >190 mg/dL.

4. Patients age 40 to 75, without diagnosed cardiovascular disease or diabetes, but with a 10-years risk of cardiovascular events ≥7.5%.

For patients >40 years without clinical atherosclerotic cardiovascular disease, the AHA/ACC risk calculator is available online (**http://tools.acc.org/ASCVD-Risk-Estimator/**), or as an application that can be downloaded. Major risk factors for atherosclerosis include cigarette smoking, diabetes mellitus, hypertension, elevated total cholesterol and low-density lipoprotein cholesterol (LDL-C), low high-density lipoprotein cholesterol (HDL-C), and older age.

When lifestyle modifications are not enough to reach the LDL goal, multiple lipid-lowering medications are available. Table 2–2 lists their effects on lipids and their potential side effects. **Statins** are generally very well tolerated, but the most common side effect is **myopathy**, which may manifest as muscle tenderness with elevated creatine kinase (CK) levels. Low-grade myalgias occur in <10% of patients, but severe myopathy is reported in 0.5% of statin-treated patients. Less commonly, **elevated liver enzymes**, or even severe hepatitis, have been reported. When these drugs are used, routine clinical or laboratory monitoring for these effects is advisable. After initiating statins, LDL cholesterol should be checked after 6 weeks, and every 6 to 12 months thereafter, to monitor medication adherence.

Table 2–2 • DRUGS FOR HYPERLIPIDEMIA			
Drug Class	**Therapeutic Effects**	**Side Effects**	**Monitoring**
HMG-CoA reductase inhibitors ("statins")	**Lower LDL 25%-60%** Lower TG 10%-25% Raise HDL 5%-10%	Myalgias, possible hepatotoxicity	Monitor LFTs and creatine kinase
Nicotinic acid (eg, niacin)	Lower TG 25%-35% Lower LDL 15%-25% **Raise HDL 15%-30%**	Flushing, tachycardia, glucose intolerance, ↑ uric acid	Flushing may be relieved by aspirin
Bile acid resins (cholestyramine, colestipol)	**Lower LDL 20%-30%** Raise HDL 5%	Constipation, nausea, GI discomfort	Binds fat-soluble vitamins, bloating, constipation
Fibric acid derivatives (gemfibrozil, fenofibrate)	**Lower TG 25%-40%** Raise HDL 5%-15%	Gallstones, nausea, increased LFTs	Dyspepsia, gallstones, myalgias (caution if used with statins)
Cholesterol absorption inhibitor (ezetimibe)	**Lower LDL 15%**	Diarrhea, GI upset	Monitor LFTs. No evidence yet that ↓ CV risk

Abbreviation: CV, cardiovascular; GI, gastrointestinal; HDL, high-density lipoprotein; LDL, low-density lipoprotein; LFT, liver function test; TG, triglycerides.
(Data from Rader DJ, Hobbs HH. Disorders of lipoprotein metabolism. In: Braunwald E, Fauci AS, Kasper KL, et al, eds. Harrison's Principles of Internal Medicine, 17th ed. New York: McGraw-Hill, 2008:2428.)

CASE CORRELATION

- See also Case 1 (Health Maintenance) and Case 3 (Acute Myocardial Infarction).

COMPREHENSION QUESTIONS

2.1 A 35-year-old man with no history of cardiac or other vascular disease asks how often he should have routine cholesterol screening. Which of the following is the best answer?

A. Every 3 months

B. Annually

C. Every 5 years

D. Every 7 to 10 years

2.2 A 48-year-old man presents to your clinic following a health fair screening of his cholesterol level because he was told that it is high. He has diet-controlled diabetes mellitus, plays tennis, exercises three to five times per week, and appears to be in good physical condition. He is a nonsmoker and has no family history of cardiovascular disease. His profile is total cholesterol 212 mg/dL, HDL 35 mg/dL, LDL 138 mg/dL, and triglycerides 175 mg/dL. Following a review of this patient's profile, which of the following would you recommend?

   A. Administer gemfibrozil.

   B. Administer HMG-CoA reductase inhibitor (statin).

   C. Administer low-dose niacin and slowly increase to achieve 3 g daily.

   D. Suggest he continues his current diet and exercise program.

2.3 Which of the following patients is the best candidate for lifestyle modification alone rather than lipid-lowering medications?

   A. A 60-year-old diabetic male smoker with a recent myocardial infarction: cholesterol 201 mg/dL, HDL 47 mg/dL, and LDL 138 mg/dL

   B. A 62-year-old diabetic man: cholesterol 210 mg/dL, HDL 27 mg/dL, and LDL 146 mg/dL

   C. A 57-year-old asymptomatic woman: cholesterol 235 mg/dL, HDL 92 mg/dL, and LDL 103 mg/dL

   D. A 39-year-old man with nephrotic syndrome: cholesterol 285 mg/dL, HDL 48 mg/dL, LDL 195 mg/dL

ANSWERS

2.1 **C.** The recommended interval for cholesterol screening in this population of healthy adults is every 5 years. Cholesterol levels do not change rapidly over a person's lifetime. A rapid change should prompt investigation for an underlying secondary cause.

2.2 **B.** In this scenario, although this 48-year-old man is very active with an exercise program, the key is that he has diabetes. A patient with diabetes is at high risk for development of atherosclerotic cardiovascular disease, and should be started on statins according to 2013 AHA/ACC guidelines.

2.3 **C.** Patient A is at highest risk for future events because he has established CHD and diabetes, he smokes, and he recently had a myocardial infarction. Patient B has diabetes, a CHD equivalent. Besides lifestyle modifications, he should start drug therapy to lower his LDL and raise his HDL. Patient C has very high HDL, which is protective, and probably contributes to her elevated total cholesterol. Patient D has nephrotic syndrome causing hyperlipidemia, which may be treated by reduction of proteinuria using angiotensin-converting enzyme (ACE) inhibitors but often requires drug therapy such as statins.

CLINICAL PEARLS

▶ Patients with established cardiovascular disease should be treated with statins, regardless of baseline LDL-C level.

▶ Diabetic patients age 40 to 75, and those with very high LDL-C >190 mg/dL (such as those with familial hypercholesterolemia) are at high risk for cardiovascular events, and should be treated with statins.

▶ LDL cholesterol is the primary target of lipid-lowering therapy; treatment reduces coronary events and death in patients with and without established coronary heart disease. Current guidelines recommend consideration of LDL-lowering drug therapy in patients >40 years, with estimated 10-year risk >7.5%.

▶ The major side effects of statins are myopathy and, less commonly hepatocellular injury.

REFERENCES

Expert Panel on Detection, Evaluation, and Treatment of High Blood Cholesterol in Adults. Executive summary of the third report of the National Cholesterol Education Program Expert Panel on Detection, Evaluation, and Treatment of High Blood Cholesterol in Adults (Adult Treatment Panel III). *JAMA*. 2001;285:2486-2497.

Libby P. In: Kasper DL, Fauci AS, Hauser SL, et al., eds. *Harrison's Principles of Internal Medicine*. 19th ed. New York, NY: McGraw-Hill Education; 2015: Chapter 291*e*, 1578.

Rader DJ, Hobbs HH. Disorders of lipoprotein metabolism. In: Kasper DL, Fauci AS, Hauser SL, et al., eds. *Harrison's Principles of Internal Medicine*. 19th ed. New York, NY: McGraw-Hill; 2015: 2435-2449.

Stone NJ, Robinson JG, Lichtenstein AH, et al. 2013 ACC/AHA guideline on the treatment of blood cholesterol to reduce atherosclerotic cardiovascular risk in adults: a report of the American College of Cardiology/American Heart Association Task Force on Practice Guidelines *Circulation*. published online November 12, 2013.

A 56-year-old man comes to the emergency department (ED) complaining of chest discomfort. He describes the discomfort as a severe, retrosternal pressure sensation that had awakened him from sleep 3 hours earlier. He previously had been well but has a medical history of hypercholesterolemia and a 40-pack-year history of smoking. On examination, he appears uncomfortable and diaphoretic, with a heart rate of 116 bpm, blood pressure of 166/102 mm Hg, respiratory rate of 22 breaths per minute, and oxygen saturation of 96% on room air. Jugular venous pressure appears normal. Auscultation of the chest reveals clear lung fields, a regular rhythm with an S_4 gallop, and no murmurs or rubs. A chest radiograph shows clear lungs and a normal cardiac silhouette. The electrocardiogram (ECG) is shown in Figure 3–1.

▶ What is the most likely diagnosis?
▶ What is the next step in therapy?

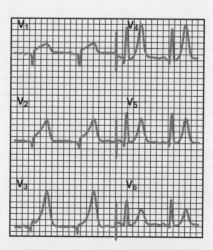

Figure 3–1. Electrocardiogram. (Reproduced, with permission, from Braunwald E, Fauci AS, Kasper DL, et al., eds. *Harrison's Principles of Internal Medicine,* 16th ed. New York: McGraw-Hill, 2005:1316.)

ANSWERS TO CASE 3:

Myocardial Infarction, Acute

Summary: This is a 56-year-old man with risk factors for coronary atherosclerosis (smoking and hypercholesterolemia) who has chest pain typical of cardiac ischemia, that is, retrosternal pressure sensation. Cardiac examination reveals an S_4 gallop, which may be seen with myocardial ischemia because of relative noncompliance of the ischemic heart, as well as hypertension, tachycardia, and diaphoresis, which all may represent sympathetic activation. The duration of the pain and the ECG findings suggest an acute myocardial infarction (MI).

- **Most likely diagnosis:** Acute ST-segment elevation MI.

- **Next step in therapy:** Administer aspirin and a beta-blocker, and assess whether he is a candidate for rapid reperfusion of the myocardium, that is, treatment with thrombolytics or percutaneous coronary intervention.

ANALYSIS

Objectives

1. Know the diagnostic criteria for acute MI.

2. Know which patients should receive thrombolytics or undergo percutaneous coronary intervention, which may reduce mortality.

3. Be familiar with the complications of MI and their treatment options.

4. Understand post-MI risk stratification and secondary prevention strategies.

Considerations

The three most important issues for this patient are: (1) the **suspicion of acute MI** based on the clinical and ECG findings, (2) deciding whether the patient has indications or contraindications for **thrombolytics or primary percutaneous coronary intervention**, and (3) **excluding other diagnoses** that might mimic acute MI but would not benefit from or might be worsened by anticoagulation or thrombolysis (eg, acute pericarditis, aortic dissection).

APPROACH TO:

Suspected Acute MI

DEFINITIONS

ACUTE CORONARY SYNDROME: Spectrum of acute cardiac ischemia ranging from **unstable angina** (ischemic pain at rest or at lower threshold of exertion or new onset of chest pain) to **acute MI** (death of cardiac tissue), usually precipitated by thrombus formation in a coronary artery with an atherosclerotic plaque.

ACUTE MYOCARDIAL INFARCTION: Death of myocardial tissue because of inadequate blood flow.

NON–ST-SEGMENT ELEVATION MYOCARDIAL INFARCTION (NSTEMI): MI, but without ST-segment elevation as defined below. It may have other ECG changes, such as ST-segment depression or T-wave inversion. NSTEMI will have elevated cardiac biomarkers. The pathophysiology is subendocardial ischemia and can cause cardiac muscle dysfunction and shock.

PCI: Percutaneous coronary intervention (angioplasty and/or stenting).

ST-SEGMENT ELEVATION MYOCARDIAL INFARCTION (STEMI): MI as defined as in acute myocardial infarction, with ST-segment elevation more than 0.1 mV in two or more contiguous leads, and elevated cardiac biomarkers. STEMI has the pathophysiology of transmural cardiac muscle ischemia and can therefore cause cardiac dysfunction and pump failure (cardiogenic shock) acutely.

THROMBOLYTICS: Drugs such as tissue plasminogen activator (tPA), streptokinase, and reteplase (recombinant plasminogen activator [r-PA]), which act to lyse fibrin thrombi in order to restore patency of the coronary artery when PCI is contraindicated or is not available.

CLINICAL APPROACH

Pathophysiology

Acute coronary syndromes, which exist on a continuum ranging from **unstable angina pectoris** to **NSTEMI** to **STEMI**, usually are caused by **in situ thrombosis** at the site of a ruptured atherosclerotic plaque in a coronary artery. Occasionally, they are caused by embolic occlusion, coronary vasospasm, vasculitis, aortic root or coronary artery dissection, or cocaine use (which promotes both vasospasm and thrombosis). The resultant clinical syndrome is related to both the degree of atherosclerotic stenosis in the artery and to the duration and extent of sudden thrombotic occlusion of the artery. If the occlusion is incomplete or if the thrombus undergoes spontaneous lysis, unstable angina occurs. If the occlusion is complete and remains for more than 30 minutes, infarction occurs. In contrast, the mechanism of chronic stable angina usually is a flow-limiting stenosis caused by atherosclerotic plaque that causes ischemia during exercise without acute thrombosis (Table 3–1).

DIAGNOSTIC CRITERIA FOR ACUTE MI

History

Chest pain is the cardinal feature of MI, even though it is not universally present. It is of the same character as angina pectoris—described as heavy, squeezing, or crushing—and is localized to the retrosternal area or epigastrium, sometimes with radiation to the arm, lower jaw, or neck. **In contrast to stable angina, however, it persists for more than 30 minutes and is not relieved by rest.** The pain often is accompanied by sweating, nausea, vomiting, and/or the sense of impending doom. In a patient older than 70 years or who is diabetic, an acute MI may be painless or associated with only vague discomfort, but it may be heralded by the sudden onset of dyspnea, pulmonary edema, or ventricular arrhythmias.

Table 3–1 • CLINICAL MANIFESTATIONS OF CORONARY ARTERY DISEASE		
Vessel Architecture	**Blood Flow**	**Clinical Manifestation**
Early plaque	Unobstructed	Asymptomatic
Critical coronary artery stenosis >70%	Blood flow limited during exertion	Stable angina
Unstable plaque rupture	Platelet thrombus begins to form and spasm limits blood flow at rest	Unstable angina
Unstable platelet thrombus on ruptured plaque	Transient or incomplete vessel occlusion (lysis occurs)	Non–ST-segment elevation (subendocardial) myocardial infarction
Platelet thrombus on ruptured plaque	Complete vessel occlusion (no lysis)	ST-segment elevation (transmural) myocardial infarction

Physical Findings

There are **no specific physical findings** in a patient with an acute MI. Many patients are anxious and diaphoretic. Cardiac auscultation may reveal an S_4 gallop, reflecting myocardial noncompliance because of ischemia; an S_3 gallop, representing severe systolic dysfunction; or a new apical systolic murmur of mitral regurgitation caused by ischemic papillary muscle dysfunction.

Electrocardiogram

The ECG is often critical in diagnosing acute MI and guiding therapy. A series of ECG changes reflect the evolution of the infarction (Figure 3–2).

1. The earliest changes are tall, positive, **hyperacute T waves** in the ischemic vascular territory.

2. This is followed by **elevation of the ST segments** (myocardial "injury pattern").

3. Over hours to days, **T-wave inversion** frequently develops.

4. Finally, diminished R-wave amplitude or **Q waves** occur, representing significant myocardial necrosis and replacement by scar tissue, and they are what one seeks to prevent in treating the acute MI.

Sometimes when acute ischemia is limited to the **subendocardium**, **ST-segment depression**, rather than ST-segment elevation, develops. **ST-segment elevation is typical of acute transmural ischemia**, that is, a greater degree of myocardial involvement than in NSTEMI.

From the ECG we can localize the ischemia related to a vascular territory supplied by one of the three major coronary arteries. **STEMI** is defined as ST-segment elevation more than 0.1 mV in two or more contiguous leads (ie, in the same vascular territory) and/or a new left bundle branch block (LBBB) (which obscures usual ST-segment analysis). As a general rule, **leads II, III, and aVF** correspond to the **inferior** surface of the heart supplied by the **right coronary artery** (RCA), leads V_2 to V_4 correspond to the **anterior** surface supplied by the **left anterior descending**

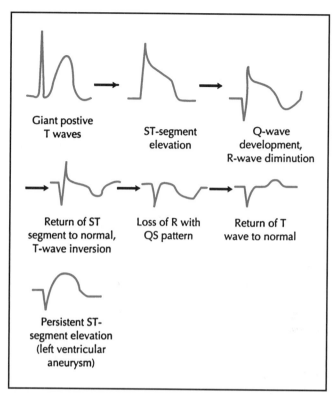

Giant postive
T waves

ST-segment
elevation

Q-wave
development,
R-wave diminution

Return of ST
segment to normal,
T-wave inversion

Loss of R with
QS pattern

Return of T
wave to normal

Persistent ST-
segment elevation
(left ventricular
aneurysm)

Figure 3–2. Temporal evolution of ECG changes in acute myocardial infarction. Note tall hyper-acute T waves and loss of R-wave amplitude, followed by ST-segment elevation, T-wave inversion, and development of Q waves. Persistent ST-segment elevation suggests left ventricular aneurysm. (Reproduced from Alpert JS. *Cardiology for the Primary Care Physician,* 2nd ed. Current Medicine/Current Science, 1998: pp 219–229. With kind permission from Current Medicine Group, LLC.)

coronary artery (LAD), and **leads I, aVL, V$_5$, and V$_6$** correspond to the **lateral** surface, supplied by the **left circumflex coronary artery** (LCX).

Cardiac Biomarkers

Certain proteins, referred to as cardiac biomarkers, are released into blood from necrotic heart muscle after an acute MI. Creatine phosphokinase (CK) level rises within 4 to 8 hours and returns to normal by 48 to 72 hours. Creatine phosphokinase is found in skeletal muscle and other tissues, but the creatine kinase myocardial band (CK-MB) isoenzyme is not found in significant amounts outside of heart muscle, so elevation of this fraction is more specific for myocardial injury. Cardiac-specific troponin I (cTnI) and cardiac-specific troponin T (cTnT) are more specific to heart muscle and are the preferred markers of myocardial injury. These protein levels rise approximately from 3 to 5 hours after infarct. Cardiac-specific troponin I levels may remain elevated for 7 to 10 days and cTnT levels for 10 to 14 days. They are very sensitive and fairly specific indicators of myocardial injury, and their levels may be elevated with even small amounts of myocardial necrosis. Generally, two sets of normal troponin levels 6 to 8 hours apart exclude MI.

The diagnosis of **acute MI** is made by finding **at least two of the following three features:** typical **chest pain persisting for more than 30 minutes,** typical **ECG findings,** and **elevated cardiac biomarker levels.** Because of the urgency in initiating treatment, diagnosis often rests upon the clinical history and the ECG findings, while determination of cardiac biomarker levels is pending. During the initial evaluation, one must consider and exclude other diagnoses that typically present with chest pain but would be worsened by the anticoagulation or thrombolysis usually used to treat acute MI. **Aortic dissection** often presents with **unequal pulses or blood pressures in the arms,** a **new murmur of aortic insufficiency,** or a **widened mediastinum** on chest x-ray film. Acute pericarditis often presents with chest pain and a pericardial friction rub, but the ECG findings show **diffuse ST-segment elevation** rather than those limited to a vascular territory.

TREATMENT OF ACUTE MI

Once an acute MI has been diagnosed based on history, ECG, or cardiac enzyme levels, several therapies are initiated. Because the process is caused by acute thrombosis, antiplatelet agents such as **aspirin** and anticoagulation with **heparin** are used. To limit infarct size, **beta-blockers** are used to decrease myocardial oxygen demand, and **nitrates** are given to increase coronary blood flow. All of these therapies appear to reduce mortality in patients with acute MI. In addition, morphine may be given to reduce pain and the consequent tachycardia, and patients are placed on supplemental oxygen (Figure 3–3).

Because prompt restoration of myocardial perfusion reduces mortality in STEMI, a decision should be made as to whether the patient can either receive thrombolytics or undergo primary PCI. Where it is readily available, primary PCI is the preferred therapy for most patients, as it is more effective than fibrinolysis in opening occluded arteries, and is associated with better clinical outcomes.

Individuals with ST-segment elevation MI benefit from thrombolytics, with a lower mortality, greater preservation of myocardial function, and fewer complications; patients without ST-segment elevation do not receive the same mortality benefit. Because myocardium can be salvaged only before it is irreversibly injured ("time is muscle"), patients **benefit maximally** when the drug is given early, for example, **within 1 to 3 hours after the onset of chest pain,** and the relative benefits decline with time. Because systemic coagulopathy may develop, the **major risk of thrombolytics is bleeding,** which can be potentially disastrous, for example, intracranial hemorrhage. The risk of hemorrhage is relatively constant, so the risk begins to outweigh the benefit by 12 hours, at which time most infarctions are completed, that is, the at-risk myocardium is dead.

Thrombolytic therapy is indicated if all of the following criteria are met:

1. Clinical complaints are consistent with ischemic-type chest pain.

2. ST-segment elevation more than 1 mm in at least two anatomically contiguous leads.

Figure 3–3. Algorithm for assessment and treatment of chest pain.

3. There are no contraindications to thrombolytic therapy.

4. Patient is younger than 75 years (greater risk of hemorrhage if >75).

Patients with STEMI should not receive thrombolytics if they have a clear contraindication, such as recent major surgery, active internal bleeding or suspected aortic dissection, severe hypertension, or a prior history of a hemorrhagic stroke.

Percutaneous coronary intervention is effective in restoring perfusion in patients with acute STEMI and has been shown in multiple trials to provide a greater survival benefit than thrombolysis and to have a lower risk for serious bleeding when performed by experienced operators in dedicated medical centers. **If patients with an acute STEMI present within 2 to 3 hours of symptom onset and receive PCI ideally within 90 minutes, then PCI is the recommended reperfusion therapy.** PCI also can be used in patients with a contraindication to thrombolytic therapy or who are hypotensive or in cardiogenic shock, for whom thrombolytics offer no survival benefit. PCI is accomplished by cardiac catheterization, in which a guidewire is inserted into the occluded coronary artery and a small balloon threaded over the guidewire and inflated in an attempt to open the blockage and restore blood flow. Sometimes intraluminal expandable stents are deployed, which may improve vessel patency. Use of primary PCI may be limited by the availability of the facilities and personnel required to perform the procedure in a timely fashion.

COMPLICATIONS OF ACUTE MI

Mortality in acute MI usually is a result of ventricular arrhythmias, or myocardial pump failure and resultant cardiogenic shock.

Life-threatening **ventricular arrhythmias,** such as **ventricular tachycardia (VT)** and **ventricular fibrillation (VF),** are common, especially in the first 24 hours. Historically, the majority of deaths from acute MI occurred in the first hour and was caused by VT/VF. This has diminished in recent years with earlier and more aggressive treatment of ischemia and arrhythmias. Premature ventricular contractions (PVCs) are very common but generally they are not treated with antiarrhythmic agents unless they occur very frequently, are sustained, or induce hemodynamic compromise. Sustained VT (>30 seconds) and VF are life threatening because they prevent coordinated ventricular contraction and thus often cause pulselessness and cardiovascular collapse. They are treated with **defibrillation,** followed by infusion of intravenous antiarrhythmics such as **amiodarone.** Electrolyte deficiency, such as hypokalemia or hypomagnesemia, which can potentiate ventricular arrhythmias, should be corrected. One benign ventricular arrhythmia that is generally not suppressed by antiarrhythmics is the **accelerated idioventricular rhythm.** This is a wide-complex escape rhythm between 60 and 110 bpm that frequently accompanies reperfusion of the myocardium but causes no hemodynamic compromise.

Supraventricular or atrial tachyarrhythmias are much less common after acute MI, but they can worsen ischemia and cause infarct extension as a consequence of the rate-related increase in myocardial oxygen demand. When they cause hemodynamic instability, they also are treated with immediate DC cardioversion. Other frequent rhythm disturbances are bradyarrhythmias. **Sinus bradycardia** is frequently seen in inferior MI because the right coronary artery supplies the sinoatrial node, but the condition generally requires no treatment unless it causes hypotension. If the heart rate is slow enough to cause cardiac output and blood pressure to fall, intravenous **atropine** usually is administered.

Bradyarrhythmias can be caused by atrioventricular (AV) conduction disturbances. **First-degree AV block** (PR interval prolongation) and **Mobitz I second-degree AV block** (gradual prolongation of the PR interval before a nonconducted P wave) often are caused by AV nodal dysfunction, for example, nodal ischemia caused by inferior MI. Patients who are symptomatic can be treated with **atropine**.

AV conduction disturbances can be caused by dysfunction below the AV node, within the bundles of His, and typically produce a widened QRS complex. Examples include **Mobitz II second-degree AV block** (nonconducted P waves not preceded by PR prolongation) and **third-degree AV block** (complete AV dissociation with no P-wave conduction). Third-degree AV block also can be caused by AV nodal dysfunction. These arrhythmias are described more fully in Cases 8-9. Conduction disturbances caused by involvement of the bundles of His include **LBBB** or **right bundle branch block (RBBB) with left anterior hemiblock**. All of these conduction disturbances have a worse prognosis than does AV nodal dysfunction because they are generally seen with anterior infarction in which a significant amount of myocardium is damaged. When symptomatic bradycardias such as third-degree AV block develop, they may be treated with external pacing but can require placement of a **temporary transvenous pacemaker if the patient is in cardiogenic shock from complete heart block. Patients in persistent complete heart block will require placement of a permanent pacemaker.**

CARDIAC PUMP FAILURE AND CARDIOGENIC SHOCK

Cardiogenic shock in acute MI usually is the most severe form of left ventricular (LV) pump failure, manifested by end-organ hypoperfusion. Ischemic reduction in ventricular diastolic compliance may lead to transient pulmonary congestion, associated with elevated left-sided filling pressures. Extensive myocardial necrosis and less contracting heart muscle may cause systolic failure and reduced cardiac output. Patients with hypotension frequently are evaluated by pulmonary artery (Swan-Ganz) catheterization to assess hemodynamic parameters. **Cardiogenic shock** is diagnosed when the patient has **hypotension** with systolic arterial pressure less than 80 mm Hg, **markedly reduced cardiac index** less than **1.8 L/min/m²**, and **elevated LV filling pressure** (measured indirectly with a pulmonary capillary wedge pressure >18 mm Hg). Clinically, such patients appear hypotensive, with cold extremities because of peripheral vasoconstriction, pulmonary edema, and elevated jugular venous pressure, reflecting high left- and right-sided filling pressures. Supportive treatment includes hemodynamic monitoring, adequate ventilation and oxygenation, and blood pressure support with vasopressors such as dobutamine and dopamine. These patients also may require mechanical assistance to augment blood pressure while providing afterload reduction, using intra-aortic balloon counterpulsation. Cardiogenic shock may require urgent revascularization with primary PCI or coronary artery bypass surgery.

Hypotension may also be seen in patients with **right ventricular (RV) infarction,** which is a complication of right coronary artery occlusion and inferior infarction.

In this case, LV function is not impaired, but LV filling is dramatically reduced because of the right-sided ventricular failure (the left heart can only pump out what it receives from the right heart). These patients can be recognized clinically as **hypotensive, with markedly elevated jugular venous pressure but clear lung fields** and no pulmonary edema seen radiographically (in contrast to the pulmonary edema seen in patients with hypotension to LV failure), and the diagnosis confirmed by observation of ST-segment elevation in a right-sided ECG. In this setting, RV function is impaired and highly dependent on adequate preload, so treatment requires support consisting of volume replacement with crystalloid or colloid solution. Patients with RV dysfunction or failure may require inotropic support to increase blood delivery to the left ventricle. Diuretics or nitrates that might lower the preload can be disastrous in these patients by causing hypotension and cardiovascular collapse, and thus should be avoided.

A number of **mechanical problems** can complicate acute MI, usually within the first week. The most common is **papillary muscle dysfunction** caused by LV ischemia or infarction, leading to **mitral regurgitation** that may be hemodynamically significant. This is in contrast with **papillary muscle rupture**, which produces a flail mitral leaflet and acute mitral regurgitation with development of heart failure and cardiogenic shock. Development of acute heart failure and shock in association with a **new holosystolic murmur also may signify ventricular septal rupture.** Transthoracic echocardiography can be used to distinguish among these conditions. In all of them, stabilization of cardiogenic shock is accomplished using afterload reduction with intravenous nitroglycerin or nitroprusside and sometimes with intra-aortic balloon counterpulsation until definitive, urgent, surgical repair can be accomplished. Other modalities of mechanical circulatory support may be used for temporary support in cardiogenic shock, including the TandemHeart or venous-arterial extracorporeal membrane oxygenation (ECMO).

The most catastrophic mechanical complication is **rupture of the ventricular free wall.** As blood fills the pericardium, cardiac tamponade develops rapidly, with sudden pulselessness, hypotension, and loss of consciousness. This complication nearly always is fatal.

Late complications that occur several weeks after an acute MI include development of a **ventricular aneurysm,** which should be suspected if ST-segment elevation persists weeks after the event, as well as **Dressler syndrome,** an immune phenomenon characterized by **pericarditis, pleuritis, and fever.** Dressler syndrome may remit and relapse, and it is treated with anti-inflammatory drugs, including nonsteroidal anti-inflammatory drugs (NSAIDs) and sometimes prednisone.

POST-MI RISK STRATIFICATION

The goal is to identify patients who are at high risk for subsequent cardiac events and who might benefit from revascularization. The initial evaluation involves noninvasive testing. **Submaximal exercise stress testing** is generally performed in stable patients before hospital discharge to detect residual ischemia and ventricular ectopy and to provide a guideline for exercise in the early recovery period. **Evaluation of LV systolic function,** usually with echocardiography, is routinely performed. High-risk patients include those with impaired systolic function, large areas of ischemic myocardium on stress testing or postinfarction angina, or ventricular ectopy who might benefit from coronary angiography to evaluate for revascularization. Percutaneous coronary intervention can be performed to reduce anginal symptoms, and **coronary artery bypass surgery** should be considered for patients with **multivessel atherosclerotic stenosis** and **impaired systolic function** because the surgery may reduce symptoms and prolong survival. Post-STEMI patients with **LV dysfunction** (LV ejection fraction <40%) are at **increased risk for sudden cardiac death** from **ventricular arrhythmias** and may benefit from placement of an implantable cardioverter-defibrillator (ICD).

SECONDARY PREVENTION OF ISCHEMIC HEART DISEASE

Medical therapy to reduce modifiable risk factors is the cornerstone of post-MI care. In addition to symptom relief, the major goal of medical therapy is to prevent cardiac events: fatal or nonfatal MI. By far, the **most important risk factor is smoking cessation.** Quitting tobacco use can reduce the risk of fatal or nonfatal cardiac events by more than 50%, more than any other medical or surgical therapy available. A number of other therapies reduce the risk of recurrent cardiovascular events and prolong survival in patients with coronary artery disease. Antiplatelet agents such as **aspirin** and **clopidogrel** reduce the risk of thrombus formation, **beta-blockers** reduce myocardial oxygen demand and may help suppress ventricular arrhythmias, and cholesterol-lowering agents such as **statins** reduce the number of coronary events and prolong survival. Patients with established coronary artery disease (CAD) should have a low-density lipoprotein (LDL) cholesterol level less than 70 mg/dL. **Angiotensin-converting enzyme (ACE) inhibitors** are recommended for all patients after STEMI but are most important for patients with impaired systolic function (ejection fraction <40%), diabetes, or hypertension.

CASE CORRELATION

- See also Case 2 (Hypercholesterolemia), Case 10 (Acute Pericarditis), and Case 13 Limb Ischemia, Peripheral Vascular Disease)

COMPREHENSION QUESTIONS

3.1 A 36-year-old woman has severe burning chest pain that radiates to her neck. The pain occurs particularly after meals, especially when she lies down, and is not precipitated by exertion. She is admitted for observation. Serial ECG and troponin I levels are normal. Which of the following is the best next step?

  A. Stress thallium treadmill test

  B. Initiation of a proton pump inhibitor

  C. Coronary angiography

  D. Initiation of an antidepressant such as a selective serotonin reuptake inhibitor

  E. Referral to a psychiatrist

3.2 A 56-year-old man is admitted to the hospital for chest pain of 2-hour duration. His heart rate is 42 bpm, with sinus bradycardia on ECG, as well as ST-segment elevation in leads II, III, and aVF. Which of the following is the most likely diagnosis?

A. He is likely in good physical condition with increased vagal tone.

B. He likely has suffered an inferior wall MI.

C. He likely has an LV aneurysm.

D. The low heart rate is a reflection of a good cardiac ejection fraction.

3.3 A 59-year-old diabetic woman had suffered an acute anterior wall MI. Five days later, she gets into an argument with her husband and complains of chest pain. Her initial ECG shows no ischemic changes, but serum cardiac troponin I levels are drawn and return mildly elevated at this time. Which of the following is the best next step?

A. Use thrombolytic therapy.

B. Treat with percutaneous coronary intervention.

C. Perform coronary artery bypass.

D. Perform serial ECGs and obtain CK-MB.

E. Prepare the patient for dialysis.

3.4 A 59-year-old male smoker complains of severe substernal squeezing chest pain of 30-minute duration. The paramedics have given sublingual nitroglycerin and oxygen by nasal cannula. His blood pressure is 110/70 mm Hg and heart rate is 90 bpm on arrival to the ER. The ECG is normal. Which of the following is the best next step?

A. Echocardiography

B. Thallium stress test

C. Aspirin

D. Coronary angiography

E. Coronary artery bypass

ANSWERS

3.1 **B.** It is appropriate to evaluate chest pain to first rule out cardiac ischemia. One of the most common causes of "chest pain" particularly in a younger patient is gastroesophageal reflux or esophageal spasm. This patient has classic symptoms of reflux esophagitis and is best treated with a proton pump inhibitor. If the chest pain has the characteristics of angina pectoris (substernal location, precipitated by exertion, relieved by rest or nitroglycerin), it should be investigated with a stress test or coronary angiography.

3.2 **B.** A 56 year old woman is admitted to the hospital with a 2 hour history of chest pain. Sinus bradycardia is often seen with inferior wall MI, because the right coronary artery supplies the inferior wall of the left ventricle and the sinoatrial node. The ischemic changes in leads II, III, and aVF are in the region of the inferior leads. Understanding which leads reflect which portion of the heart allows for an understanding of the aspect of the heart that is affected. Also understanding the area of the heart perfused by the various coronary arteries allows for correlation of associated symptoms or therapy.

3.3 **D.** Diabetic patients can have myocardial ischemia or infarction with atypical or absent symptoms. Clinical suspicion and a liberal use of cardiac enzymes are required. Troponin levels often remain elevated for 7 to 10 days and should not be used to diagnose reinfarction, especially if the levels are trending downward. New ECG findings or rapidly rising markers such as serum myoglobin or CK-MB can be used in this setting.

3.4 **C.** Aspirin is the first agent that should be used after oxygen and nitroglycerin. Aspirin use decreases mortality in the face of an acute coronary event. Because initial ECGs and cardiac enzymes may be normal in an acute MI, serial studies are needed to definitively rule out MI. Clinical assessment to exclude other causes of chest pain should be undertaken. The other answer choices are aimed toward diagnostic tests and may be important, but the first and foremost priority should be to "save myocardium."

CLINICAL PEARLS

▶ Acute coronary syndromes (unstable angina or acute myocardial infarction) occur when a thrombus forms at the site of rupture of an atherosclerotic plaque and acutely occludes a coronary artery.

▶ Acute myocardial infarction is diagnosed based on the presence of at least two of three criteria: typical symptoms, ECG findings, and cardiac enzymes. Initial ECG and enzyme levels may be normal, so serial studies are necessary.

▶ Early reperfusion with PCI or thrombolytics reduces mortality and preserves ventricular function in patients who have ST-segment elevation, have no contraindications, and receive treatment within the first 6 to 12 hours.

▶ The goal of secondary prevention after myocardial infarction is to prevent recurrent cardiac events and death. Smoking cessation, aspirin and clopidogrel, beta-blockers, ACE inhibitors, and statins all reduce the rate of events and mortality.

▶ After myocardial infarction, PCI can be performed to reduce ischemia and anginal symptoms. Bypass surgery may be indicated for patients with multivessel stenosis and impaired systolic function to reduce symptoms and prolong survival.

▶ The ECG can indicate the location of the ischemia or infarction: anterior (leads V_2 through V_4), lateral (leads I, aVL, V_5, and V_6), inferior (leads II, III, and aVF), and posterior (R waves in leads V_1 and V_2).

▶ STEMI is characterized by ischemic discomfort along with ST-segment elevation on ECG. Unstable angina and NSTEMI will not have ST-segment elevation, but NSTEMI is diagnosed by positive cardiac biomarkers.

REFERENCES

Antman EM, Loscalzo J. ST-segment elevation myocardial infarction. In: Longo DL, Fauci AS, Kasper, DL, et al., eds. *Harrison's Principles of Internal Medicine.* 18th ed. New York, NY: McGraw-Hill; 2012:2021-2035.

Antman EM, Selwyn AP, Loscalzo, J. Ischemic heart disease. In: Longo DL, Fauci AS, Kasper, DL, et al., eds. *Harrison's Principles of Internal Medicine.* 18th ed. New York, NY: McGraw-Hill; 2012:1998-2015.

Kushner FG, Hand M, Smith SC Jr, et al. 2009 focused update of the ACC/AHA 2004 guidelines for the management of patients with ST-elevation myocardial infarction. *Circulation.* 2009;120:2271.

Tatum JL, Jesse RL, Kontos MC, et al. Comprehensive strategy for the evaluation and triage of the chest pain patient. *Ann Emerg Med.* 1997;29:116-125.

A 72-year-old man presents to the clinic complaining of several weeks of worsening exertional dyspnea. Previously, he had been able to work in his garden and mow the lawn, but now he feels short of breath after walking 100 ft. He does not have chest pain when he walks, although in the past, he has experienced episodes of retrosternal chest pressure with strenuous exertion. Once recently he had felt light-headed, as if he were about to faint while climbing a flight of stairs, but the symptom passed after he sat down. He has been having some difficulty in sleeping at night and has to prop himself up with two pillows. Occasionally, he wakes up at night feeling quite short of breath, which is relieved within minutes by sitting upright and dangling his legs over the bed. His feet have become swollen, especially by the end of the day. He denies any significant medical history, takes no medications, and prides himself on the fact that he has not seen a doctor in years. He does not smoke or drink alcohol.

On physical examination, he is afebrile, with a heart rate of 86 bpm, blood pressure of 115/92 mm Hg, and respiratory rate of 16 breaths per minute. Examination of the head and neck reveals pink mucosa without pallor, a normal thyroid gland, and distended neck veins. Bibasilar inspiratory crackles are heard on examination. On cardiac examination, his heart rhythm is regular with a normal S_1 and a second heart sound that splits during expiration, an S_4 at the apex, a nondisplaced apical impulse, and a late-peaking systolic murmur at the right upper sternal border that radiates to his carotids. The carotid upstrokes have diminished amplitude.

▶ What is the most likely diagnosis?
▶ What test would confirm the diagnosis?

ANSWERS TO CASE 4:

Congestive Heart Failure due to Critical Aortic Stenosis

Summary: A 72-year-old man complains of several weeks of worsening exertional dyspnea. He has experienced angina-like chest pressure with strenuous exertion and near-syncope while climbing a flight of stairs, and now he has symptoms of heart failure (HF) such as orthopnea and paroxysmal nocturnal dyspnea. Heart failure is also suggested by physical signs of volume overload (pedal edema, elevated jugular venous pressure, and crackles suggesting pulmonary edema). The cause of his heart failure may be aortic valvular stenosis, given the late systolic murmur radiating to his carotid, the paradoxical splitting of his second heart sound, and the diminished carotid upstrokes.

- **Most likely diagnosis:** Congestive heart failure (CHF), possibly as a result of aortic stenosis.

- **Diagnostic test:** Echocardiogram to assess the aortic valve area as well as the left ventricular systolic function.

ANALYSIS

Objectives

1. Know the causes of chronic heart failure (eg, ischemia, hypertension, valvular disease, alcohol abuse, cocaine, and thyrotoxicosis).

2. Recognize impaired systolic function versus diastolic dysfunction.

3. Be familiar with the treatment of acute and chronic heart failure.

4. Be familiar with the evaluation of aortic stenosis and the indications for valve replacement.

Considerations

This is an elderly patient with symptoms and signs of aortic stenosis. The valvular disorder has progressed from previous angina and presyncopal symptoms to heart failure, reflecting worsening severity of the stenosis and worsening prognosis for survival. This patient should undergo urgent evaluation of his aortic valve surface area and coronary artery status to assess the need for valve replacement.

APPROACH TO:

Congestive Heart Failure

DEFINITIONS

ACUTE HEART FAILURE: Acute (hours, days) presentation of cardiac decompensation with pulmonary edema and low cardiac output, which may proceed to cardiogenic shock.

CHRONIC HEART FAILURE: Chronic (months, years) presence of cardiac dysfunction; symptoms may range from minimal to severe.

DIASTOLIC DYSFUNCTION: Increased diastolic filling pressures caused by impaired diastolic relaxation and decreased ventricular compliance, but with preserved ejection fraction (EF) >40% to 50%.

SYSTOLIC DYSFUNCTION: Low cardiac output caused by impaired systolic function (low ejection fraction <40%).

CARDIAC REMODELING: Changes to the heart due to increased cardiac loading (preload and afterload), which leads to cardiac dysfunction. Some medications can prevent or even reverse the remodeling.

CLINICAL APPROACH

Congestive heart failure (CHF) is a **clinical syndrome** that is produced when the heart is **unable to meet the metabolic needs of the body while maintaining normal ventricular filling pressures.** A series of **neurohumoral responses** develop, including activation of the renin-angiotensin-aldosterone axis and increased sympathetic activity, which initially may be compensatory but ultimately cause further cardiac decompensation. Symptoms may be a result of **forward failure** (low cardiac output or systolic dysfunction), including **fatigue, lethargy, and even hypotension,** or **backward failure** (increased filling pressures or diastolic dysfunction), including **dyspnea, peripheral edema, and ascites.** Some patients have isolated diastolic dysfunction with preserved left ventricular ejection fraction (LVEF >40%-50%), most often as a consequence of hypertension or simply of aging. Half of patients with CHF have impaired systolic dysfunction (LVEF <40%) with associated increased filling pressures. Some patients have isolated right-sided heart failure (with elevated jugular venous pressure, hepatic congestion, peripheral edema but no pulmonary edema), but more commonly patients have left ventricular failure (with low cardiac output and pulmonary edema) that progresses to biventricular failure. **Auscultatory findings may include an S$_4$ (atrial gallop) or an S$_3$ (ventricular gallop),** low-pitched heart sounds that are heard best with the bell of the stethoscope.

Heart failure is a **chronic and progressive disease** that can be assessed by following the patient's exercise tolerance, such as the **New York Heart Association (NYHA) functional classification** (Table 4–1). This functional classification carries prognostic significance. Individuals in class III who have low oxygen consumption during exercise have an annual mortality rate of 20%; in class IV, the rate is 60% annually. Patients with a low ventricular ejection fraction (LVEF <20%) also have very high mortality risks. Death associated with CHF may occur from the underlying disease process, cardiogenic shock, or sudden death as a result of ventricular arrhythmias.

Table 4–1 • NYHA FUNCTIONAL CLASSIFICATION
Class I: No limitation during ordinary physical activity
Class II: Slight limitation of physical activity. Develops fatigue or dyspnea with moderate exertion
Class III: Marked limitation of physical activity. Even light activity produces symptoms
Class IV: Symptoms at rest. Any activity causes worsening

Table 4–2 • SELECTED CAUSES OF CONGESTIVE HEART FAILURE
Myocardial injury, or other chemotherapeutic agents
• Adriamycin
• Alcohol use
• Cocaine
• Ischemic cardiomyopathy (atherosclerotic coronary artery disease)
• Rheumatic fever
• Viral myocarditis
Chronic pressure overload
• Aortic stenosis
• Hypertension
Chronic volume overload
• Mitral regurgitation
Infiltrative diseases
• Amyloidosis
• Hemochromatosis
Chronic tachyarrhythmia or bradyarrhythmia

Although heart failure has many causes (Table 4–2), identification of the underlying treatable or reversible causes of disease is essential. For example, heart failure related to tachycardia, alcohol consumption, or viral myocarditis may be reversible with removal of the inciting factor. In patients with underlying multivessel atherosclerotic coronary disease and a low ejection fraction, revascularization with coronary artery bypass grafting improves cardiac function and prolongs survival. For patients with heart failure, appropriate investigation is guided by the history but may include echocardiography to assess ejection fraction and valvular function, cardiac stress testing, or coronary angiography as indicated, and, in some cases, endomyocardial biopsy.

The three major treatment goals for patients with chronic heart failure are relief of symptoms, preventing disease progression, and a reduction in mortality risk. The heart failure symptoms, which are mainly caused by low cardiac output and fluid overload, usually are relieved with dietary sodium restriction and loop diuretics. Because heart failure has such a substantial mortality, however, measures in an attempt to halt or reverse disease progression are necessary. Reversible causes should be aggressively sought and treated. Use of **angiotensin-converting enzyme (ACE) inhibitors or angiotensin receptor blockers (ARBs) and some beta-blockers, such as carvedilol (CAR), metoprolol, or bisoprolol, have been shown to reduce mortality in patients with impaired systolic function and moderate to severe symptoms. In patients who cannot tolerate ACE inhibition (or in black patients in whom ACE inhibitors appear to confer less benefit), the use of hydralazine with nitrates has been shown to decrease mortality. Aldosterone antagonists such as spironolactone may be added to patients with NYHA class III or IV heart failure with persistent symptoms, but patients should be monitored for hyperkalemia. Digoxin can be added to these regimens for persistent symptoms, but it provides no survival benefit.**

The mechanisms of the various agents are as follows:

Beta-blockers: Prevent and reverse adrenergically mediated intrinsic myocardial dysfunction and remodeling.

ACE inhibitors: Reduce preload and afterload, thereby reducing right atrial, pulmonary arterial, and pulmonary capillary wedge pressures along with systemic vascular resistance, and prevent remodeling. These **agents are the initial drugs of choice in treating CHF since there is a survival advantage with their use.**

Nitrates and nitrites: (not as commonly used) Reduce preload and clear pulmonary congestion.

Diuretics: Used to decrease preload, used especially acutely.

Digoxin: Acts to improve the cardiac contractility somewhat.

Aldosterone antagonists: Block the action of aldosterone.

Some devices may also be useful in reducing symptoms and mortality in patients with heart failure. Patients with depressed ejection fraction and advanced symptoms often have a widened QRS >120 ms, indicating dyssynchronous ventricular contraction. Placement of a biventricular pacemaker, called **cardiac resynchronization therapy (CRT)**, to stimulate both ventricles to contract simultaneously can improve symptoms and reduce mortality. Since patients with class II-III HF and depressed EF <35% have elevated risk of sudden cardiac death due to ventricular arrhythmias, placement of an **implantable cardiac defibrillator (ICD)** should be considered.

In patients with **acute decompensated heart failure**, the initial treatment goals are to **stabilize the patient's hemodynamic derangements** and to **identify and treat reversible factors** that may have precipitated the decompensation, such as arrhythmias or myocardial ischemia. Regarding hemodynamics, if patients appear to have elevated LV filling pressures, they often require intravenous vasodilators such as nitroglycerin infusion, and patients with decreased cardiac output may require inotropes such as dobutamine, and if hypotensive, they may require vasoconstrictors such as dopamine.

Aortic Stenosis

The history and physical findings presented in the scenario suggest that this patient's heart failure may be a result of aortic stenosis. This is the **most common symptomatic valvular abnormality in adults.** The large majority of cases occur in men. The causes of the valvular stenosis vary depending on the typical age of presentation: stenosis in patients **younger than 30 years** usually is caused by a **congenital bicuspid valve;** in patients 30 to 70 years old, it usually is caused by congenital stenosis or acquired rheumatic heart disease; and in patients **older than 70 years,** it **usually is caused by degenerative calcific stenosis.**

Typical physical findings include a **narrow pulse pressure,** a **harsh late-peaking systolic murmur** heard best at the right second intercostal space with radiation to the carotid arteries, and a delayed slow-rising carotid upstroke (*pulsus parvus et tardus*). The electrocardiography (ECG) often shows left ventricular hypertrophy.

Doppler echocardiography reveals a thickened abnormal valve and can define severity as assessed by the aortic valve area and by estimating the transvalvular pressure gradient. As the valve orifice narrows, the pressure gradient increases in an attempt to maintain cardiac output. Severe aortic stenosis is defined as a valve area less than 1 cm^2 (normal 3-4 cm^2) and mean pressure gradient more than 40 mm Hg.

Symptoms of aortic stenosis develop as a consequence of the resulting left ventricular hypertrophy as well as the diminished cardiac output caused by the flow-limiting valvular stenosis. The first symptom typically is **angina pectoris**, that is, retrosternal chest pain precipitated by exercise and relieved by rest. As the stenosis worsens and cardiac output falls, patients may experience **syncopal episodes**, typically precipitated by exertion. Finally, because of the low cardiac output and high diastolic filling pressures, patients develop clinically apparent **heart failure** as described earlier. The prognosis for patients worsens as symptoms develop, with mean survival with angina, syncope, or heart failure of 5 years, 3 years, and 2 years, respectively.

Patients with severe stenosis who are symptomatic should be considered for aortic valve replacement. Preoperative cardiac catheterization is routinely performed to provide definitive assessment of aortic valve area and the pressure gradient, as well as to assess the coronary arteries for significant stenosis. In patients who are not good candidates for valve replacement, the stenotic valve can be enlarged using balloon valvuloplasty, but this will provide only temporary relief of symptoms, as there is a high rate of restenosis. Percutaneous transcatheter aortic valve replacement (TAVR) is a new technique that has been developed for patients who are assessed as having unacceptably high surgical risk, and catheter-based aortic valves have now been approved for use in Europe and the United States.

COMPREHENSION QUESTIONS

4.1 A 55-year-old man is noted to have moderately severe congestive heart failure with impaired systolic function. Which of the following drugs would most likely lower his risk of mortality?

A. Angiotensin-converting enzyme inhibitors

B. Loop diuretics

C. Digoxin

D. Aspirin

4.2 In the United States, which of the following is most likely to have caused the congestive heart failure in the patient described in Question 4.1?

A. Diabetes

B. Atherosclerosis

C. Alcohol

D. Rheumatic heart disease

4.3 A 75-year-old man is noted to have chest pain with exertion and has been passing out recently. On examination he is noted to have a harsh systolic murmur.
Which of the following is the best therapy for his condition?

A. Coronary artery bypass

B. Angioplasty

C. Valve replacement

D. Carotid endarterectomy

4.4 A 55-year-old man is noted to have congestive heart failure and states that he is
comfortable at rest but becomes dyspneic even with walking to the bathroom.
On echocardiography, he is noted to have an ejection fraction of 47%. Which
of the following is the more accurate description of this patient's condition?

A. Diastolic dysfunction

B. Systolic dysfunction

C. Dilated cardiomyopathy

D. Pericardial disease

ANSWERS

4.1 **A.** Angiotensin-converting enzyme inhibitors and beta-blockers decrease the
risk of mortality for patients who have CHF with impaired systolic function.
For this reason, these agents are the initial therapies of choice to treat CHF.
They both prevent and can even, in some circumstances, reverse the **cardiac
remodeling.**

4.2 **B.** In the United States, the most common cause of CHF associated with
impaired systolic function is ischemic cardiomyopathy due to coronary
atherosclerosis.

4.3 **C.** The symptoms of aortic stenosis classically progress through angina, syncope, and, finally, congestive heart failure, which has the worse prognosis for
survival. This patient's systolic murmur is consistent with aortic stenosis. An
evaluation should include echocardiography to confirm the diagnosis, and
then aortic valve replacement.

4.4 **A.** When the ejection fraction exceeds 40%, there is likely diastolic dysfunction, with stiff ventricles. The stiff thickened ventricles do not accept blood
very readily. This patient has symptoms with mild exertion that are indicative
of functional class III. The worst class is level IV, manifested as symptoms at
rest or with minimal exertion. ACE inhibitors are important agents in patients
with diastolic dysfunction.

CLINICAL PEARLS

▶ Congestive heart failure is a clinical syndrome that is always caused by some underlying heart disease, most commonly ischemic cardiomyopathy as a result of atherosclerotic coronary disease, or hypertension.

▶ Heart failure can be caused by impaired systolic function (ejection fraction <40%) or impaired diastolic function (with preserved systolic function).

▶ Chronic heart failure is a progressive disease with a high mortality. A patient's functional class, that is, his or her exercise tolerance, is the best predictor of mortality and often guides therapy.

▶ The primary goals of therapy are to relieve congestive symptoms with salt restriction, diuretics, and vasodilators. Angiotensin-converting enzyme inhibitors, beta-blockers, and aldosterone antagonists can decrease mortality.

▶ Cardiac resynchronization therapy (CRT) and placement of an implantable cardioverter defibrillator (ICD) can reduce symptoms and improve mortality in patients with advanced heart failure and low ejection fraction <35%.

▶ Aortic stenosis produces progressive symptoms such as angina, exertional syncope, and heart failure, with increasingly higher risk of mortality. Valve replacement should be considered for patients with symptoms and severe aortic stenosis, for example, an aortic valve area less than 1 cm^2.

REFERENCES

Carabello BA. Clinical practice: aortic stenosis. *N Engl J Med*. 2002;346:677-682.

Jessup M, Brozena S. Heart failure. *N Engl J Med*. 2003;348:2007-2018.

Lejemtel TH, Sonnenblick EH, Frishman WH. Diagnosis and management of heart failure. In: Fuster V, Alexander RX, O'Rourke RA, eds. *Hurst's the Heart*. 10th ed. New York, NY: McGraw-Hill; 2001:6.

Mann DL. Heart failure and cor pulmonale. In: Longo DL, Fauci AS, Kasper DL, et al., eds. *Harrison's Principles of Internal Medicine*. 18th ed. New York, NY: McGraw-Hill; 2012:1901-1915.

A 42-year-old man is brought to the emergency department (ED) by ambulance after a sudden onset of severe retrosternal chest pain that began an hour ago while he was at home mowing the lawn. He describes the pain as sharp, constant, and unrelated to movement. It was not relieved by three doses of sublingual nitroglycerin administered by the paramedics while en route to the hospital. He has never had symptoms like this before. His only medical history is hypertension, for which he takes enalapril. There is no cardiac disease in his family. He does not smoke, drink alcohol, or use illicit drugs. He is a basketball coach at a local high school, and is usually physically very active.

On physical examination, he is a tall man with long arms and legs who appears uncomfortable and diaphoretic; he is lying on the stretcher with his eyes closed. He is afebrile, with a heart rate of 118 bpm, and blood pressure of 156/64 mm Hg in the right arm and 188/74 mm Hg in the left arm. His head and neck examination is unremarkable. His chest is clear to auscultation bilaterally, and incidental note is made of pectus excavatum. His heart rate is tachycardic and regular, with a soft, early diastolic murmur at the right sternal border, and his pulses are bounding. His abdominal examination is benign, and neurologic examination is nonfocal. His chest x-ray shows a widened mediastinum.

▶ What is the most likely diagnosis?
▶ What is your next step?

ANSWERS TO CASE 5:

Aortic Dissection, Marfan Syndrome

Summary: A 42-year-old man is brought in to the ED with severe chest pain, which was unrelieved by nitroglycerin. His blood pressure is elevated but asymmetric in his arms, and he has a new murmur of aortic insufficiency. The chest x-ray shows a widened mediastinum. All of these features strongly suggest aortic dissection as the cause of his pain. He is tall with pectus excavatum and other features suggestive of Marfan syndrome, which may be the underlying cause of his dissection.

- **Most likely diagnosis:** Aortic dissection.

- **Next step:** Administer an intravenous beta-blocker to lower blood pressure and arterial shear stress, then perform a noninvasive imaging procedure, such as transesophageal echocardiography (TEE), computed tomography (CT) angiography, or magnetic resonance imaging (MRI).

ANALYSIS

Objectives

1. Learn the clinical and radiographic features of aortic dissection as well as complications of dissection.

2. Know the risk factors for aortic dissection.

3. Understand the management of dissection and the indications for surgical versus medical treatment.

4. Learn about other aortic diseases, such as abdominal aortic aneurysm (AAA), the role of surveillance, and indications for surgical repair.

Considerations

Most patients with chest pain seek medical attention, because of the concern about a myocardial infarction (MI). Differentiating other conditions of chest pain is important because some underlying conditions, such as aortic dissection, could be worsened by the treatment of MI, for example, by anticoagulation with heparin or use of thrombolytics. In hypertensive patients with dissection, urgent blood pressure lowering is indicated to limit propagation of the dissection.

APPROACH TO:

Aortic Aneurysm and Dissection

DEFINITIONS

ABDOMINAL AORTIC ANEURYSM: Defined as a pathologic dilation to more than 1.5 times the normal diameter of the aorta. Aneurysms can occur anywhere in the thoracic or abdominal aorta, but the large majority occurs in the abdomen, below the renal arteries.

AORTIC DISSECTION: Tear or ulceration of the aortic intima that allows pulsatile aortic flow to dissect longitudinally along elastic planes of the media, creating a false lumen or channel for blood flow. Sometimes referred to as a "dissecting aneurysm," although that term is misleading because the dissection typically produces the aneurysmal dilation rather than the reverse.

CLINICAL APPROACH

The aorta is the largest conductance vessel in the body. It receives most of the shear forces generated by the heart with every heartbeat throughout the lifetime of an individual. The wall of the aorta is composed of three layers: the intima, the media, and the adventitia. These specialized layers allow the aortic wall to distend under the great pressure created by every heartbeat. Some of this kinetic energy is stored as potential energy, thus allowing forward flow to be maintained during the cardiac cycle. One must consider the great tensile stress that the walls of this vessel face when considering the pathologic processes that affect it.

Cystic degeneration of the elastic media predisposes patients to aortic dissection. This occurs in various connective tissue disorders that cause cystic medial degeneration, such as Marfan syndrome and Ehlers-Danlos syndrome. Other factors predisposing to aortic dissection are hypertension, aortic valvular abnormalities such as aortic stenosis and congenital bicuspid aortic valve, coarctation of the aorta, pregnancy, and atherosclerotic disease. Aortic dissection may occur iatrogenically after cardiac surgery or catheterization.

A dissection occurs when there is a sudden intimal tear or rupture followed by the formation of a dissecting hematoma within the aortic media, separating the intima from the adventitia and propagating distally. The presence of hypertension and associated shear forces are the most important factors causing propagation of the dissection. Aortic dissection can produce several devastating or fatal complications. It can produce an intraluminal intimal flap, which can occlude branch arteries and cause organ ischemia or infarction. The hematoma may rupture into the pericardial sac, causing cardiac tamponade, or into the pleural space, causing exsanguination. It can produce severe acute aortic regurgitation leading to fulminant heart failure.

The clinical features of aortic dissection typically include a **sudden onset of ripping or tearing pain in the chest, which often radiates to the back** and may radiate to the neck or extremities as the dissection extends (Table 5–1). Differentiating the pain of dissection from the pain of myocardial ischemia or infarction is essential because **the use of anticoagulation or thrombolytics in a patient with a dissection may be devastating.** In contrast to anginal pain, which often builds over minutes, the pain of dissection is **often maximal at onset.** In addition, myocardial ischemia pain usually is relieved with nitrates, whereas the pain of dissection is not. Also, because most dissections begin very close to the aortic valve, a dissection may produce the **early diastolic murmur of aortic insufficiency;** if it occludes branch arteries, it can produce dramatically different pulses and blood pressures in the extremities. Most patients

Table 5–1 • CLINICAL MANIFESTATION OF AORTIC DISSECTION	
Complication	Mechanism
Horner syndrome	Compression of the superior cervical ganglion
Myocardial infarction	Occlusion of coronary artery ostia
Hemopericardium, pericardial tamponade	Thoracic dissection with retrograde flow into the pericardium
Aortic regurgitation	Thoracic dissection involving the aortic root
Bowel ischemia, hematuria	Dissection involving the mesenteric arteries or renal arteries
Hypertension, different blood pressures in arms	Thoracic dissection involving brachiocephalic artery
Hemiplegia	Carotid artery involvement

with dissection are hypertensive; if hypotension is present, one must suspect aortic rupture, cardiac tamponade, or dissection of the subclavian artery supplying the arm where the blood pressure is being measured. Often a widened superior mediastinum is noted on plain chest film because of dissection of the ascending aorta.

When aortic dissection is suspected, confirming the diagnosis with an imaging study is essential. Conventional aortography was the traditional diagnostic "gold standard," but in recent years, very sensitive noninvasive studies, such as TEE, dynamic CT scanning, and MRI, have gained widespread use. Because of the emergent nature of the condition, the best initial study is the one that can be obtained and interpreted quickly in the given hospital setting.

Several classification schemes describe the different types of aortic dissections. Figure 5–1 shows the Stanford classification. Type A dissection always involves the ascending aorta but can involve any other part. Type B dissection does not involve the ascending aorta but can involve any other part.

Two-thirds of aortic dissections originate in the ascending aorta a few centimeters above the aortic valve. The classification system is important because it guides therapy. Virtually all **type A (proximal or ascending) dissections require urgent surgical therapy** with replacement of the involved aorta and sometimes the aortic valve. Without surgery, the mortality rate for type A dissections is 90%. Type B dissections do not involve the ascending aorta and typically originate in the aortic arch distal to the left subclavian artery. Type B dissections usually are first managed medically, and surgery usually is performed only for complications such as rupture or ischemia of a branch artery of the aorta.

The aim of medical therapy is to prevent propagation of the dissection by reducing mean arterial pressure and the rate of rise (dP/dT) of arterial pressure, which correlates with arterial shear forces. Intravenous vasodilators, such as **sodium nitroprusside** to lower blood pressure to a goal systolic pressure <120 mm Hg can be administered, along with **intravenous beta-blockers**, such as metoprolol or esmolol as a continuous infusion, to reduce shear forces and try to achieve a heart rate of 60 bpm. Alternatively, one can administer intravenous labetalol, which accomplishes both tasks.

Figure 5–1. Classification of aortic aneurysms. (Reproduced, with permission, from Doroghazi RM, Slater EE. Aortic dissection. In: Braunwald E, Fauci AS, Kasper DL, et al, eds. *Harrison's Principles of Internal Medicine,* 17th ed. New York: McGraw-Hill, 2008:1566.)

In marked contrast to the dramatic presentation of dissection of the thoracic aorta, patients with **AAA are typically asymptomatic;** their **AAAs** often are detected by physical examination, with detection of a midline pulsatile mass, or are noted incidentally on ultrasound or other imaging procedure. The AAA usually is defined as a dilation of the aorta with a diameter more than 3 cm. It is found in 1.5% to 3% of older adults but in 5% to 10% of higher-risk patients, such as those with known atherosclerotic disease. It is a degenerative condition typically found in older men (>50 years), most commonly in smokers, who often have atherosclerotic disease elsewhere, such as coronary artery disease or peripheral vascular disease. **It is recommended that men between the ages of 65 and 75 who have a history of smoking should be screened for AAA with ultrasound.**

The feared complication of AAA is spontaneous rupture. If the AAA ruptures anteriorly into the peritoneal cavity, the patient usually exsanguinates and dies within minutes. If the AAA ruptures posteriorly and the bleeding is confined to the retroperitoneum, the peritoneum can produce local tamponade, and the patient presents with severe lower back or midabdominal pain. Overall, the mortality rate of ruptured AAA is 80%, with 50% of patients dead before they reach the hospital.

The risk of rupture is related to the size of the aneurysm: the annual rate of rupture is low if the aneurysm is smaller than 5 cm but is at least 10% to 20% for 6-cm aneurysms. The risk of rupture must be weighed against the surgical risk of elective repair, which traditionally required excision of the diseased aorta and replacement with a Dacron graft, although endovascular treatment with placement of an aortic stent graft is now commonly performed. **Operative repair of AAAs is indicated for aneurysms 5.5 cm or greater** in diameter or those expanding more than 0.5 cm per year, or if the aneurysm is symptomatic. As for surveillance of AAAs, the current recommendations are that patients undergo some sort of imaging of the aneurysm (MRI, CT scan, or ultrasound study) at 3- to 12-month intervals, depending on the risk of rupture.

> ## CASE CORRELATION
> - See also Case 3 (Myocardial Infarction), Case 6 (Hypertension), and Case 7 (Hypertensive Encephalopathy).

COMPREHENSION QUESTIONS

5.1 A 59-year-old man complains of severe chest pain that radiates to his back. His brachial pulses appear unequal between his right and left arms. He appears hemodynamically stable. On chest radiography, he has a widened mediastinum. Which of the following is the best next step?

A. Initiate thrombolytic therapy.

B. Obtain CT of chest with intravenous contrast.

C. Initiate aspirin and heparin.

D. Measure serial cardiac enzyme levels.

5.2 A 45-year-old woman with new-onset aortic regurgitation is found to have aortic dissection of the ascending aorta and aortic arch by echocardiography. She is relatively asymptomatic. Which of the following is the best management?

A. Oral atenolol therapy and monitor the dissection

B. Angioplasty

C. Surgical repair of the dissection

D. Oral warfarin (Coumadin) therapy

5.3 A healthy 75-year-old man undergoing an ultrasound examination for suspected gallbladder disease is found incidentally to have a 4.5-cm abdominal aneurysm of the aorta. Which of the following is the best management for this patient?

A. Surgical repair of the aneurysm

B. Serial ultrasound examinations every 6 months

C. Urgent MRI

D. Beta-agonist therapy

5.4 A 45-year-old man is concerned because his father died of a ruptured abdominal aortic aneurysm. On evaluation, he is found to have a bicuspid aortic valve. Which of the following is the most accurate statement regarding his condition?

A. He is at risk for an aortic aneurysm of the ascending aorta.

B. He is at risk for an abdominal aortic aneurysm.

C. He is not at increased risk for aortic aneurysms.

D. He should have surgical correction of the aortic valve.

ANSWERS

5.1 **B.** This clinical presentation of severe chest pain radiating to the back, unequal brachial BPs or pulse strengths, and a widened mediastinum on CXR is consistent with acute aortic dissection. A CT scan of the chest is a quick imaging test to confirm the aortic dissection. Thrombolytic therapy or anticoagulation can worsen the process.

5.2 **C.** Surgery is urgently required in the event of aortic root or other proximal (type A) dissections. Unrecognized and hence untreated aortic dissection can quickly lead to exsanguination and death. Medical therapy such as beta-blockers can help to decrease the risk of dissection while getting the patient urgently to the operating room.

5.3 **B.** When an AAA reaches 5.5 cm or greater, surgery is usually required, because of the high risk of aneurysm rupture. For asymptomatic aneurysms smaller than 5 cm, the 5-year risk of rupture is less than 1% to 2%, so serial noninvasive monitoring is an alternative strategy.

5.4 **C.** Risk factors for AAA include smoking, hypertension, and peripheral vascular disease. A bicuspid aortic valve is usually asymptomatic and does not place the patient at risk for **abdominal** aortic aneurysms, although this valvular disorder is a risk factor for the development of aortic stenosis or dissection.

CLINICAL PEARLS

▶ Hypertension is an underlying factor that predisposes to aortic dissection in the majority of cases. Other patients at risk include those with Marfan syndrome, patients with congenital aortic anomalies, or otherwise normal women in the third trimester of pregnancy.

▶ Chest pain in the presence of a widened mediastinum on chest x-ray should suggest aortic dissection.

▶ Medical therapy for aortic dissection includes intravenous beta-blockers such as metoprolol, esmolol, or labetalol to lower cardiac contractility, arterial pressure, and shear stress, thus limiting propagation of the dissection.

▶ Men between the ages of 65 and 75 with a smoking history should be screened for AAA by ultrasound.

▶ Urgent surgical repair is indicated for type A (ascending) aortic dissections. Uncomplicated, stable, type B (transverse or descending) aortic dissections can be managed medically.

▶ Aortic dissection may be complicated by rupture, occlusion of any branch artery of the aorta, or retrograde dissection with hemopericardium and cardiac tamponade.

▶ The risk of rupture of abdominal aortic aneurysms increases with size. Aneurysms larger than 5.5 cm should undergo elective surgical repair; those smaller than 5 cm can be monitored with serial ultrasonography or other imaging procedure.

REFERENCES

Brewster DC, Cronenwett JL, Hallett JW Jr, et al. Guidelines for the treatment of abdominal aortic aneurysm. *J Vasc Surg.* 2003;37:1106-1117.

Creager MA, Loscalzo J. Diseases of the aorta. In: Longo DL, Fauci AS, Kasper DL, et al., eds. *Harrison's Principles of Internal Medicine.* 18th ed. New York, NY: McGraw-Hill; 2012:2060-2066.

Erbel R, Alfonso F, Boileau C, et al. Diagnosis and management of aortic dissection. *Eur Heart J.* 2001;22:1642-1681.

Powell JT, Greenhalgh RM. Clinical practice: small abdominal aortic aneurysms. *N Engl J Med.* 2003;348:1895-1901.

A 56-year-old man comes into your clinic as a new patient. Seven years ago at a work-related health screening, he was diagnosed with hypertension and hyper-cholesterolemia. At that time, he saw a physician who prescribed a diuretic, and encouraged him to lose some weight and to diet and exercise. Since that time, he has not followed up with any physician. Last month, he had a routine optometry examination, and was told he had evidence of hypertensive retinopathy, and he was instructed to follow up with a physician. He brings the optometry report to this visit, which describes arteriovenous crossing defects and increased arteriolar light reflex. He denies chest pain, shortness of breath, dyspnea on exertion, or paroxysmal nocturnal dyspnea. He smokes one pack of cigarettes per day and has done so since he was 15 years old. He typically drinks two glasses of wine with dinner. On examination, the patient is obese, and you calculate his body mass index (BMI) as 30 kg/m². His blood pressure is 168/98 mm Hg in the right arm and 170/94 mm Hg in the left arm, and his heart rate is 84 bpm. He has no thyromegaly or carotid bruits. Cardiac examination reveals an S_4 gallop. No cardiac murmurs are auscultated. Lung and abdomen examinations are normal.

▶ What are your next steps?

ANSWER TO CASE 6:

Hypertension, Outpatient

Summary: A 56-year-old hypertensive man is being evaluated as a new patient. His blood pressures are in the range of 170/95 mm Hg. Funduscopic examination reveals hypertensive retinopathy. His fourth heart sound is consistent with a thickened, noncompliant ventricle. In addition, he has multiple cardiovascular risk factors, including his age, obesity, and smoking.

- **Next steps:**

   1. Laboratory evaluation and a baseline electrocardiogram (ECG) to assess for end-organ damage.

   2. Assess patient's overall cardiovascular risk status, including lipid profile.

   3. Rule out secondary causes of hypertension.

ANALYSIS

Objectives

   1. Understand the initial evaluation of a patient with hypertension.

   2. Be familiar with the most common antihypertensive medications, and indications and cautions regarding their usage.

   3. Be familiar with the various causes of secondary hypertension and when to pursue these diagnoses.

Considerations

This is a 56-year-old man with severe hypertension who has evidence on physical examination of hypertensive end-organ damage, that is, hypertensive retinopathy and left ventricular hypertrophy as well as multiple risk factors for atherosclerotic disease. The most likely diagnosis is essential hypertension, but secondary causes still must be considered. Although you have measured his blood pressure (BP) only once in your clinic, he has been told before that he is hypertensive, and he already appears to have end-organ damage of hypertension. His blood pressure is above 160/100 mm Hg, which places him in **stage II hypertension, which warrants starting him on two-drug therapy without further delay.**

APPROACH TO:
Hypertension

DEFINITIONS

ESSENTIAL HYPERTENSION: Also known as idiopathic or primary hypertension. It has no known cause, yet it comprises approximately 80% to 95% of all cases of hypertension.

LIFESTYLE MODIFICATION: A cornerstone in the treatment of hypertension, consisting of regular aerobic activity, weight loss, decreased salt intake, and adherence to a Dietary Approaches to Stop Hypertension (DASH)-type dietary plan. Alcohol consumption should be moderated, no more than two glasses of wine per day for men and one glass per day for women.

PREHYPERTENSION: Blood pressures 120 to 139/80 to 89 mm Hg.

STAGE I HYPERTENSION: Blood pressures 140 to 159/90 to 99 mm Hg.

STAGE II HYPERTENSION: Blood pressures more than 160/100 mm Hg.

SECONDARY HYPERTENSION: Elevated arterial blood pressure with a known underlying cause, such as renal artery stenosis or primary aldosteronism. Prevalence is approximately 5% to 20% of all cases of hypertension.

DASH DIET: Diet rich in fruits, vegetables, legumes, and low-fat dietary products, and low in snacks, sweets, meat, and saturated fat.

CLINICAL APPROACH

Initial Evaluation and Management

Hypertension can first be staged, to guide the intensity of medical intervention, by measuring blood pressures on two or more occasions. Underlying causes of hypertension must then be considered. Essential or idiopathic hypertension is the most common form of hypertension, comprising 80% to 95% of cases, but approximately 5% to 20% of cases of hypertension are caused by secondary causes (Table 6–1). To identify the secondary (and potentially reversible) causes of hypertension, the clinician must be aware of the clinical and laboratory manifestations of the processes. A secondary cause of hypertension, and thus more extensive testing, is indicated when patients have any of the following clinical features: age of onset before 25 or after 55, presenting with malignant hypertension, refractory hypertension requiring three or more antihypertensive medications, hypertension that has suddenly become uncontrolled, a rising creatinine level with the use of angiotensin-converting enzyme (ACE) inhibitors, or other clinical signs of a secondary cause.

Table 6–1 • SECONDARY CAUSES OF HYPERTENSION
Renal diseases   • Parenchymal (glomerulonephritis, polycystic kidney disease, renal tumors)   • Renovascular (atherosclerosis or fibromuscular dysplasia)
Endocrine   • Primary aldosteronism   • Cushing syndrome   • Pheochromocytoma   • Hyperthyroidism   • Growth hormone excess (acromegaly)
Miscellaneous   • Obstructive sleep apnea   • Coarctation of the aorta   • Increased intravascular volume (posttransfusion)   • Hypercalcemia   • Medications (sympathomimetics, glucocorticoids, high-dose estrogen, NSAIDs)

OTHER CARDIAC RISK FACTORS AND EVALUATION FOR TARGET ORGAN DAMAGE

Cardiovascular risk factors and hypertensive target organ damage should be identified. The major risk factors of cardiovascular disease are age, cigarette smoking, dyslipidemia, diabetes mellitus, obesity, kidney disease, and a family history of premature cardiovascular disease. Target organ damage of hypertension includes left ventricular hypertrophy, nephropathy, retinopathy, and cerebrovascular disease. A complete history and physical examination, including funduscopic examination, auscultation of the major arteries for bruits, palpation of the abdomen for enlarged kidneys, masses, or an enlarged abdominal aorta, evaluation of the lower extremities for edema and perfusion, and a neurologic examination should be standard. Some initial laboratory testing is also indicated (Table 6–2). Counseling patients on lifestyle changes is important at any blood pressure level and includes weight loss, limitation of alcohol intake, increased aerobic physical activity, reduced sodium intake (<6 g NaCl or 2.3 g sodium), cessation of smoking, and adherence to a DASH diet.

Therapy

Initial therapy should be based on the stage or degree of hypertension. For all patients with hypertension, lifestyle modifications should be instituted. For those

Table 6–2 • BASIC TESTS FOR INITIAL EVALUATION OF HYPERTENSION
Urinalysis, to evaluate for hematuria, and albumin/creatinine ratio to screen for proteinuria
Serum sodium, potassium, calcium, and creatinine to estimate glomerular filtration rate
Fasting glucose; total, HDL, and LDL cholesterol; triglycerides to evaluate cardiovascular risk
Electrocardiogram
Consider thyroid-stimulating hormone, echocardiogram, and evaluation for secondary causes of hypertension, as guided by history and clinical findings

with **prehypertension** (blood pressure 120-139/80-89 mm Hg), lifestyle modifications are the only interventions indicated unless they have another comorbid condition, such as heart failure or diabetes, which necessitates use of an antihypertensive. Patient with **stage I hypertension** (blood pressure 140-159/90-99 mm Hg) should be started on a single antihypertensive agent, whereas those with **stage II hypertension** (blood pressure >160/100 mm Hg) usually will need at least two antihypertensives in combination.

For most patients with hypertension, the **degree of blood pressure reduction** is the major determinant of cardiovascular risk reduction, rather than the class of antihypertensive drug used. Each of the major classes of antihypertensives (thiazide diuretics, long-acting calcium channel blockers, ACE inhibitors, or angiotensin II receptor blockers [ARBs]) seem to be equally efficacious when used as monotherapy. Thiazide diuretics or long-acting calcium channel blockers should be used as initial monotherapy in black patients, and an ACE inhibitor or ARB should be used for initial monotherapy in patients with diabetic nephropathy or those with nondiabetic chronic kidney disease complicated by proteinuria. Beta-blockers are not recommended for initial monotherapy unless there is a specific indication, such as ischemic heart disease. If patients have markedly elevated blood pressures at baseline (stage II hypertension), a single agent will often not be able to achieve good blood pressure control, and they will often require combination therapy with two or more agents. Whatever drug class is used, a long-acting formulation that provides 24-hour efficacy is preferred over short-acting agents for better compliance and more consistent blood pressure control. A list of oral antihypertensive drugs is extensive (Table 6–3).

For some patients, there are specific compelling indications to use specific drug classes. **ACE inhibitors or ARBs are the agents of choice in hypertensive patients with diabetes or systolic heart failure.** Beta-blockers would be first-line agents in patients with hypertension and coronary artery disease, or a history of tachyarrhythmias. Alpha-blockers may be considered in men with hypertension and benign prostatic hypertrophy. Most patients ultimately need more than one drug to control their blood pressure. It is critical to tailor the treatment to the patient's personal, financial, lifestyle, and medical factors, and to periodically review compliance and adverse effects.

Goal blood pressures have been the subject of academic debate. In 2013, the Eighth Joint National Committee (JNC 8) released evidence-based guidelines on treatment thresholds, goals, and medications in the management of hypertension. The target blood pressure is <140/90 mm Hg for the general hypertensive population under age 60, and <150/90 for patients aged 80 or older. Some guidelines recommend lower targets of <130/80 for patients with diabetes, atherosclerosis, or chronic kidney disease but overly aggressive blood pressure control may not be advantageous (observations of a "J-curve" effect of increased cardiovascular risk at blood pressures that are either too high or too low). In 2015, the National Institutes of Health (NIH)-sponsored **SPRINT trial** showed that for patients age 50 or older, with at least one other cardiovascular risk factor, a target blood pressure of **120 mm Hg** (rather than 140 mm Hg) produced a 30% risk reduction in cardiovascular events, stroke, and cardiovascular death. The effects of this study on blood pressure guidelines remain to be determined.

Table 6–3 • PARTIAL LISTING OF ORAL ANTIHYPERTENSIVE AGENTS

Category	Agents	Mechanisms of Action	Side Effects	Indications	Contraindications/ Cautions
Diuretic	Thiazide diuretic: **Hydrochlorothiazide, chlorthalidone**	Sodium diuresis, volume depletion, possible lower peripheral vascular resistance	Hypokalemia, hyponatremia, carbohydrate intolerance, hyperuricemia, hyperlipidemia	Initial monotherapy or as combination with ACEI/ARB	Diabetes mellitus, gout, hypokalemia
	Potassium sparing: **spironolactone, eplerenone**	Competitive inhibitor of aldosterone, causing renal sodium loss	**Hyperkalemia,** gynecomastia	CHF with systolic dysfunction	Renal failure, hyperkalemia
Antiadrenergic	Clonidine	Stimulation of alpha-2 vasomotor center of brain	Postural hypotension, drowsiness, dry mouth, **rebound hypertension** with abrupt withdrawal		History of medication noncompliance (risk of rebound hypertension)
	Beta-blocker: **Metoprolol, atenolol**	Block sympathetic effect of heart and kidneys (renin)	**Bronchospasm,** hyperlipidemia, depression, erectile dysfunction	Angina, post-MI, tachyarrhythmia	Asthma, 2nd- or 3rd-degree heart block, sick sinus syndrome
	Alpha-beta blocker: **Carvedilol**	Same as beta-blockers and also direct vasodilation	Similar to beta-blockers	Post-MI, CHF with systolic dysfunction	Similar to beta-blockers
Vasodilator	Hydralazine	Arterial vasodilation, produces reflex tachycardia	Headache, tachycardia, angina, lupus-like syndrome		Severe coronary artery disease

ACE inhibitor	**Lisinopril, captopril, enalapril,** ramipril	Inhibit conversion of angiotensin I to angiotensin II (powerful vasoconstrictor)	Orthostatic hypotension, **cough,** angioedema, **hyperkalemia,** acute renal failure	Post-MI, CHF with systolic dysfunction, diabetes, proteinuric chronic kidney disease	Renal failure, bilateral renal artery stenosis, pregnancy
Angiotensin receptor antagonist	**Losartan, valsartan, candesartan, irbesartan**	Competitive inhibition of the angiotensin II receptor	Similar to ACE inhibitors but no cough or angioedema	Same as ACE inhibitors	Same as ACE inhibitors
Calcium channel antagonist	Dihydropyridines: **Amlodipine, nifedipine, felodipine**	Blockade of L-channels, reducing intracellular calcium and causing vasodilation	Tachycardia, flushing, gastrointestinal side effects, hyperkalemia, **edema**		May worsen peripheral edema
	Nondihydropyridine: **Diltiazem, verapamil**	Similar to dihydropyridines	**Heart block,** constipation	Post-MI, supraventricular tachycardia	Heart failure, 2nd- or 3rd-degree heart block

(Data from Kasper DL, Fauci AS, Hauser SL, et al. Harrison's Principles of Internal Medicine. 19th ed. New York, NY: McGraw-Hill; 2015: 1624.)

SELECTED CAUSES OF SECONDARY HYPERTENSION

The most common cause of secondary hypertension is renal disease (**renal parenchymal or renovascular**). Renal artery stenosis is caused by atherosclerotic disease with hemodynamically significant blockage of the renal artery in older patients or by fibromuscular dysplasia in younger adults. The clinician must have a high index of suspicion, and further testing may be indicated, for instance, in an individual with diffuse atherosclerotic disease. Potassium level may be low or borderline low in patients with renal artery stenosis caused by secondary hyperaldosteronism. A captopril-enhanced radionuclide renal scan often is helpful in establishing the diagnosis; other diagnostic tools include magnetic resonance angiography and spiral computed tomography. Surgical or angioplastic correction of the vascular occlusion may be considered.

Polycystic kidney disease is inherited as an autosomal dominant trait. The classic clinical findings are positive family history of polycystic kidney disease, bilateral flank masses, flank pain, elevated blood pressure, and hematuria. Other causes of chronic renal disease very commonly lead to hypertension.

Other causes of secondary hypertension include **primary hyperaldosteronism**, which typically will cause hypertension and hypokalemia. Anabolic steroids, sympathomimetic drugs, tricyclic antidepressants, oral contraceptives, nonsteroidal anti-inflammatory agents, and illicit drugs, such as cocaine, as well as licit ones, such as caffeine and alcohol, are included in possible secondary causes of hypertension.

Obstructive sleep apnea is another fairly common cause of hypertension. The cause of obstructive sleep apnea is a critical narrowing of the upper airway that occurs when the resistance of the upper airway musculature fails against the negative pressure generated by inspiration. In most patients, this is a result of a reduced airway size that is congenital or perhaps complicated by obesity. These patients frequently become hypoxic and hypercarbic multiple times during sleep, which, among other things, eventually can lead to systemic vasoconstriction, systolic hypertension, and pulmonary hypertension.

Hyperthyroidism may also cause hypertension. The patient will have a widened pulse pressure with increased systolic blood pressure and decreased diastolic blood pressure, as well as a hyperdynamic precordium. The patient may have warm skin, tremor, and thyroid gland enlargement or a palpable thyroid nodule. A low level of serum thyroid-stimulating hormone (TSH) and elevated levels of thyroid hormones (such as free T_4) are diagnostic.

Glucocorticoid excess states, including **Cushing syndrome**, and iatrogenic (treatment with glucocorticoids) states usually present with thinning of the extremities with truncal obesity, round moon face, supraclavicular fat pad, purple striae, acne, and possible psychiatric symptoms. An excess of corticosteroids can cause secondary hypertension because many glucocorticoid hormones have mineralocorticoid activity. Dexamethasone suppression testing of the serum cortisol level aids in the diagnosis of Cushing syndrome.

Coarctation of the aorta is a congenital narrowing of the aortic lumen and usually is diagnosed in younger patients by finding hypertension along with discordant upper and lower extremity blood pressures. Coarctation of the aorta can cause leg claudication, cold extremities, and diminished or absence of femoral pulses as a result of decreased blood pressure in the lower extremities.

Carcinoid syndrome is caused by overproduction of serotonin. Carcinoid tumors arise from the enterochromaffin cells located in the gastrointestinal tract and in the lungs. Clinical manifestations include cutaneous flushing, headache, diarrhea, and bronchial constriction with wheezing, and often, hypertension.

Pheochromocytoma is a catecholamine-releasing tumor that typically produces hypertension. Clinical manifestations include headaches, palpitations, diaphoresis, and chest pain. Other symptoms include anxiety, nervousness, tremor, pallor, malaise, and occasionally nausea and/or vomiting. Symptoms typically are paroxysmal and associated with hypertension.

CASE CORRELATION

- See also Case 7 (Hypertensive Encephalopathy).

COMPREHENSION QUESTIONS

6.1 A 30-year-old woman is noted to have blood pressures in the 160/100 mm Hg range. She also has increased obesity, especially around her abdomen, which also shows some striae. She has been bruising very easily and has increased hair growth on her face and chest. Which of the following is the most likely diagnosis?

    A. Hyperthyroidism

    B. Coarctation of the aorta

    C. Cushing syndrome

    D. Pheochromocytoma

6.2 A 45-year-old man is diagnosed with essential hypertension based on two blood pressures of 150/100 and 156/102 mm Hg during two separate visits. Which of the following would most likely provide prognostic information regarding this patient?

    A. Vascular biopsy

    B. End-organ effects from hypertension

    C. Patient's enrollment in a clinical trial

    D. Measurement of serum homocysteine levels

6.3 A 34-year-old woman contemplating pregnancy is diagnosed with stage I hypertension, and after an evaluation is noted to have no complications. Which of the following antihypertensive classes may be appropriate for this individual?

   A. Labetolol

   B. Angiotensin-receptor blockers

   C. Direct rennin inhibitors

   D. Angiotensin-receptor blockers

   E. Hydrochlorothiazine

6.4 A 45-year-old man with type 2 diabetes is noted to have blood pressures of 145/90 and 150/96 mm Hg on two separate occasions. Which of the following is the best initial therapy for this patient?

   A. Hydrochlorothiazide

   B. ACE inhibitor

   C. Beta-blocker

   D. Clonidine

ANSWERS

6.1 **C.** The central obesity, abdominal striae, hirsutism, and easy bruisability are consistent with Cushing syndrome, a disease of adrenal steroid overproduction.

6.2 **B.** Prognosis in hypertension depends on the patient's other cardiovascular risks and observed end-organ effects (such as left ventricular hypertrophy) from the hypertension.

6.3 **A.** Labetolol is widely used in pregnant women, and is considered safe for the fetus. ACE inhibitors or ARBs and direct renin inhibitors are contraindicated in all stages of pregnancy. HCTZ can cause thrombocytopenia in teh fetus and is not recommended in pregnancy. Methyldopa is an older agent and not as effective as labetolol.

6.4 **B.** For diabetics, in general, the antihypertensive agent of choice is the ACE inhibitor. If the blood pressure is uncontrolled, then a thiazide diuretic may be added. ACE inhibitors provide a survival advantage to diabetics with hypertension.

CLINICAL PEARLS

▶ In general, the diagnosis of hypertension requires two or more blood pressure measurements on at least two visits.

▶ Cardiovascular disease risk evaluation consists of identifying target organ dysfunction and cardiovascular risk factors, such as diabetes and hyperlipidemia.

▶ Most patients with hypertension have essential hypertension, but secondary causes of hypertension should be evaluated when clinically indicated.

▶ Renal diseases, including renovascular hypertension, are the most common causes of secondary hypertension.

▶ Lifestyle modifications consisting of dietary changes, exercise, and moderation of alcohol intake are indicated to address hypertension control and lower overall cardiovascular risk.

▶ For most patients, the degree of blood pressure reduction is the major determinant of cardiovascular risk reduction, rather than the class of antihypertensive drug used.

REFERENCES

Kotchen TA. Hypertensive vascular disease. In: Kasper DL, Fauci AS, Hauser SL, et al., eds. *Harrison's Principles of Internal Medicine*. 19th ed. New York, NY: McGraw-Hill; 2015:1611-1627.

James PA, Oparil S, Carter BL, et al. 2014 evidence-based guideline for the management of high blood pressure in adults: report from the panel members appointed to the Eighth Joint National Committee (JNC 8). *JAMA*. 2014;311(5):507-520.

Mancia G, Fagard R, Narkiewicz K, et al. 2013 ESH/ESC Guidelines for the management of arterial hypertension: the Task Force for the management of arterial hypertension of the European Society of Hypertension (ESH) and of the European Society of Cardiology (ESC). *J Hypertens*. 2013;31(7):1281-1357.

The SPRINT Research Group. A randomized trial of intensive versus standard blood pressure control. *N Engl J Med*. 2015;373:2103-2116.

A 39-year-old man is brought to the emergency center (EC) by ambulance after he was found wandering in the street in a disoriented state. He is confused and agitated, and further history is obtained from his wife. She reports that for the last several months he has been complaining of intermittent headaches and palpitations, and he had experienced feelings of light-headedness and flushed skin when playing basketball. Three weeks ago, he was diagnosed with hypertension and was started on clonidine twice per day. He took the clonidine for 2 weeks, but because the drug made him feel sedated, he was instructed by his physician 5 days ago to stop the clonidine and to begin metoprolol twice daily. On examination, he is afebrile, with heart rate 110 bpm, respiratory rate of 26 bpm, oxygen saturation of 98%, and blood pressure of 215/132 mm Hg, equal in both arms. He is agitated and diaphoretic, and he is looking around the room but does not appear to recognize his wife. His pupils are dilated but reactive, and he has papilledema and scattered retinal hemorrhages. He has no thyromegaly. Heart, lung, and abdominal examinations are normal. His pulses are bounding and equal in his arms and legs. He moves all of his extremities well, his reflexes are brisk and symmetric, and he is slightly tremulous. A noncontrast computed tomography (CT) of the head is read as negative for hemorrhage. Laboratory studies include a normal leukocyte count and a hemoglobin level of 16.5 g/dL. Serum sodium level is 139 mEq/L, potassium 4.7 mEq/L, chloride 105 mEq/L, HCO_3 29 mEq/L, blood urea nitrogen (BUN) 32 mg/dL, and creatinine 1.3 mg/dL. Urinalysis is normal, and a urine drug screen is negative. Lumbar puncture is performed, and the cerebrospinal fluid (CSF) has no red or white blood cells, no xanthochromia, and normal protein and glucose.

▶ What is the most likely diagnosis?
▶ What is the underlying etiology?
▶ What is the next step?

ANSWERS TO CASE 7:
Hypertensive Encephalopathy/Pheochromocytoma

Summary: A 39-year-old man recently diagnosed with hypertension is now in the EC in an acute confusional state, and with critically elevated blood pressures. He has been having episodes of palpitations, headaches, and light-headedness. His medication was recently changed from clonidine to metoprolol. His examination is significant for dilated pupils, papilledema, and bounding peripheral pulses. The urine drug screen is negative. The CT scan of the head and CSF studies show no evidence of intracranial hemorrhage or infection.

- **Most likely diagnosis:** Hypertensive encephalopathy.

- **Possible etiology:** Pheochromocytoma, consider clonidine rebound hypertension.

- **Next step:** Admit to the intensive care unit (ICU), immediately lower blood pressure with a parenteral agent, and closely monitor the arterial pressure.

ANALYSIS

Objectives

1. Learn the definition and management of hypertensive emergencies and urgencies.

2. Understand the relationship between systemic blood pressure and cerebral blood flow.

3. Know how to diagnose and medically treat a patient with a pheochromocytoma.

Considerations

This is a relatively young man with severely elevated blood pressures who presents with **altered mental status.** Use of illicit drugs, such as cocaine and amphetamines, must be considered, but this patient's drug screen was negative. **Hypertensive encephalopathy,** a symptom complex of **severely elevated blood pressures, confusion, increased intracranial pressure, and/or seizures,** is a diagnosis of exclusion, meaning other causes for the patient's acute mental decline, such as stroke, subarachnoid hemorrhage, meningitis, or mass lesions, must be ruled out. Knowing the specific etiology of the patient's hypertension is not necessary to treat his encephalopathy; urgent blood pressure lowering is indicated. However, it is not necessary, and it **may be harmful to *normalize* the blood pressure too quickly,** because it may cause cerebral hypoperfusion. **Parenteral medications should be used to lower the blood pressure to 160/100 to 110 mm Hg range.** The patient has tachycardia, hypertension, diaphoresis, dilated pupils, and a slight tremor, all signs of a hyperadrenergic state. Pheochromocytoma must be considered as a possible underlying etiology of his hypertension. His antihypertensive medication changes may also be contributory—perhaps clonidine rebound.

APPROACH TO:
Hypertensive Crises

DEFINITIONS

HYPERTENSIVE URGENCY: Acute elevation in blood pressure to greater than 180 mm Hg systolic pressure and/or greater than 110 mm Hg diastolic pressure without evidence of end-organ damage.

HYPERTENSIVE EMERGENCY: Acute elevation in blood pressure with associated end-organ damage.

CLINICAL APPROACH

Hypertensive crises are critical elevations in blood pressure, which usually are classified as either hypertensive emergencies or urgencies. The presence of **acute end-organ damage** constitutes a **hypertensive emergency**, whereas the absence of such complications is considered **hypertensive urgency**. Examples of acute end-organ damage include hypertensive encephalopathy, myocardial ischemia or infarction associated with markedly elevated blood pressure, aortic dissection, stroke, declining renal function with proteinuria, and pulmonary edema secondary to acute left ventricular failure.

Hypertensive emergencies require immediate reduction in blood pressure over minutes to hours, typically with intravenous medications and close monitoring in an intensive care unit. Hypertensive urgencies also require prompt medical attention, but the blood pressure can be lowered over 1 to 2 days and can be monitored in the outpatient setting for patients with reliable follow-up.

Hypertensive crises are uncommon but occur most often in patients with an established history of essential hypertension, that is, hypertension without an apparent underlying cause. A crisis may be precipitated by use of sympathomimetic agents, such as cocaine, or by conditions that produce excess sympathetic discharge, such as clonidine withdrawal. Hypertensive crises also result from underlying diseases that cause hypertension, such as renovascular disease (eg, renal artery stenosis), renal parenchymal disease (eg, glomerulonephritis), and pheochromocytoma.

Although the pathophysiology is not completely understood, abrupt rises in vascular resistance are met with endothelial compensation by the release of vasodilator molecules such as nitric oxide. If the increase in arterial pressure persists, the endothelial response is overwhelmed and decompensates, leading to a further rise in pressure and endothelial damage and dysfunction.

Cerebral blood flow is a good example of vascular compensation by vasodilation or vasoconstriction in response to changes in arterial pressure (Figure 7–1). In normotensive adults, cerebral blood flow remains relatively constant over a range of mean arterial pressures between 60 and 120 mm Hg because cerebral vasoconstriction limits excessive cerebral perfusion. As the mean arterial pressure increases beyond the normal range of cerebral autoregulation, there is cerebrovascular endothelial dysfunction and increased permeability of the blood-brain barrier, leading to vasogenic edema and the formation of microhemorrhages. Patients then

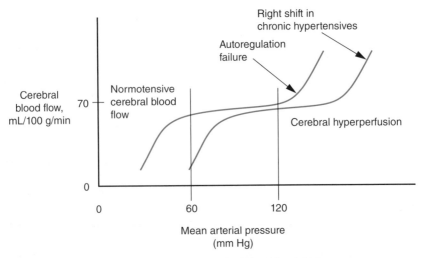

Figure 7–1. Cerebral blood flow autoregulation. Cerebral blood flow is fairly constant over a range of blood pressures. Chronic hypertensive patients have an adaptive mechanism that shifts the curve to the right.

manifest symptoms of hypertensive encephalopathy, such as lethargy, confusion, headaches, or vision changes. Typical imaging findings on magnetic resonance imaging (MRI) include posterior leukoencephalopathy, usually in the parietooccipital regions, which may or may not be seen on CT scanning. Without therapy, the condition can lead to seizures, coma, and death.

The **definition of hypertensive emergency does not require numerical thresholds** of arterial pressure but **is based on end-organ effects.** Autoregulation failure can occur in previously normotensive individuals at blood pressures as low as 160/100 mm Hg; however, individuals with long-standing hypertension frequently develop adaptive mechanisms (eg, cerebral arterial autoregulation) and may not show clinical manifestations until the blood pressure rises to above 220/110 mm Hg. Thus, **emergent treatment of hypertensive encephalopathy** (and indeed all hypertensive emergencies) should **focus on the symptoms** rather than the numbers. In fact, it may be dangerous to "normalize" the blood pressure of patients with chronic hypertension. As a consequence of the right shift in the autoregulation curve, rapid lowering of blood pressures may lead to decreased perfusion to the brain, resulting in cerebral ischemia or infarction, or similar renal or coronary hypoperfusion. Usually, a reasonable goal is reduction of mean arterial pressures by no more than 25% or to a diastolic blood pressure of 100 to 110 mm Hg over a period of minutes to hours.

Treatment of **hypertensive emergencies usually necessitates parenteral medication without delay;** direct blood pressure monitoring with an arterial catheter often is necessary. One of the most commonly used medications for treating hypertensive emergencies is **sodium nitroprusside.** It has the advantage of nearly instantaneous onset of action, and its dose can be easily titrated for a smooth reduction in blood pressure. However, its metabolite may accumulate, resulting in **cyanide or thiocyanate toxicity** when it is given for more than 2 to 3 days. Certain clinical situations may favor the use of other medications. Intravenous loop diuretics and vasodilators such as nitroglycerin decrease the preload (central venous pressure) in acute pulmonary edema. Myocardial ischemia or infarction is treated with intravenous nitroglycerin to improve coronary perfusion and beta-blockers to reduce blood pressure, heart rate, and myocardial oxygen demand. Patients with aortic dissection benefit from medications that reduce the shear forces affecting the aorta, which will help limit propagation of the dissection. A useful technique in treating these individuals is the use of intravenous nitroprusside to lower the arterial blood pressure and a beta-blocker to blunt reflex tachycardia. Alternatively, intravenous labetalol, a combined alpha- and beta-blocker, alone can be used. **Patients presenting with acute cerebral infarction generally should not have acute blood pressure lowering unless the systolic blood pressure is greater than 220 mm Hg because of the possibility of worsening cerebral ischemia.**

The vast majority of hypertension has no discernible cause, so-called essential hypertension. Some patients have secondary causes, such as renal artery stenosis, hyperaldosteronism, or pheochromocytoma. This patient's history of paroxysmal hypertension with headaches, palpitations, and hyperadrenergic state (flushing, dilated pupils, diaphoresis) suggests the diagnosis of **pheochromocytoma.** Pheochromocytomas are catecholamine-producing tumors that arise from chromaffin cells of the adrenal medulla. Other symptoms may include episodic anxiety, tremor, and orthostatic hypotension caused by volume contraction from pressure-induced natriuresis. Although uncommon, accounting for only 0.01% to 0.1% of hypertensive individuals, these tumors have important therapeutic considerations.

The diagnosis is established by measuring increased concentrations of catecholamines or their metabolites in either urine or plasma. Usually, **a 24-hour urine collection** is assayed for **metanephrines, vanillylmandelic acid (VMA), and catecholamines.** One-time measurement of plasma free metanephrines is a convenient and fairly sensitive screening test. After the biochemical tests document the excess catecholamines, the next step is to locate the tumor for surgical removal. Approximately 90% of pheochromocytomas are in the adrenal gland, usually identified by computed tomography or magnetic resonance imaging. If the initial imaging is unrevealing, scintigraphic localization with ^{123}I-metaiodobenzylguanidine (^{123}I-MIBG) or an octreotide (somatostatin-analog) scan is indicated, because this radioisotope is preferentially taken up in catecholamine-producing tumors.

The treatment of choice for these tumors is surgical resection, but it is critical to reverse the acute and chronic effects of the excess catecholamines prior to excision. **Alpha-adrenergic blocking agents, such as phenoxybenzamine, an irreversible, long-acting agent, started a week prior to surgery help to prevent hypertensive exacerbations,** which are especially worrisome during surgery. To expand the commonly seen contracted blood volume, a liberal salt diet is initiated. Sometimes, a beta-blocking agent is started, but **only after alpha-blockade is established.** The products of pheochromocytomas stimulate both the alpha- and beta-adrenergic receptors; thus, using a beta-blocker alone may worsen the hypertension because of unopposed alpha-adrenergic stimulation. Also, beta-blockade may result in acute pulmonary edema, especially in the presence of cardiomyopathy secondary to chronic catecholamine exposure.

Less than 10% of pheochromocytomas are familial, and these tend to be bilateral. One should consider screening for the presence of the *RET* protooncogene seen in multiple endocrine neoplasia type II (MEN II) or the *VHL* gene for von Hippel-Lindau syndrome, or screening family members for these diseases as well as for familial pheochromocytoma and neurofibromatosis.

COMPREHENSION QUESTIONS

7.1 A 50-year-old man with chronic hypertension presents at the clinic having run out of his medications, lisinopril and amlodipine, for more than a month. He is asymptomatic and has a blood pressure of 200/104 mm Hg. Which of the following is the best management?

A. Admit in the hospital and initiate intravenous nitroprusside.

B. Prescribe clonidine 0.1 mg TID and recheck the blood pressure in 24 to 48 hours.

C. Restart his angiotensin-converting enzyme (ACE) inhibitor and calcium channel blocker and recheck blood pressure in 24 to 48 hours.

D. Refer to a social worker and do not prescribe any antihypertensive agent.

7.2 An 80-year-old woman without a history of hypertension undergoes surgery for a hip fracture. Her blood pressure on postoperative day 1 is 178/110 mm Hg. She is asymptomatic except for hip pain. Which of the following is the best next step?

A. Transfer the patient to the intensive care unit, obtain cardiac enzyme levels, and lower the blood pressures to the 140/90 mm Hg range.

B. Control the pain and monitor the blood pressure.

C. Start the patient on a beta-blocker and monitor the blood pressure.

D. Restrict visitors and turn down television, alarms, and other noise.

7.3 A 61-year-old man with coronary artery disease complains of progressive orthopnea and pedal edema. He is hospitalized with a blood pressure of 190/105 mm Hg. Cardiac enzyme levels and the electrocardiography (ECG) are normal. Intravenous furosemide has been administered. Which of the following is the best next step?

A. Prescribe a beta-blocker to decrease myocardial oxygen demands.

B. Start intravenous dopamine.

C. Observe his clinical status.

D. Start an ACE inhibitor.

7.4 A 58-year-old woman with aphasia and right arm weakness of 8 hours' duration is seen in the ER. CT scan shows no intracranial hemorrhage. Her blood pressure is 162/98 mm Hg. Which of the following is the best next step?

A. Normalize the blood pressure with beta-blockade.

B. Admit to ICU with sodium nitroprusside.

C. Normalize the blood pressure with an ACE inhibitor.

D. Observe the blood pressure.

ANSWERS

7.1 **C.** This man has a hypertensive urgency—elevated blood pressures without end-organ symptoms. The appropriate treatment is reinitiation of blood pressure medications and reassessment in 24 to 48 hours. Clonidine would not be a good maintenance therapy given questions regarding his compliance with treatment and the risk of rebound hypertension.

7.2 **B.** Elevated blood pressures without symptoms may occur acutely after surgery, particularly as a consequence of postoperative pain. Blood pressure medications are usually not indicated when they are below the malignant range, but rather, pain control is the primary treatment. Lowering the blood pressure excessively can lead to orthostatic hypotension when the patient gets out of bed.

7.3 **D.** Elevated blood pressures may exacerbate congestive heart failure and must be treated. Generally, beta-blockers are avoided when patients are volume overloaded because beta-blockers decrease myocardial contractility. ACE inhibition reduces afterload, and oral nitrates or IV nitroglycerine reduce preload, and are used to treat acute heart failure.

7.4 **D.** In general, blood pressure should not be acutely decreased (unless >220 mm Hg systolic) in an individual suspected of having an ischemic stroke because of the concern for cerebral hypoperfusion and worsening brain ischemia. If thrombolytic therapy is considered, blood pressure should be controlled to <185/100 mm Hg, but this patient's symptom duration precludes that consideration. In contrast, patients with intracerebral hemorrhage require urgent blood pressure decrease to values of 140 mm Hg systolic or less to decrease the propagation of the hemorrhage.

CLINICAL PEARLS

▶ A hypertensive emergency is defined as an episode of elevated blood pressure associated with acute end-organ damage or dysfunction and requires immediate lowering of the blood pressure.

▶ Asymptomatic patients with elevated blood pressure usually can be started on an oral regimen and reassessed as outpatients in 24 to 48 hours.

▶ The cerebral autoregulation curve of individuals with chronic hypertension is shifted to the right. Nevertheless, marked elevations in mean arterial pressure can exceed the ability of cerebral vessels to constrict, causing hyperperfusion, cerebral edema, and hypertensive encephalopathy.

▶ Pheochromocytomas may cause paroxysmal blood pressure elevations, in association with episodic headaches, palpitations, and diaphoresis.

▶ Preoperative blood pressure control in pheochromocytoma can be achieved with the use of alpha-blockers such as phenoxybenzamine. Beta-blockers used alone can, paradoxically, increase blood pressure because of unopposed alpha-adrenergic effects.

REFERENCES

Dluhy RG, Lawrence JE, Williams GH. Endocrine hypertension. In: Larsen PR, Kronenberg HM, Melmed S, Polonsky KS, eds. *Williams' Textbook of Endocrinology.* 10th ed. Philadelphia, PA: WB Saunders; 2003:555-562.

Kotchen TA. Hypertensive vascular disease. In: Longo DL, Fauci AS, Kasper DL, et al., eds. *Harrison's Principles of Internal Medicine.* 18th ed. New York, NY: McGraw-Hill; 2012:2066-2076.

Neumann HP. Pheochromocytoma. In: Longo DL, Fauci AS, Kasper DL, et al., eds. *Harrison's Principles of Internal Medicine.* 18th ed. New York, NY: McGraw-Hill; 2012:2962-2967.

Pacak K, Linehan WM, Eisenhofer G, et al. Recent advances in the diagnosis, localization, and treatment of pheochromocytoma. *Ann Intern Med.* 2001;134:315-329.

Vaughan CJ, Delanty N. Hypertensive emergencies. *Lancet.* 2000;356:411-417.

A 26-year-old woman originally from Nigeria presents to the emergency center (EC) complaining of the sudden onset of palpitations and severe shortness of breath and coughing. She reports that she has experienced several episodes of palpitations in the past, often lasting a day or two, but never with dyspnea like this. She has a history of rheumatic fever at the age of 14. She is now 20 weeks' pregnant with her first child and takes prenatal vitamins. She denies the use of any other medications, tobacco, alcohol, or illicit drugs.

On examination, her heart rate is between 110 and 130 bpm and is irregularly irregular, with blood pressure of 92/65 mm Hg, respiratory rate of 24 breaths per minute, and oxygen saturation of 94% on room air. She appears uncomfortable, with labored respirations. She is coughing, producing scant amounts of frothy sputum with a pinkish tint. She has ruddy cheeks and a normal jugular venous pressure. She has bilateral inspiratory crackles in the lower lung fields. On cardiac examination, her heart rhythm is irregularly irregular with a loud S_1 and low-pitched diastolic murmur at the apex. Her apical impulse is nondisplaced. Her uterine fundus is palpable at the umbilicus, and she has no peripheral edema. An electrocardiogram (ECG) is obtained (Figure 8–1).

V_1

Figure 8–1. Electrocardiogram. (Reproduced, with permission, from Braunwald E, Fauci AS, Kasper DL, et al, eds. *Harrison's Principles of Internal Medicine,* 16th ed. New York: McGraw-Hill, 2005:1345.)

▶ What is the most likely diagnosis?
▶ What is your next step?

ANSWERS TO CASE 8:
Atrial Fibrillation, Mitral Stenosis

Summary: This 26-year-old woman, with a history of rheumatic fever during adolescence, is now in the second trimester of pregnancy and presents with acute onset of palpitations. She is found to have atrial fibrillation (AF) with a rapid ventricular response. She has a diastolic rumble suggestive of mitral stenosis, which is the likely cause of her atrial fibrillation as a result of left atrial enlargement. Because of the increased blood volume associated with pregnancy and the onset of tachycardia and loss of atrial contraction, the atrial fibrillation has caused her to develop pulmonary edema.

- **Most likely diagnosis:** Atrial fibrillation caused by mitral stenosis.

- **Next step:** Cardiac rate control with intravenous beta-blockers.

ANALYSIS
Objectives

1. Know the causes of atrial fibrillation.
2. Understand the management of acute atrial fibrillation with rapid ventricular response.
3. Understand the rationale for anticoagulation in chronic atrial fibrillation.
4. Know the typical cardiac lesions of rheumatic heart disease and the physical findings in mitral stenosis.
5. Understand the physiologic basis of Wolff-Parkinson-White (WPW) syndrome and the special considerations in atrial fibrillation.

APPROACH TO:
Atrial Fibrillation

DEFINITIONS

ATRIAL FIBRILLATION: Abnormal irregular heart rhythm with chaotic generation of electrical signals in the atria of the heart.

DC CARDIOVERSION: Converting an abnormal rhythm of the heart to normal sinus rhythm by applying direct current electrical shock.

CLINICAL APPROACH

AF is the most common arrhythmia for which patients seek treatment; it occurs in acute, paroxysmal, and chronic forms. During AF, disordered atrial depolarization,

Table 8–1 • CAUSES OF ATRIAL FIBRILLATION
Structural heart disease (hypertension, mitral valve disease)
Ischemic heart disease
Pericarditis or pericardial injury (postsurgical)
Pulmonary disease (especially pulmonary embolism)
Hyperthyroidism
Stress or increased sympathetic tone (acute illness, pheochromocytoma)
Alcohol consumption (holiday heart syndrome, alcoholic cardiomyopathy)
Sick sinus syndrome (tachy-brady syndrome)

often at rates exceeding 300 to 400 bpm, produces an irregular ventricular response, depending on the number of impulses that are conducted through the atrioventricular (AV) node. The ECG is characterized by **absence of discrete P waves** and an **irregularly irregular ventricular contraction.** The incidence of AF increases with age, affecting 5% to 10% of patients older than 75 years. Although many patients can maintain a normal activity level and remain essentially asymptomatic with chronic AF, there are several causes of morbidity from this arrhythmia: it may trigger a rapid ventricular rate leading to myocardial ischemia or exacerbation of heart failure in patients with heart disease, and **thrombus formation** in the noncontractile atria can lead to systemic embolization (AF is a common cause of stroke).

Anything that causes atrial dilation or excessive sympathetic tone can lead to AF, but the **two most common causes** of AF are **hypertension and coronary atherosclerosis.** The common causes of AF are listed in Table 8–1.

Acute AF with rapid ventricular response must be addressed quickly. The four major goals are: (1) hemodynamic stabilization, (2) rate control, (3) anticoagulation, and (4) possible conversion to sinus rhythm. If a patient is **hemodynamically unstable** (hypotensive, angina pectoris, pulmonary edema), **urgent direct current (DC) cardioversion** is indicated. If the patient is hemodynamically stable, **ventricular rate control** can generally be achieved with **intravenous beta-blockers, calcium channel blockers, or digoxin,** which slow conduction through the AV node. Once the ventricular rate has been controlled, consideration can be given to reversing the underlying causes (eg, thyrotoxicosis, use of adrenergic stimulants, or worsening heart failure) so that patients can undergo **cardioversion** to sinus rhythm. This may occur spontaneously or after correction of underlying abnormalities, or it may require pharmacologic or electrical cardioversion. If the duration of **AF exceeds 48 hours, the risk of intra-atrial thrombus formation increases.**

Rate control alone (ie, the use of agents to maintain a slow ventricular response rate) is often effective in managing the symptoms of atrial fibrillation, and it has been shown to be at least as effective as rhythm control for long-term outcomes.

If patients are unstable or persistently symptomatic, however, they may require efforts to terminate the atrial fibrillation, and restore sinus rhythm. **The most effective method of terminating AF is electrical cardioversion.** After cardioversion, the return of coordinated atrial contraction in the presence of an atrial thrombus may result in clot embolization, leading to a cerebral infarction or other distant ischemic event. Therefore, after 24 to 48 hours of AF, patients should receive 3 to 4 weeks of warfarin therapy prior to and after cardioversion to reduce the risk of thromboembolic phenomena. Alternatively, low-risk patients can undergo transesophageal echocardiography to exclude the presence of an atrial appendage thrombus prior to cardioversion. Postcardioversion anticoagulation is still required for 4 weeks, because even though the rhythm returns to sinus, the atria do not contract normally for some time. Pharmacologic antiarrhythmic agents, such as propafenone, sotalol, and amiodarone may be used to try to maintain sinus rhythm.

Many patients with AF cannot be cardioverted and be expected to remain in sinus rhythm. **Two important prognostic factors** are **left atrial dilation** (atrial diameter >4.5 cm predicts failure of cardioversion) and duration of AF. The longer the patient is in fibrillation, the more likely the patient is to stay there ("atrial fibrillation begets atrial fibrillation") as a consequence of electrical remodeling of the heart. In patients with chronic AF, the management goals are rate control, using drugs to reduce AV nodal conduction (such as digitalis or beta-blockers) as described earlier, and anticoagulation.

Patients with chronic AF who are not anticoagulated have a 1% to 5% per year incidence of clinically evident embolization such as stroke. Risk-assessment tools such as the **CHA_2DS_2-VASc score** (CHF, Hypertension, Age $\geq$75, Diabetes mellitus, Stroke/transient ischemic attack/thromboembolism, Vascular disease [prior myocardial infarction, peripheral arterial disease, or aortic plaque], Age 65-74, Sex category [female gender]) can be used to estimate stroke risk and need for anticoagulation. CHA_2DS_2-VASc score correlates with increasing event rate with increasing score. For chronic AF caused by valvular disease such as mitral stenosis, the annual risk of stroke is substantially higher. AF that develops in patients younger than 60 years without evidence of structural heart disease, hypertension, or other factors for stroke is termed **lone AF**, and the **risk of stroke is very low**, so anticoagulation with warfarin is not used. Instead, aspirin may be used.

Anticoagulation reduces the risk of stroke in patients with chronic AF by two-thirds. New oral anticoagulants such as dabigatran and rivaroxaban have been developed for use in atrial fibrillation, but the oral vitamin K antagonist warfarin remains the most widely used medication for this purpose. Warfarin does not produce a predictable dose-related response; therefore, the level of anticoagulation needs to be monitored by regular laboratory testing using the international normalized ratio (INR). In AF not caused by valvular disease, the goal INR is 2 to 3.

The major complication of warfarin therapy is bleeding as a consequence of excessive anticoagulation. The risk of bleeding increases as the INR increases. If the INR is markedly elevated (eg, INR 6-9) but there is no apparent bleeding, the values will return to normal over several days if the warfarin is held. For higher levels of INR (such as >9) but without bleeding, vitamin K can be administered. If clinically significant bleeding is present, warfarin toxicity can be rapidly reversed with administration of vitamin K and fresh frozen plasma to replace clotting factors and provide intravascular volume replacement.

RHEUMATIC HEART DISEASE

In the case presented in the scenario, the cause of this patient's AF appears to be mitral stenosis. Because she has a history of acute rheumatic fever, her mitral stenosis almost certainly is a result of rheumatic heart disease. **Rheumatic heart**

disease is a late sequela of acute rheumatic fever, usually becoming symptomatic many years after the original attack. Valvular thickening, fibrosis, and calcifications lead to valvular stenosis. The **mitral valve is most frequently involved.** The aortic valve may also develop stenosis, but usually in combination with the mitral valve. The right side of the heart is rarely involved.

Most cases of **mitral stenosis** in adults are secondary to **rheumatic heart disease,** especially in the developing world. Congenital mitral stenosis is also commonly seen. The physical signs of mitral stenosis are a **loud S_1** and an **opening snap following S_2.** The S_2-OS (mitral valve opening snap) interval narrows as the severity of the stenosis increases. There is a **low-pitched diastolic rumble** after the opening snap, heard best at the apex with the bell of the stethoscope. Because of the stenotic valve, pressure in the left atrium is increased, leading to left atrial dilation and, ultimately, to pulmonary hypertension. Pulmonary hypertension can cause hemoptysis and signs of right-sided heart failure such as peripheral edema. When AF develops, the rapid ventricular response produces pulmonary congestion as a consequence of shortened diastolic filling time. Rate control with intravenous beta-blockers or calcium channel blockers is essential to relief of pulmonary symptoms. In this case, the mitral stenosis likely became symptomatic due to the patient's pregnancy, with increased blood volume and increased cardiac output of up to 30% to 50%.

WOLFF-PARKINSON-WHITE SYNDROME

Another cause of AF is the **Wolff-Parkinson-White (WPW) syndrome.** In patients with this condition, AF may be life threatening. In addition to the AV node, patients with WPW have an **accessory pathway** that provides an alternate route for electrical communication between the atria and ventricles, leading to **preexcitation,** that is, early ventricular depolarization that begins prior to normal AV nodal conduction. A portion of ventricular activation occurs over the accessory pathway, with the remaining occurring normally through the His-Purkinje system. This preexcitation is recognized on the ECG as a **delta wave,** or early upslurring of the R wave, which both **widens the QRS complex** and **shortens the PR interval,** which represents the normal AV nodal conduction time (Figure 8–2). Some patients with the ECG abnormalities of WPW syndrome are asymptomatic; others have recurrent tachyarrhythmias. Most of the tachycardia is caused by paroxysmal supraventricular tachycardia; one-third of patients will have AF. AF with conduction to the ventricles over an accessory pathway is a special case for two reasons. First, when conducted through the accessory pathway, the **widened QRS** may look like ventricular tachycardia, except that it will have the **irregular RR interval of AF.** Second, because the AV conduction is occurring through the accessory pathway rather than through the AV node, the ventricular rate may be very rapid, and the usual AV nodal–blocking drugs given for ventricular rate control will not affect the accessory pathway. In fact, **beta-blockers, verapamil,** and other AV nodal–blocking agents can, **paradoxically, increase the ventricular rate** and **should be avoided in WPW patients with AF.** If hemodynamically unstable, **DC cardioversion** should be performed. If hemodynamically stable, the agent of choice is procainamide or amiodarone, to slow conduction and convert the rhythm to sinus.

Figure 8–2. Electrocardiogram revealing the delta wave of Wolff-Parkinson-White syndrome. (Reproduced, with permission, from Stead LG, Stead SM, Kaufman MS. *First Aid for the Medicine Clerkship,* 2nd ed. New York: McGraw-Hill, 2006:44.)

CASE CORRELATION

- See also Case 11 (Pericardial Effusion) and Case 4 (Congestive Heart Failure).

COMPREHENSION QUESTIONS

8.1 A 28-year-old woman has been told she has rheumatic heart disease, specifically mitral stenosis. Which of the following murmurs is most likely present?

A. Diastolic rumble at apex of the heart

B. Early diastolic decrescendo at right upper sternal border

C. Holosystolic murmur at apex

D. Late-peaking systolic murmur at right upper sternal border

8.2 A 48-year-old woman is noted to have atrial fibrillation with a ventricular heart rate of 140 bpm. She is feeling dizzy and dyspneic with a systolic blood pressure of 75/48 mm Hg. Which of the following is the most appropriate next step?

A. Intravenous digoxin

B. DC cardioversion

C. Vagal maneuvers

D. Intravenous diltiazem (Cardizem)

8.3 A third-year medical student has been reading about the dangers of excessive anticoagulation and bleeding potential. He reviews the charts of several patients with atrial fibrillation currently taking Coumadin. Which of the following patients is best suited to have anticoagulation discontinued?

A. A 45-year-old man who has normal echocardiographic findings and no history of heart disease or hypertension, but a family history of hyperlipidemia

B. A 62-year-old man with mild chronic hypertension and dilated left atrium, but normal ejection fraction

C. A 75-year-old woman who is in good health except for a prior stroke, from which she has recovered nearly all function

D. A 52-year-old man with orthopnea and paroxysmal nocturnal dyspnea

8.4 A 59-year-old woman has been placed on warfarin (Coumadin) after being found to have had chronic atrial fibrillation. She is noted to have an INR of 5.8, is asymptomatic, and has no overt bleeding. Which of the following is the best management for this patient?

A. Transfuse with erythrocytes.

B. Give vitamin K.

C. Give fresh frozen plasma.

D. Hold warfarin.

8.5 A 45-year-old woman is noted to have dizziness, pounding of the chest, and fatigue of 3 hours' duration. On examination, she is noted to have a blood pressure (BP) of 110/70 mm Hg and heart rate of 180 bpm. She is noted on ECG to have atrial fibrillation, and a prior baseline ECG showed delta waves. The ED physician counsels the patient regarding cardioversion, but the patient declines. Which of the following is the best therapy for her condition?

A. Digoxin

B. Angiotensin-converting enzyme (ACE) inhibitor

C. Calcium channel blocker

D. Procainamide

ANSWERS

8.1 **A.** A diastolic rumble at the cardiac apex suggests mitral stenosis. The early diastolic decrescendo murmur is typical of aortic regurgitation; holosystolic murmur at the apex is typical of mitral regurgitation; and late-peaking systolic murmur at the upper sternal border is typical of aortic stenosis.

8.2 **B.** This individual has significant symptoms and hypotension caused by the atrial fibrillation and rapid ventricular rate; consequently, DC cardioversion is the treatment of choice.

8.3 **A.** Clinical factors associated with a higher risk for embolic stroke include congestive heart failure, hypertension, age >75, diabetes, or prior stroke. Echocardiographic factors include dilated left atrium or the presence of an atrial thrombus. The man in answer A has "lone atrial fibrillation" with a $CHADS_2$ score <2, and has a low risk for stroke and thus would not benefit from anticoagulation.

8.4 **D.** The target INR with warfarin is 2 to 3; thus, 5.8 is markedly elevated. However, because she has no overt bleeding and is asymptomatic, holding the warfarin until the INR reaches the acceptable range is a reasonable approach. Patients with overt bleeding require more urgent intervention such as clotting factors.

8.5 **D.** This patient has atrial fibrillation but with WPW as indicated by the delta wave. In this setting, the typical agents used to treat atrial fibrillation that slow the AV node are contraindicated since the conduction through the accessory pathway could actually accelerate. DC cardioversion is an option; however in a hemodynamically stable patient, procainamide may be used since it will slow propagation through the accessory pathway. Because this patient declines cardioversion, procainamide is the best choice.

CLINICAL PEARLS

▶ The most common causes of atrial fibrillation are hypertension, atherosclerotic heart disease, pericardial or pulmonary disease, and hyperthyroidism.

▶ Acute atrial fibrillation is treated with direct current cardioversion if the patient is unstable. If the patient is stable, initial management is ventricular rate control with an atrioventricular nodal–blocking agent, such as beta-blockers, diltiazem, or verapamil.

▶ Patients with chronic atrial fibrillation generally require long-term anticoagulation to prevent embolic strokes. An exception is "lone atrial fibrillation."

▶ CHA_2DS_2-VASc score can help with risk stratification for both thromboembolic events and need for long-term anticoagulation with score of 0 being low risk, 1 equal to intermediate risk (0.6%), and 2 being high risk (3%) for stroke or thromboembolic events.

▶ Wolff-Parkinson-White syndrome is a ventricular preexcitation syndrome with a delta wave, short PR interval (<0.12 seconds), and prolonged QRS interval (>0.12 seconds). WPW is associated with paroxysmal tachycardias, including AF. AF in WPW syndrome is treated with DC cardioversion or with procainamide. AV nodal–blocking agents can, paradoxically, increase the ventricular rate.

▶ Auscultatory findings in mitral stenosis include a loud S_1 and an opening snap (OS) following the sound of second heart sound (S_2). The interval between S_2 and OS varies inversely with the severity of the stenosis.

REFERENCES

Marchlinski F. The tachyarrhythmias. In: Longo DL, Fauci AS, Kasper DL, et al., eds. *Harrison's Principles of Internal Medicine.* 18th ed. New York, NY: McGraw-Hill; 2012:1878-1900.

Feldman T. Rheumatic mitral stenosis. On the rise again. *Postgrad Med.* 1993;93:93-104.

Lip GY, Nieuwlaat R, Pisters R, Lane DA, Crijns HJ. Refiningh clinical risk stratification for predicting stroke and thromboembolism in atrial fibrillation using a novel risk factor-based approach. *Chest.* 2010;137(2):263-272.

O'Gara P, Loscalzo P. Valvular heart disease. In: Longo DL, Fauci AS, Kasper DL, et al., eds. *Harrison's Principles of Internal Medicine.* 18th ed. New York, NY: McGraw-Hill; 2012:1929-1950.

Snow V, Weiss KB, LeFevre M, et al. Management of newly detected atrial fibrillation: a clinical practice guideline from the American Academy of Family Physicians and the American College of Physicians. *Ann Intern Med.* 2003;139:1009-1017.

Van Gelder IC, Hagens VE, Bosker HA, et al. A comparison of rate control and rhythm control in patients with recurrent persistent atrial fibrillation. *N Engl J Med.* 2002;347:1834-1840.

A 72-year-old man is brought to the emergency department after fainting while in church. He had stood up to sing a hymn and then fell to the floor. His wife, who witnessed the episode, reports that he was unconscious for approximately 2 or 3 minutes. When he woke up, he was groggy for another minute or two, and then seemed himself. No abnormal movements were noted. This has never happened to him before, but his wife does report that for the last several months he has had to curtail activities, such as mowing the lawn, because he becomes weak and feels light-headed. His only medical history is osteoarthritis of his knees, for which he takes acetaminophen.

On examination, he is alert, talkative, and smiling. He is afebrile, his heart rate is regular at 35 bpm, and his blood pressure is 118/72 mm Hg, which remains unchanged on standing. He has contusions on his face, left arm, and chest wall, but no lacerations. His chest is clear to auscultation, and his heart rhythm is regular but bradycardic with a nondisplaced apical impulse. He has no focal deficits. Laboratory examination shows normal blood counts, renal function, and serum electrolyte levels, and negative cardiac enzymes. His rhythm strip is shown in Figure 9–1.

▶ What is the most likely diagnosis?
▶ What is your next step?

Figure 9–1. Electrocardiogram. (Reproduced, with permission, from Stead LG, Stead SM, Kaufman MS. *First Aid for the Medicine Clerkship,* 2nd ed. New York: McGraw-Hill, 2006:46.)

ANSWERS TO CASE 9:

Syncope—Heart Block

Summary: A 72-year-old man presents with a witnessed syncopal episode, which was brief and not associated with seizure activity. He has experienced decreasing exercise tolerance recently because of weakness and presyncopal symptoms. He is bradycardic, with third-degree atrioventricular (AV) block on electrocardiogram (ECG). Arrows in Figure 9–1 point to P waves.

- **Most likely diagnosis:** Syncope as a consequence of third-degree AV block.

- **Next step:** Placement of temporary transcutaneous or transvenous pacemaker and evaluation for placement of a permanent pacemaker.

ANALYSIS

Objectives

1. Know the major causes of syncope and important historical clues to the diagnosis.

2. Understand the basic evaluation of syncope based on the history.

3. Recognize vasovagal syncope and carotid sinus hypersensitivity.

4. Be able to diagnose and know the management of first-, second-, and third-degree AV block.

Considerations

There are two major considerations to the management of this patient: the cause and the management of his AV block. He should be evaluated for myocardial infarction and structural cardiac abnormalities. If this evaluation is negative, he may simply have conduction system disease as a consequence of aging. Regarding temporary management, atropine or isoproterenol can be used when the conduction block is at the level of the AV node, but in this case, the heart rate is less than 40 bpm, and the QRS is widened, suggesting the defect is below the AV node, in the bundles of His. A permanent pacemaker likely is required.

APPROACH TO:

Syncope

DEFINITIONS

SYNCOPE: A transient loss of consciousness and postural tone with subsequent spontaneous recovery.

VASOVAGAL SYNCOPE: Fainting due to excessive vagal tone causing impaired autonomic responses such as hypotension without appropriate rise in heart rate or vasomotor tone.

CLINICAL APPROACH

Syncope is a very common phenomenon, resulting in 5% to 10% of emergency center visits and subsequent hospitalizations. The causes are varied, but they all result in transiently diminished cerebral perfusion leading to loss of consciousness. The prognosis is quite varied, ranging from a benign episode in an otherwise young, healthy person with a clear precipitating event, such as emotional stress, to a more serious occurrence in an older patient with cardiac disease. In the latter situation, syncope has been referred to as "sudden cardiac death, averted." For that reason, higher-risk patients routinely undergo hospitalization and sometimes extensive evaluation to determine the cause.

Traditionally, the etiologies of syncope have been divided into neurologic and cardiac. However, this probably is not a useful classification, because neurologic diseases are uncommon causes of syncopal episodes. Syncope is essentially never a result of transient ischemic attacks (TIAs), because syncope reflects global cerebral hypoperfusion, and TIAs are a result of regional ischemia. Vertebrobasilar insufficiency with resultant loss of consciousness is often discussed yet rarely seen in clinical practice. Seizure episodes are a common cause of transient loss of consciousness, and distinguishing seizure episodes from syncopal episodes based on history often is quite difficult. Loss of consciousness associated with seizure typically lasts longer than 5 minutes, with a prolonged postictal period, whereas patients with syncope usually become reoriented quickly. To further complicate matters, the same lack of cerebral blood flow that produced the loss of consciousness can lead to postsyncopal seizure activity. Seizures are best discussed elsewhere, so our discussion here is confined to syncope.

The only neurologic diseases that commonly cause syncope are disturbances in **autonomic function** leading to **orthostatic hypotension as occurs in diabetes, parkinsonism, or idiopathic dysautonomia.** For patients in whom a definitive diagnosis of syncope can be ascertained, the causes usually are excess vagal activity, orthostatic hypotension, or cardiac disease—either arrhythmias or outflow obstructions. Table 9–1 lists the most common causes of syncope. By far, **the most useful evaluation for diagnosing the cause of syncope is the patient's history.** Because, by definition, the patient was unconscious, the patient may only be able to report preceding and subsequent symptoms, so finding a witness to describe the episode is extremely helpful.

Vasovagal syncope refers to excessive vagal tone causing impaired autonomic responses, that is, a fall in blood pressure without appropriate rise in heart rate or vasomotor tone. This is, by far, the **most common cause of syncope** and is the usual cause of a "fainting spell" in an otherwise healthy young person. Episodes often are precipitated by physical or emotional stress, or by a painful experience. There is usually a clear precipitating event by history and, often, prodromal symptoms such as nausea, yawning, or diaphoresis. The episodes are brief, lasting seconds to minutes, with a rapid recovery. Syncopal episodes also can be triggered by physiologic activities that increase vagal tone, such as **micturition**, defecation, or coughing in otherwise healthy people. Vasovagal syncope needs to be differentiated from orthostatic hypotension.

Carotid sinus hypersensitivity is also **vagally mediated.** This usually occurs in older men, and episodes can be triggered by turning the head to the side, by wearing

Table 9–1 • CAUSES OF SYNCOPE
CARDIOGENIC
Cardiac arrhythmias
• Bradyarrhythmias
• Sinus bradycardia, sinoatrial block, sinus arrest, sick sinus syndrome
• Atrioventricular block
• Tachyarrhythmias
• Supraventricular tachycardia with structural cardiac disease
• Atrial fibrillation associated with the Wolff-Parkinson-White syndrome
• Atrial flutter with 1:1 atrioventricular conduction
• Ventricular tachycardia
Other cardiopulmonary etiologies
• Pulmonary embolism
• Pulmonary hypertension
• Atrial myxoma
• Myocardial disease (massive myocardial infarction)
• Left ventricular myocardial restriction or constriction
• Pericardial constriction or tamponade
• Aortic outflow tract obstruction (aortic valvular stenosis, hypertrophic obstructive cardiomyopathy)
NONCARDIOGENIC
Vasovagal (vasodepressor, neurocardiogenic)
Postural (orthostatic) hypotension
• Drug induced (especially antihypertensive or vasodilator drugs)
• Peripheral neuropathy (diabetic, alcoholic, nutritional, amyloid)
• Idiopathic postural hypotension
• Neurologic disorder (Shy-Drager syndrome)
• Physical deconditioning
• Sympathectomy
• Acute dysautonomia (Guillain-Barré syndrome variant)
• Decreased blood volume (adrenal insufficiency, acute blood loss, etc)
• Carotid sinus hypersensitivity
Situational
• Cough, Valsalva
• Micturition, defecation
• Hypoglycemia
• Generalized anxiety, panic disorder, somatization

a tight collar, or even by shaving the neck over the area. Pressure over one or both carotid sinuses causes excess vagal activity with resultant cardiac slowing and can produce sinus bradycardia, sinus arrest, or even AV block. Less commonly, carotid sinus pressure can cause a fall in arterial pressure without cardiac slowing. When recurrent syncope as a result of bradyarrhythmias occurs, a demand pacemaker is often required.

Patients with **orthostatic hypotension** typically report symptoms related to positional changes, such as rising from a seated or recumbent position, and **the postural drop in systolic blood pressure by more than 20 mm Hg** can be demonstrated on examination. This can occur because of hypovolemia (hemorrhage, anemia, diarrhea or vomiting, Addison disease) or with adequate circulating volume but impaired autonomic responses. The most common reason for this autonomic impairment probably is iatrogenic as a result of antihypertensive or other medications, especially in elderly persons. It also can be caused by autonomic insufficiency seen in diabetic neuropathy, in a syndrome of chronic idiopathic orthostatic hypotension in older men, or the primary neurologic conditions mentioned previously. Multiple events that all are unwitnessed (not corroborated) or that occur only in periods of emotional upset suggest **factitious** symptoms.

Etiologies of **cardiogenic syncope** include rhythm disturbances and structural heart abnormalities. Certain structural heart abnormalities will cause obstruction of blood flow to the brain, resulting in syncope. These include aortic stenosis or hypertrophic obstructive cardiomyopathy (HOCM). Syncope due to cardiac outflow obstruction can also occur with massive pulmonary embolism and severe pulmonary hypertension. Syncope caused by cardiac outflow obstruction typically presents during or immediately after exertion. An echocardiogram often is obtained to elucidate such abnormalities.

Arrhythmias, usually bradyarrhythmias, are the most common cardiac cause of syncope. Sinus bradycardia most often due to degenerative sinoatrial node dysfunction and AV node blocks (see section on Heart Block) are bradyarrhythmic causes of syncope. Sick sinus syndrome (SSS) in elderly patients is one of the most common causes for pacemaker placement. Patients with SSS may experience sinus bradycardia or arrest, alternating with a supraventricular tachycardia, most often atrial fibrillation (tachycardia-bradycardia syndrome). Tachyarrhythmias such as atrial fibrillation or flutter, supraventricular tachycardia (SVT), ventricular tachycardia (VT), or ventricular fibrillation (VF) are more likely to produce palpitations than syncope. Often, the rhythm abnormality is apparent by routine ECG, or, if it occurs paroxysmally, it can be recorded using a 24-hour Holter monitor or an event monitor. Sometimes evaluation requires invasive electrophysiologic studies to assess sinus node or AV node function or to induce supraventricular or ventricular arrhythmias.

Heart Block

There are three types of AV node block, all based on ECG findings. **First-degree AV block** is a prolonged PR interval longer than 200 ms (>1 large box). This is a conduction delay in the AV node. Prognosis is good, and there is usually no need for pacing. **Second-degree AV block** comes in two types. Mobitz type I (Wenckebach) is a progressive **lengthening of the PR interval**, until a dropped beat is produced. The resulting P wave of the dropped beat is not followed by a QRS complex. This phenomenon is caused by abnormal conduction in the AV node and may be the result of inferior myocardial infarction. Prognosis is good, and there is generally no need for pacing unless the patient is symptomatic (ie, bradycardia, syncope, heart failure, asystole >3 seconds). On the other hand, **Mobitz type II produces dropped beats without lengthening of the PR interval.** This is usually caused by a block within the bundle of His. Permanent pacing is often indicated in these patients because the Mobitz type II AV block may later progress to complete heart block. **Third-degree AV block** is a complete heart block, where the sinoatrial (SA) node and AV node fire at independent rates. The atrial rhythm is faster than the ventricular escape rhythm. Permanent pacing is indicated in these patients, especially when associated with symptoms such as exercise intolerance or syncope.

> ## CASE CORRELATION
>
> - See also Case 8 (Atrial Fibrillation), Case 36 (Transient Ischemic Attack), and Case 39 (Dizziness/Benign Positional Vertigo).

COMPREHENSION QUESTIONS

9.1 An 18-year-old woman is brought to the emergency center because she fainted at a rock concert. She apparently recovered spontaneously, did not exhibit any seizure activity, and has no medical history. Her heart rate is 90 bpm and blood pressure 110/70 mm Hg. The neurologic examination is normal. The pregnancy test is negative, and an ECG shows normal sinus rhythm. Which of the following is the most appropriate management?

A. Admit to hospital for cardiac evaluation.

B. Obtain an outpatient echocardiogram.

C. Use 24-hour Holter monitor.

D. Reassure the patient and discharge home.

9.2 A 67-year-old woman has diabetes and mild hypertension. She is noted to have some diabetic retinopathy, and she states that she cannot feel her legs. She has recurrent episodes of light-headedness when she gets up in the morning. She comes in now because she had fainted this morning. Which of the following is the most likely cause of her syncope?

A. Carotid sinus hypersensitivity

B. Pulmonary embolism

C. Autonomic neuropathy

D. Critical aortic stenosis

9.3 A 74-year-old man with no prior medical problems faints while shaving. He has a quick recovery and has no neurologic deficits. His blood sugar level is normal, and an ECG shows a normal sinus rhythm. Which of the following is the most useful diagnostic test of his probable condition?

A. Carotid massage

B. Echocardiogram

C. Computed tomographic (CT) scan of head

D. Serial cardiac enzymes

9.4 A 49-year-old man is admitted to the intensive care unit (ICU) with a diagnosis of an inferior myocardial infarction. His heart rate is 35 bpm and blood pressure 90/50 mm Hg. His ECG shows a Mobitz type I heart block. Which of the following is the best next step?

A. Atropine

B. Transvenous pacer

C. Lidocaine

D. Observation

ANSWERS

9.1 **D.** A young patient without a medical history, without a seizure activity, and with a history suggestive of emotionally mediated vasovagal syncope has an excellent prognosis.

9.2 **C.** This diabetic patient has evidence of microvascular disease, including peripheral neuropathy, and likely has autonomic dysfunction. Although this is the most likely etiology, one must be concerned about a possible cardiac issue, since the patient had numerous cardiovascular risk factors.

9.3 **A.** He likely has carotid hypersensitivity; thus, careful carotid massage (after auscultation to ensure no bruits are present) may be given in an attempt to reproduce the symptoms. Carotid massage in an older patient should be used with caution because it may lead to cerebral ischemia, emboli of a plaque, or to atrial fibrillation.

9.4 **A.** This patient's bradycardia is severe, probably a result of the inferior myocardial infarction. Atropine is the agent of choice in this situation. Mobitz type I block has a good prognosis (vs complete heart block), so transvenous pacing is not usually required.

CLINICAL PEARLS

▶ Vasovagal syncope is the most common cause of syncope in healthy young people. It often has a precipitating event, prodromal symptoms, and an excellent prognosis.

▶ Carotid sinus hypersensitivity causes bradyarrhythmias in older patients with pressure over the carotid bulb and sometimes requires a pacemaker.

▶ Syncope caused by cardiac outflow obstruction, such as aortic stenosis, occurs during or after exertion.

▶ Syncope is a very common problem, affecting nearly one-third of the adult population at some point, but a specific cause is identified in less than half of cases.

▶ Permanent pacing usually is indicated for symptomatic bradyarrhythmias (eg, sick sinus syndrome), Mobitz II atrioventricular block, or third-degree heart block.

REFERENCES

Freeman R, Carlson MD. Syncope. In: Longo DL, Fauci AS, Kasper DL, et al., eds. *Harrison's Principles of Internal Medicine*. 18th ed. New York, NY: McGraw-Hill; 2012:171-177.

Kapoor WN. Syncope. *N Engl J Med*. 2000;343:1856-1862.

Spragg DD, Tomaselli GF. The bradyarrhythmias. In: Longo DL, Fauci AS, Kasper DL, et al., eds. *Harrison's Principles of Internal Medicine*. 18th ed. New York, NY: McGraw-Hill; 2012:1867-1877.

A 27-year-old woman presents to the emergency center complaining of retrosternal chest pain for the past 2 days. The pain is constant, not associated with exertion, worsens when she takes a deep breath, and is relieved by sitting up and leaning forward. She denies any shortness of breath, nausea, or diaphoresis.

On examination, her temperature is 99.4°F, heart rate is 104 bpm, and blood pressure 118/72 mm Hg. She is sitting forward on the stretcher, with shallow respirations. Her conjunctivae are clear and her oral mucosa is pink, with two aphthous ulcers. Her neck veins are not distended; her chest is clear to auscultation and is mildly tender to palpation. Her heart rhythm is regular, with a harsh leathery sound over the apex heard during systole and diastole. Her abdominal examination is benign, and her extremities show warmth and swelling of the proximal interphalangeal (PIP) joints of both hands.

Laboratory studies are significant for a white blood cell (WBC) count of 2100 cells/mm^3, hemoglobin concentration 10.4 g/dL with mean corpuscular volume (MCV) 94 fL, and platelet count 78,000/mm^3. Her blood urea nitrogen (BUN) and creatinine levels are normal. Urinalysis shows 10 to 20 WBCs and 5 to 10 red blood cells (RBCs) per high-powered field (hpf). A urine drug screen is negative.

Chest x-ray is read as normal, with a normal cardiac silhouette and no pulmonary infiltrates or effusions. The electrocardiogram (ECG) is shown in Figure 10–1.

▶ What is the most likely diagnosis?

Figure 10–1. Electrocardiogram. (Reproduced, with permission, from Stead LG, Stead SM, Kaufman MS. *First Aid for the Medicine Clerkship*, 2nd ed. New York: McGraw-Hill, 2006:33)

ANSWER TO CASE 10:
Acute Pericarditis Caused by Systemic Lupus Erythematosus

Summary: A 27-year-old woman presents with nonexertional pleuritic chest pain that is relieved with sitting forward. In addition, she has a pericardial friction rub and ECG changes consistent with acute pericarditis. She has no radiographic evidence of a large pericardial effusion and no clinical signs of cardiac tamponade. Regarding the etiology of her pericarditis, she has pancytopenia and an active urinary sediment, which could be caused by infection but may also represent a connective tissue disease such as systemic lupus erythematosus (SLE).

- **Most likely diagnosis:** Acute pericarditis as a consequence of SLE.

ANALYSIS

Objectives

1. Know the clinical and ECG features of pericarditis and be able to recognize a pericardial friction rub.

2. Know the causes of pericarditis and its treatment.

3. Know the diagnostic criteria for SLE.

4. Know the major complications of SLE and its treatment.

Considerations

In patients with chest pain, one of the primary diagnostic considerations is always myocardial ischemia or infarction. This is particularly true when the ECG is abnormal with changes that may represent myocardial injury, such as ST-segment elevation. However, other conditions may produce ST-segment elevation, such as acute pericarditis. ECG findings can help distinguish between these two diagnoses.

APPROACH TO:
Acute Pericarditis

DEFINITIONS

ACUTE PERICARDITIS: An inflammation of the pericardial sac surrounding the heart.

PERICARDIAL FRICTION RUB: Harsh, high-pitched, scratchy sound, with variable intensity, usually best heard at the left sternal border by auscultation, due to pericarditis.

CLINICAL APPROACH

Acute pericarditis can result from a multitude of disease processes, but the most common causes are listed in Table 10–1.

There is a wide spectrum of clinical presentations, from subclinical or inapparent inflammation, to the classic presentation of acute pericarditis with chest pain, to subacute or chronic inflammation, persisting for weeks to months. Most patients with acute pericarditis seek medical attention because of **chest pain**. The classic description is a sudden onset of substernal chest pain, which worsens on inspiration and with recumbency, that often radiates to the trapezius ridge, and is improved by sitting and leaning forward. Other clinical features vary according to the cause of the pericarditis, but most patients are thought to have viral infection and often present with low-grade fever, malaise, or upper respiratory illness symptoms.

A **pericardial friction rub** is pathognomonic and virtually 100% specific for acute pericarditis. The sensitivity of this sign varies, though, because friction rubs tend to come and go over hours. Classically, a rub is a harsh, high-pitched, scratchy sound, with variable intensity, usually best heard at the left sternal border. It can have one, two, or three components: presystolic (correlating with atrial systole), systolic, and diastolic. The large majority of rubs are triphasic (all three components) or biphasic, having a systolic and either an early or late diastolic component. In these cases, it usually is easy to diagnose the pericardial friction rub and acute pericarditis. When the rub is monophasic (just a systolic component), it often is difficult to distinguish a pericardial friction rub from a harsh murmur, making bedside diagnosis difficult and uncertain. In these cases, one should look for ECG evidence of pericarditis (Table 10–2) and perform serial examinations because the rub may vary with time.

The classic ECG findings in **acute pericarditis** as seen in this patient include **diffuse ST-segment elevation** in association with PR-segment depression. The opposite findings (PR-segment elevation and ST-segment depression) are often seen in leads aVR and V_1. Because of the presentation with chest pain and ST-segment elevation on ECG, acute pericarditis may be confused with acute myocardial infarction (MI). This is potentially a serious problem because if the patient is treated with **thrombolytics** for infarction, the patient may develop **pericardial hemorrhage and cardiac tamponade**. Several clinical features can help to differentiate

Table 10-1 • COMMON CAUSES OF ACUTE PERICARDITIS
Idiopathic pericarditis: specific diagnosis unidentified, presumably either viral or autoimmune and requires no specific management
Infectious: viral, bacterial, tuberculous, parasitic
Vasculitis: autoimmune diseases, postradiation therapy
Hypersensitivity/immunologic reactions, eg, Dressler syndrome
Diseases of contiguous structures, eg, during transmural myocardial infarction
Metabolic disease, eg, uremia, Gaucher disease
Trauma: penetrating or nonpenetrating chest injury
Neoplasms: usually thoracic malignancies such as breast, lung, or lymphoma

(Data from Spodick DH. Acute pericarditis: Current concepts and practice. JAMA 2003;289:1150–1153.)

Table 10-2 • PERICARDITIS VERSUS MYOCARDIAL INFARCTION

ECG Findings	Acute Pericarditis	Acute MI
ST-segment elevation	Diffuse: in limb leads as well as V_2-V_6	Regional (vascular territory), eg, inferior, anterior, or lateral
PR-segment depression	Present	Usually absent
Reciprocal ST-segment depression	Absent	Typical, eg, ST-segment depression inferiorly with anterior ischemia (ST-segment elevation)
QRS complex changes	Absent	Loss of R-wave amplitude and development of Q waves

the two conditions: acute ischemia is more likely to have a gradual onset of pain with crescendo pattern, it usually is described as a heavy pressure or squeezing sensation rather than the sharp pain of pericarditis, it typically does not vary with respiration, and it is relieved with nitrates, whereas the pain of pericarditis is not. In addition, several ECG features can help to make the distinction (Table 10–2). Also, if the ECG reveals arrhythmias or conduction abnormalities, the condition is much more likely to represent ischemia rather than pericarditis.

Most patients with acute viral or idiopathic pericarditis have excellent prognoses. Treatment is mainly symptomatic, with aspirin or another nonsteroidal anti-inflammatory drug (NSAID), such as indomethacin, for relief of chest pain. Colchicine or corticosteroids may be used for refractory symptoms. In most patients, symptoms typically resolve within days to 2 to 3 weeks. Any form of pericarditis can cause pericardial effusion and bleeding; however, the most serious consequence would be cardiac tamponade. It is a common misconception that a pericardial friction rub cannot coexist with an effusion (both are very common in uremic pericarditis). Therefore, it is important to monitor these patients for signs of developing hemodynamic compromises, such as cardiac tamponade.

Our patient is very young and has no significant previous medical history. The presence of symmetric arthritis as well as laboratory findings suggests a systemic disease, such as SLE, as the cause of her pericarditis. SLE is a systemic inflammatory disease that mainly affects women. It is characterized by autoimmune multiorgan involvement, such as pericarditis, nephritis, pleuritis, arthritis, and skin disorders. To diagnose SLE, the patient must meet 4 of the 11 criteria listed in Table 10–3 (96% sensitive and 96% specific).

Our patient has serositis (pericarditis), oral ulcers, hematologic disorders (leukopenia, lymphopenia, and thrombocytopenia), arthritis, and renal involvement (hematuria)—she clearly meets the criteria for SLE. Although the patient in the scenario, like most lupus patients, sought medical attention because of the pain of arthritis or serositis, both these problems are generally manageable or self-limited. The arthritis is generally nonerosive and nondeforming, and the serositis usually resolves spontaneously without sequelae. The major complication of SLE usually is related to renal involvement, which can cause hypertension, chronic renal failure, nephrotic syndrome, or end-stage renal disease. In the past, renal disease was the most common cause of death of SLE patients, but now it can be treated with powerful immunosuppressants, such as high-dose corticosteroids or

Table 10–3 • DIAGNOSTIC CRITERIA FOR SLE
Malar rash: fixed erythema, flat or raised over the malar area, that tends to spare nasolabial folds
Discoid rash: erythematous raised patches with adherent keratotic scaling and follicular plugging
Photosensitivity: skin rash as a result of exposure to sunlight
Oral or vaginal ulcers: usually painless
Arthritis: nonerosive, involving two or more peripheral joints with tenderness, swelling, and effusion
Serositis: usually pleuritis or pericarditis
Renal involvement: persistent proteinuria or cellular casts
Neurologic disorder: seizure or psychosis
Hematologic disorder: hemolytic anemia or leukopenia (<4000/mm^3) on two or more occasions, or lymphopenia (<1500/mm^3) on two or more occasions, or thrombocytopenia (<100 000/mm^3)
Immunologic disorder: positive anti-double-stranded DNA, anti-Smith Ab, antiphospholipid Ab
Antinuclear antibody (ANA): positive ANA in absence of drugs known to induce ANA

Ab, antibody.

cyclophosphamide. Other serious complications of lupus include central nervous system (CNS) disorders, which are highly variable and unpredictable and can include seizures, psychosis, stroke syndromes, and cranial neuropathies. In addition to renal failure and CNS involvement, the most common causes of death in SLE patients are infection (often related to the immunosuppression used to treat the disease) and vascular disease, for example, myocardial infarction.

CASE CORRELATION

- See also Case 3 (Myocardial Infarction, Acute), Case 5 (Aortic Dissection), and Case 20 (Peptic Ulcer Disease) as a differential diagnosis of chest pain.

COMPREHENSION QUESTIONS

10.1 A 68-year-old man with a history of end-stage renal disease is admitted to the hospital for chest pain. On examination, a pericardial friction rub is noted. His ECG shows diffuse ST-segment elevation. Which of the following is the best definitive treatment?

   A. NSAIDs

   B. Dialysis

   C. Steroids

   D. Kayexalate (sodium polystyrene sulfonate)

10.2 The patient described in Question 10.1 is hospitalized, but there is a delay in initiating treatment. You are called to the bedside because he has become hypotensive with systolic blood pressure of 85/68 mm Hg, a heart rate of 122 bpm, and pulsus paradoxus. A repeat ECG is unchanged from admission. Which of the following is the most appropriate immediate intervention?

A. Draw blood cultures and initiate broad-spectrum antibiotics for suspected sepsis.

B. Intravenous furosemide for fluid overload.

C. Echocardiographic-guided pericardiocentesis.

D. Percutaneous coronary intervention for acute myocardial infarction.

10.3 A 25-year-old woman complains of pain in her PIP and metacarpophalangeal (MCP) joints and reports a recent positive antinuclear antibody (ANA) laboratory test. Which of the following clinical features would **not** be consistent with a diagnosis of SLE?

A. Pleural effusion

B. Malar rash

C. Sclerodactyly

D. Urinary sediment with RBC casts

ANSWERS

10.1 **B.** Uremic pericarditis is considered a medical emergency and an indication for urgent dialysis.

10.2 **C.** The clinical picture suggests the patient has developed pericardial tamponade, which may be life threatening and often requires urgent pericardiocentesis.

10.3 **C.** Sclerodactyly, which is thickened and tight skin of the fingers and toes, is a classic feature of patients with scleroderma (who may also have a positive ANA test), but is not seen in SLE. The other findings (malar rash, serositis, glomerulonephritis) are typical of SLE, but not seen in scleroderma.

CLINICAL PEARLS

▶ Acute pericarditis is characterized by pleuritic chest pain, a pericardial friction rub, and ECG findings of diffuse ST-segment elevation and PR-segment depression.

▶ Pericardial friction rub does not exclude a pericardial effusion; patients with acute pericarditis should be monitored for development of effusion and tamponade.

▶ Treatment of pericarditis is directed at the underlying cause; for example, for uremic pericarditis, urgent dialysis is necessary. For viral or inflammatory causes, treatment is nonsteroidal anti-inflammatory drugs or corticosteroids for refractory cases.

▶ Systemic lupus erythematosus can be diagnosed if a patient has four of the following features: malar rash, discoid rash, photosensitivity, oral ulcers, arthritis, serositis, renal disease, neurologic manifestations, hematologic cytopenias, immunologic abnormalities (eg, false-positive Venereal Disease Research Laboratory [VDRL] test), and positive anti-nuclear antibody.

▶ The major morbidity and mortality of systemic lupus erythematosus are consequences of renal disease, central nervous system involvement, or infection.

REFERENCES

Braunwald E. Pericardial disease. In: Longo DL, Fauci AS, Kasper DL, et al., eds. *Harrison's Principles of Internal Medicine*. 18th ed. New York, NY: McGraw-Hill; 2012:1971-1978.

Hahn BH. Systemic lupus erythematosus. In: Longo DL, Fauci AS, Kasper DL, et al., eds. *Harrison's Principles of Internal Medicine*. 18th ed. New York, NY: McGraw-Hill; 2012:2724-2735.

Lange RA, Hillis LD. Acute pericarditis. *N Engl J Med*. 2004;351:2195-2202.

Spodick DH. Acute pericarditis: current concepts and practice. *JAMA*. 2003;289:1150-1153.

A 42-year-old man complains of 2 days of worsening chest pain and dyspnea. Six weeks ago, he was diagnosed with non-Hodgkin lymphoma with lymphadenopathy of the mediastinum, and he has been treated with mediastinal radiation therapy. His most recent treatment was 1 week ago. He has no other medical or surgical history, and takes no medications. His chest pain is constant and unrelated to activity. He becomes short of breath with minimal exertion. He is afebrile, heart rate is 115 bpm with a thready pulse, respiratory rate 22 breaths per minute, and blood pressure 108/86 mm Hg. Systolic blood pressure drops to 86 mm Hg on inspiration. He appears uncomfortable and is diaphoretic. His jugular veins are distended to the angle of the jaw, and his chest is clear to auscultation. He is tachycardic, his heart sounds are faint, and no extra sounds are appreciated. The chest x-ray is shown in Figure 11–1.

Figure 11–1. Chest x-ray. (Courtesy of Dr. Jorge Albin.)

▶ What is the most likely diagnosis?
▶ What is your next step in therapy?

ANSWERS TO CASE 11:

Pericardial Effusion/Tamponade Caused by Malignancy

Summary: A 42-year-old man with a thoracic malignancy and history of radiotherapy to the mediastinum now presents with chest pain, dyspnea, cardiac enlargement on chest x-ray (which could represent cardiomegaly or pericardial effusion), jugular venous distention, distant cardiac sounds, and pulsus paradoxus.

- **Most likely diagnosis:** Pericardial effusion causing cardiac tamponade.

- **Next therapeutic step:** Urgent pericardiocentesis or surgical pericardial window.

ANALYSIS

Objectives

1. Recognize pericardial tamponade; know how to check for pulsus paradoxus.

2. Know the features of cardiac tamponade, constrictive pericarditis, and restrictive cardiomyopathy and how to distinguish among them.

3. Understand the treatment of each of these conditions.

4. Know the potential cardiac complications of thoracic malignancies and radiation therapy.

Considerations

The patient described in the scenario, with his thoracic malignancy and history of radiation therapy, is at risk for diseases of the pericardium and myocardium. The jugular venous distention, distant heart sounds, and pulsus paradoxus all are suggestive of cardiac tamponade. The major diagnostic considerations in this case, each with a very different treatment, are pericardial effusion causing cardiac tamponade, constrictive pericarditis, and restrictive cardiomyopathy. All of these conditions can impede diastolic filling of the heart and lead to cardiovascular compromise. Urgent differentiation among these conditions is required, because the treatment is very different and the consequences of these diseases can be immediately fatal. Clinically, the patient's fall in systolic blood pressure with inspiration, pulsus paradoxus, is suggestive of cardiac tamponade, which would be treated by evacuating the pericardial fluid.

APPROACH TO:
Suspected Cardiac Tamponade

DEFINITIONS

PERICARDIAL EFFUSION: Fluid that fills the pericardial space, which may be due to infection, hemorrhage, or malignancy. A rapidly accumulating effusion may lead to cardiac compromise.

CARDIAC TAMPONADE: Increased pressure within the pericardial space caused by an accumulating effusion, which compresses the heart and impedes diastolic filling.

CLINICAL APPROACH

Cardiac tamponade refers to increased pressure within the pericardial space caused by an accumulating effusion, which compresses the heart and impedes diastolic filling. Because the heart can only pump out during systole what it receives during diastole, severe restrictions of diastolic filling lead to a marked decrease in cardiac output, which can cause cardiovascular collapse and death. If pericardial fluid accumulates slowly, the sac may dilate and hold up to 2000 mL (producing amazing cardiomegaly on chest x-ray) before causing diastolic impairment. If the fluid accumulates rapidly, as in a hemopericardium caused by trauma or surgery, as little as 200 mL can produce tamponade. The classic description of **Beck triad (hypotension, elevated jugular venous pressure, and small quiet heart)** is a description of **acute tamponade** with rapid accumulation of fluid, as in cardiac trauma or ventricular rupture. If the fluid accumulates slowly, the clinical picture may look more like congestive heart failure, with cardiomegaly on chest x-ray (although there should be no pulmonary edema), dyspnea, elevated jugular pressure, hepatomegaly, and peripheral edema. A high index of suspicion is required, and cardiac tamponade should be considered in any patient with hypotension and elevated jugular venous pressure.

The **most important physical sign** to look for **in cardiac tamponade** is **pulsus paradoxus.** This refers to a **drop in systolic blood pressure of more than 10 mm Hg during inspiration.** Although called "paradoxical," this drop in systolic blood pressure is actually not contrary to the normal physiologic variation with respiration; it is an exaggeration of the normal small drop in systolic pressure during inspiration. Although not a specific sign of tamponade (ie, it is often seen in patients with disturbed intrathoracic pressures during respiration, eg, those with obstructive lung disease), the paradoxical pulse is fairly sensitive for hemodynamically significant tamponade in almost all cases. To test for this, one must use a manual blood pressure cuff that is inflated above systolic pressure and deflated very slowly until the first Korotkoff sound is heard during expiration and then, finally, during both phases of respiration. The difference between these two pressure readings is the pulsus paradoxus. When the pulsus paradoxus is severe, it may be detected by palpation as a diminution or disappearance of peripheral pulses during inspiration.

Constrictive pericarditis is a complication of previous pericarditis, either acute or chronic fibrinous pericarditis. The inflammation with resultant granulation tissue forms a **thickened fibrotic adherent sac** that gradually contracts, encasing the heart and **impairing diastolic filling**. In the past, tuberculosis was the most common cause of this problem but now is rare in the United States. Currently, this is **most commonly caused by radiation therapy, cardiac surgery**, or any cause of acute pericarditis, such as **viral infection, uremia, or malignancy**. The pathophysiology of constrictive pericarditis is similar to that of cardiac tamponade in the restricted ability of the ventricles to fill during diastole because of the thickened noncompliant pericardium.

Because the process is **chronic**, patients with **constrictive pericarditis** generally do not present with acute hemodynamic collapse but rather with **chronic and slowly progressive weakness and fatigue and exertional dyspnea**. Patients commonly have what appears to be right-sided heart failure, that is, chronic lower extremity edema, hepatomegaly, and ascites. Like patients with tamponade, they have elevated jugular venous pressures, but **pulsus paradoxus usually is absent**. Examination of neck veins shows an increase in jugular venous pressure during inspiration, termed **Kussmaul sign**. This is easy to see because it is the opposite of the normal fall in pressure as a person inspires. Normally, the negative intrathoracic pressure generated by inspiration sucks blood into the heart, but because of the severe diastolic restriction, the blood cannot enter the right atrium or ventricle, so it fills the jugular vein. Another physical finding characteristic of constrictive pericarditis is a **pericardial knock**, which is a high-pitched early diastolic sound occurring just after aortic valve closure. Chest radiography frequently shows cardiomegaly and a calcified pericardium.

Restrictive cardiomyopathy, like the previous diagnoses, is primarily a problem of impaired diastolic filling, usually with preserved systolic function. This is a relatively uncommon problem in the Western world. The **most common causes are amyloidosis**, an infiltrative disease of the elderly, in which an abnormal fibrillar amyloid protein is deposited in heart muscle, or fibrosis of the myocardium following radiation therapy or open heart surgery. In **Africa**, restrictive cardiomyopathy is much more common because of a process called **endomyocardial fibrosis**, characterized by fibrosis of the endocardium along with fever and marked eosinophilia, accounting for up to 25% of deaths due to heart disease.

Clinically, it may be very difficult to distinguish restrictive cardiomyopathy from constrictive pericarditis, and various echocardiographic criteria have been proposed to try to distinguish between them. In addition, magnetic resonance imaging (MRI) can be very useful to visualize or exclude the presence of the thickened pericardium typical of constrictive pericarditis. Nevertheless, it may be necessary to obtain an **endomyocardial biopsy** to make the diagnosis. Differentiation between the two is essential because constrictive pericarditis is a potentially curable disease, whereas very little effective therapy is available for either the underlying conditions or the cardiac failure of restrictive cardiomyopathy. Table 11–1 compares features of cardiac tamponade, acute pericarditis, restrictive cardiomyopathy, and constrictive pericarditis.

Table 11–1 • FEATURES OF CARDIAC TAMPONADE, ACUTE PERICARDITIS, RESTRICTIVE CARDIOMYOPATHY, AND CONSTRICTIVE PERICARDITIS			
Disease	Pathophysiology	Clinical Features	ECG Findings
Cardiac tamponade	Increased pressure in pericardial space due to effusion, impeding diastolic filling	**Pulsus paradoxus,** hypotension, elevated jugular venous distention, small quiet heart	Low voltage diffusely, electrical alternans
Constrictive pericarditis	Inflammation and granulation tissue forms a thickened fibrotic adherent sac, commonly caused by radiation, viral infection, uremia	Absent pulsus paradoxus, **Kussmaul sign,** pericardial knock, chronic and slow progressive weakness, and exertional dyspnea	Low voltage
Acute pericarditis	Acute inflammation of the parietal pericardium and superficial myocardium	Chest pain, fever, pericardial rub	ST-segment elevation, low voltage diffusely
Restrictive cardiomyopathy	Myocardial fibrosis, hypertrophy, or infiltration leading to impaired diastolic filling	No pulsus paradoxus or Kussmaul sign; progressive exertional dyspnea and dependent edema	

Treatment

Treatment of cardiac tamponade consists of relief of the pericardial pressure, either by echocardiographically guided pericardiocentesis or a surgical pericardial window. Resection of the pericardium is the definitive treatment of constrictive pericarditis. There is no effective treatment for restrictive cardiomyopathy.

CASE CORRELATION

- See also Case 3 (Myocardial Infarction, Acute), Case 4 (Congestive Heart Failure), Case 8 (Atrial Fibrillation), and Case 10 (Acute Pericarditis).

COMPREHENSION QUESTIONS

11.1 A 35-year-old woman is noted to have a positive Kussmaul sign. Which of the following conditions does she most likely have?

A. Constrictive pericarditis

B. Cardiac tamponade

C. Dilated cardiomyopathy

D. Diabetic ketoacidosis

11.2 Which of the following is the most sensitive finding in patients with cardiac tamponade?

A. Disappearance of radial pulse during inspiration

B. Drop in systolic blood pressure more than 10 mm Hg during inspiration

C. Rise in heart rate more than 20 bpm during inspiration

D. Distant heart sounds

11.3 While awaiting pericardiocentesis, immediate supportive care of a patient with cardiac tamponade should include which of the following?

A. Diuresis with furosemide

B. Intravenous fluids

C. Nitrates to lower venous congestion

D. Morphine to relieve dyspnea

11.4 Which of the following is most likely to cause restrictive cardiomyopathy?

A. Endomyocardial fibrosis

B. Viral myocarditis

C. Beriberi (thiamine deficiency)

D. Doxorubicin therapy

ANSWERS

11.1 **A.** Kussmaul sign, an increase in neck veins with inspiration, is seen with constrictive pericarditis, due to the impaired diastolic dysfunction and inability of blood to enter the right ventricle.

11.2 **B.** Pulsus paradoxus is a sensitive although nonspecific sign for cardiac tamponade. Pulsus paradoxus is one of the more sensitive signs for hemodynamically significant cardiac tamponade; however it is relatively nonspecific. Other clinical features include hypotension, elevated jugular venous distention, and soft heart sounds.

11.3 **B.** Patients with cardiac tamponade are preload dependent, and diuretics, nitrates, or morphine may cause them to become hypotensive. In contrast, volume expansion with intravenous fluids helps maintain intravascular volume and cardiac output.

11.4 **A.** Endomyocardial fibrosis is an etiology of restrictive cardiomyopathy, common in developing countries, that is associated with eosinophilia. The other disease processes mentioned are causes of dilated cardiomyopathy.

CLINICAL PEARLS

▶ Elevated jugular venous pressure and pulsus paradoxus are features of cardiac tamponade.

▶ Kussmaul sign and right-sided heart failure are features of constrictive cardiomyopathy, but pulsus paradoxus is not.

▶ Cardiac tamponade requires urgent treatment by pericardiocentesis or a pericardial window.

▶ Constrictive pericarditis may show calcifications of the pericardium on chest x-ray or thickened pericardium on echocardiography. Definitive therapy is resection of the pericardium.

▶ Restrictive cardiomyopathy is most often caused by amyloidosis or radiation therapy. There is no effective therapy.

REFERENCES

Bertog SC, Thambidorai SK, Parakh K, et al. Constrictive pericarditis: etiology and cause-specific survival after pericardiectomy. *J Am Coll Cardiol.* 2004;43:1445-1452.

McGregor M. Pulsus paradoxus. *N Engl J Med.* 1979;301:480-482.

Spodick DH. Acute cardiac tamponade. *N Engl J Med.* 2003;349:684-690.

Wynne J, Braunwald E. Cardiomyopathy and myocarditis. In: Longo DL, Fauci AS, Kasper DL, et al., eds. *Harrison's Principles of Internal Medicine.* 18th ed. New York, NY: McGraw-Hill; 2012: 1951-1970.

A 28-year-old man comes to the emergency center complaining of 6 days of fever with shaking chills. Over the past 2 days, he has also developed a productive cough with greenish sputum, which occasionally is blood streaked. He reports no dyspnea, but sometimes he experiences chest pain with deep inspiration. He does not have headache, abdominal pain, urinary symptoms, vomiting, or diarrhea. He has no significant medical history. He smokes cigarettes and marijuana regularly, drinks several beers daily, but denies intravenous drug use.

On examination, his temperature is 102.5°F, heart rate is 109 bpm, blood pressure is 128/76 mm Hg, and respiratory rate is 23 bpm. He is alert and talkative. He has no oral lesions, and funduscopic examination reveals no abnormalities. His jugular veins show prominent V waves, and his heart rhythm is tachycardic but regular with a harsh holosystolic murmur at the left lower sternal border that becomes louder with inspiration. Chest examination reveals inspiratory rales bilaterally. On both of his forearms, he has linear streaks of induration, hyperpigmentation, and some small nodules overlying the superficial veins, but no erythema, warmth, or tenderness.

Laboratory examination is significant for an elevated white blood cell (WBC) count at 17,500/mm^3, with 84% polymorphonuclear cells, 7% band forms, and 9% lymphocytes, a hemoglobin concentration of 14 g/dL, hematocrit 42%, and platelet count 189,000/mm^3. Liver function tests and urinalysis are normal. Chest radiograph shows multiple peripheral, ill-defined nodules, some with cavitation.

▶ What is the most likely diagnosis?
▶ What is your next step?

ANSWERS TO CASE 12:

Endocarditis (Tricuspid)/Septic Pulmonary Emboli

Summary: A 28-year-old man complains of shaking chills and fever. He also has a productive cough. He denies intravenous drug use. He has a temperature of 102.5°F, heart rate of 109 bpm, and a new holosystolic murmur at the left lower sternal border, which increases with inspiration. He has linear streaks of induration on both forearms, and chest radiograph shows multiple ill-defined nodules.

- **Most likely diagnosis:** Infective endocarditis involving the tricuspid valve, with probable septic pulmonary emboli.

- **Next step:** Obtain serial blood cultures and institute empiric broad-spectrum antibiotics.

ANALYSIS

Objectives

1. Understand the differences in clinical presentation between acute and subacute, and left-sided versus right-sided endocarditis.

2. Learn the most common organisms that cause endocarditis, including "culture-negative" endocarditis.

3. Know the diagnostic and therapeutic approach to infective endocarditis, including the indications for valve replacement.

4. Understand the complications of endocarditis.

Considerations

Although this patient denied IV drug use, his track marks on the forearms are very suspicious for intravenous drug abuse. He has fever, a new heart murmur very typical of tricuspid regurgitation, and a chest radiograph suggestive of multiple septic pulmonary emboli. Serial blood cultures, ideally obtained before antibiotics are started, are essential to establish the diagnosis of infective endocarditis. The rapidity with which antibiotics are started depends on the clinical presentation of the patient: a septic, critically ill patient needs antibiotics immediately; a patient with a subacute presentation can wait many hours while cultures are obtained.

APPROACH TO:

Suspected Endocarditis

DEFINITIONS

INFECTIOUS ENDOCARDITIS: A microbial process of the endocardium, usually involving the heart valves.

JANEWAY LESIONS: Painless hemorrhagic macules on the palms and soles that are consistent with infectious endocarditis, thought to be caused by **septic emboli**, resulting in microabscesses.

OSLER NODES: Painful, palpable, erythematous lesions most often involving the pads of the fingers and toes, representing **vasculitic** lesions caused by **immune complexes**.

ROTH SPOTS: Hemorrhagic retinal lesions with white centers, due to infectious endocarditis, also thought to be an immune complex–mediated vasculitis.

CLINICAL APPROACH

The clinical presentation depends on the which valves are involved (left-sided vs right-sided), as well as the virulence of the organism. Highly virulent species, such as *Staphylococcus aureus*, produce acute infection, and less virulent organisms, such as the viridans group of streptococci, tend to produce a more subacute illness, which may evolve over weeks. **Fever is present in 95% of all cases.** For **acute endocarditis**, patients often present with high fever, acute valvular regurgitation, and embolic phenomena (eg, to the extremities or to the brain, causing stroke). **Subacute endocarditis** is more often associated with constitutional symptoms such as anorexia, weight loss, night sweats, and findings attributable to immune complex deposition and vasculitis; these include petechiae, splenomegaly, glomerulonephritis, **Osler nodes, Janeway lesions, and Roth spots.** These classic peripheral lesions, although frequently discussed, are actually seen in only 20% to 25% of cases. **Splinter hemorrhages** under the nails may also be seen, but this finding is very nonspecific.

Right-sided endocarditis usually involves the **tricuspid** valve, causing **pulmonary** emboli, rather than involving the systemic circulation. Accordingly, patients develop pleuritic chest pain, purulent sputum, or hemoptysis, and radiographs may show multiple peripheral nodular lesions, often with cavitation. The murmur of tricuspid regurgitation may not be present, especially early in the illness.

In all cases of endocarditis, the critical finding is bacteremia, which usually is sustained. The initiating event is a transient bacteremia, which may be a result of mucosal injury, as in dental extraction, or a complication of the use of intravascular catheters. Bacteria are then able to seed valvular endothelium. Previously damaged, abnormal, or prosthetic valves form vegetations, which are composed of platelets and fibrin, and are relatively avascular sites where bacteria may grow protected from immune attack.

Serial blood cultures are the most important step in the diagnosis of endocarditis. Acutely ill patients should have **three blood cultures** obtained over a **2- to 3-hour** period prior to initiating antibiotics. In **subacute** disease, **three blood cultures over a 24-hour** period maximize the diagnostic yield. Of course, if patients are critically ill or hemodynamically unstable, no delay in initiating therapy is appropriate, and cultures are obtained on presentation, even while broad-spectrum antibiotics are administered. Usually it is not difficult to isolate the infecting organism, because the hallmark of infective endocarditis is sustained bacteremia; thus, all blood cultures often are positive for the microorganism. Table 12–1 lists typical organisms, frequency of infection, and associated conditions.

Table 12–1 • ORGANISMS CAUSING ENDOCARDITIS

Organism	Frequency	Associated Conditions
Staphylococcus aureus	30%-40% of native valve infection	Intravascular catheter, intravenous drug use (tricuspid valve endocarditis)
Coagulase-negative staphylococci	30%-35% of early prosthetic valve infection	Neonates, prosthetic valves
Streptococcus viridans	40%-60% of native valve infection	Oral flora, after dental surgery
Enterococci	15%, usually in older patients	Previous genitourinary tract disease or instrumentation
Streptococcus bovis	5%-10%	Elderly patients, often with underlying GI mucosal lesion, eg, adenoma or malignancy
Candida spp	5%-10%	Intravascular catheters, intravenous drug use

Culture-negative endocarditis, an uncommon situation in which routine cultures fail to grow, is most likely a result of prior **antibiotic** treatment, **fungal** infection (fungi other than *Candida* spp often require special culture media), or **fastidious** organisms. These organisms can include *Abiotrophia* spp, *Bartonella* spp, *Coxiella burnetii*, *Legionella* spp, *Chlamydia*, and the **HACEK organisms** (*Haemophilus aphrophilus/paraphrophilus, Actinobacillus actinomycetemcomitans, Cardiobacterium hominis, Eikenella corrodens, Kingella kingae*). The clinical features, blood cultures, and echocardiography are used to diagnose cases of infective endocarditis using the highly sensitive and specific **Duke criteria**. It should be noted that transesophageal echocardiography (TEE) rather than transthoracic echocardiography (TTE) is the method of choice in assessing these vegetations. Endocarditis is considered to definitely be present if the patient satisfies two major criteria; one major and three minor criteria; or five minor criteria (Table 12–2).

Table 12–2 • DUKE CRITERIA FOR DIAGNOSIS OF ENDOCARDITIS

Major criteria
- Isolation of typical organisms (viridans streptococci, *S aureus*, enterococci, *Streptococcus bovis*, or one of the HACEK organisms) from two separate blood cultures, or persistently positive blood cultures with other organisms
- Evidence of endocardial involvement: either echocardiographic evidence of endocarditis, eg, oscillating intracardiac mass, or new valvular regurgitation

Minor criteria
- Predisposing valvular lesion or intravenous drug use
- Fever >100.4°F (38.0°C)
- Vascular phenomena: arterial or septic pulmonary emboli, mycotic aneurysm, Janeway lesions
- Immunologic phenomena: glomerulonephritis, Osler nodes, Roth spots, positive rheumatoid factor
- Positive blood cultures not meeting major criteria

One life-threatening complication of endocarditis is **congestive heart failure**, usually as a consequence of **infection-induced valvular damage**. Other cardiac complications are intracardiac abscesses and conduction disturbances caused by septal involvement by infection. Systemic arterial embolization may lead to splenic or renal infarction or abscesses. Vegetations may embolize to the coronary circulation, causing a myocardial infarction, or to the brain, causing a cerebral infarction. A **stroke syndrome** in a **febrile** patient should always suggest the possibility of **endocarditis**. Infection of the vasa vasorum may weaken the wall of major arteries and produce mycotic aneurysms, which can occur anywhere but are most common in the cerebral circulation, sinuses of Valsalva, or abdominal aorta. These aneurysms may leak or rupture, producing sudden fatal intracranial or other hemorrhage.

Antibiotic treatment is usually begun in the hospital but because of the prolonged nature of therapy is often completed on an outpatient basis when the patient is clinically stable. **Treatment generally lasts 4 to 6 weeks.** If the organism is susceptible, such as **most *Streptococcus* species, penicillin G** is the agent of choice. For *Staphylococcus* **aureus, nafcillin** is the drug of choice, often used in combination with **gentamicin** initially for synergy, to help resolve bacteremia. Therapy for intravenous drug users should be directed against *S aureus*. **Vancomycin** is used when **methicillin-resistant *S aureus* or coagulase-negative staphylococci** are present. **Ceftriaxone is the usual therapy for the HACEK** group of organisms. Deciding appropriate therapy for culture-negative endocarditis may be challenging and depends on the clinical situation.

Table 12–3 summarizes the commonly recognized indications for surgical intervention: valve excision and replacement.

Patients at high risk for developing infective endocarditis benefit from antibiotic prophylaxis prior to dental procedures. The most recent American Heart Association guidelines (2008) specify the following individuals:

- Prosthetic heart valves
- Previous infective endocarditis
- Congenital heart disease (unrepaired cyanotic coronary heart disease [CHD] including palliative shunts and conduits)
- Completely repaired CHD repaired with prosthetic material or device during the first 6 postoperative months
- Repaired CHD with residual defects at the site or adjacent to the site of a prosthetic patch or prosthetic device
- Valve regurgitation caused by a structurally abnormal valve in cardiac transplant recipients

Amoxicillin is the drug of choice for prophylaxis unless the patient is allergic to penicillin or unable to take medications by mouth. Alternatives for use in these situations include ampicillin, cephalosporins, and clindamycin.

Table 12–3 • INDICATIONS FOR SURGICAL MANAGEMENT OF ENDOCARDITIS
Intractable congestive heart failure caused by valve dysfunction, >1 serious systemic embolic episode, or large (>10 mm) vegetation with high risk for embolism
Uncontrolled infection, eg, positive cultures after 7 d of therapy
No effective antimicrobial therapy (eg, fungal endocarditis)
Most cases of prosthetic valve endocarditis, especially *S aureus* prosthetic valve infection
Local suppurative complications, eg, myocardial abscess

CASE CORRELATION

- See also Case 3 (Myocardial Infarction, Acute), Case 5 (Aortic Dissection), Case 9 (Syncope and Heart Block), and Case 42 (Fever and Sepsis).

COMPREHENSION Questions

12.1 A 68-year-old man is hospitalized with *Streptococcus bovis* endocarditis of the mitral valve and recovers completely with appropriate therapy. Which of the following is the most important next step?

A. Good dental hygiene and proper denture fitting to prevent reinfection of damaged heart valves from oral flora.

B. Repeat echocardiography in 6 weeks to ensure the vegetations have resolved.

C. Colonoscopy to look for mucosal lesions.

D. Mitral valve replacement to prevent systemic emboli such as cerebral infarction.

12.2 A 24-year-old intravenous drug user is admitted with 4 weeks of fever. He has three blood cultures positive with *Candida* spp and suddenly develops a cold blue toe. Which of the following is the appropriate next step?

A. Repeat echocardiography to see if the large aortic vegetation previously seen has now embolized.

B. Cardiovascular surgery consultation for aortic valve replacement.

C. Aortic angiography to evaluate for a mycotic aneurysm, which may be embolizing.

D. Switch from fluconazole to amphotericin B.

12.3 A patient with which of the following conditions requires antimicrobial prophylaxis before dental surgery?

A. Atrial septal defect

B. Mitral valve prolapse without mitral regurgitation

C. Previous coronary artery bypass graft

D. Previous infective endocarditis

ANSWERS

12.1 **C.** Colonoscopy is necessary because a significant number of patients with *S bovis* endocarditis have a colonic cancer or premalignant polyp, which leads to seeding of the valve by gastrointestinal (GI) flora. Heart valves damaged by endocarditis are more susceptible to infection, so good dental hygiene is important, but in this case, the organism came from the intestinal tract, not the mouth, and the possibility of malignancy is most important to address. Serial echocardiography would not add to the patient's care after successful therapy because vegetations become organized and persist for months or years without late embolization. Prophylactic valve replacement would not be indicated because the prosthetic valve is even more susceptible to reinfection than the damaged native valve and would actually increase the risk of cerebral infarction or other systemic emboli as a consequence of thrombus formation, even if adequately anticoagulated.

12.2 **B.** Fungal endocarditis, which occurs in intravenous drug users or immunosuppressed persons with indwelling catheters, frequently gives rise to large friable vegetations with a high risk of embolization (often to the lower extremities) and is very difficult to cure with antifungal medications. Valve replacement is usually necessary. Repeat echocardiography would not add to the patient's care because the clinical diagnosis of peripheral embolization is almost certain, and it would not change the management. Medical therapy with any antifungal agent is unlikely to cure this infection. Mycotic aneurysms may occur in any artery as a consequence of endocarditis and can cause late embolic complications, but in this case, the source probably is the heart.

12.3 **D.** Prior endocarditis damages valvular surfaces, and these patients are at increased risk for reinfection during a transient bacteremia, as may occur during dental procedures or some other GI or genitourinary tract procedures. All of the other conditions mentioned have a negligible risk of endocarditis, the same as in the general population, and antibiotic prophylaxis is not recommended by the American Heart Association.

CLINICAL PEARLS

▶ The diagnosis of infective endocarditis is established by using clinical criteria, the most important of which are sustained bacteremia and evidence of endocardial involvement, usually by echocardiography.

▶ Right-sided endocarditis may be difficult to diagnose because it lacks the systemic emboli seen in left-sided endocarditis, and the new murmur of tricuspid regurgitation is often not heard.

▶ Left-sided native valve endocarditis usually is caused by *Streptococcus viridans*, *S aureus*, and *Enterococcus*. The large majority of right-sided endocarditis is caused by *S aureus*.

▶ Valve replacement usually is necessary for persistent infection, recurrent embolization, or when medical therapy is ineffective, for example, in cases of large vegetations as seen in fungal endocarditis.

▶ Culture-negative endocarditis usually is caused by prior administration of antibiotics before obtaining blood cultures or by infection with fungi or fastidious organisms such as the HACEK group.

REFERENCES

Baddour LM, Wilson WR, Bayer AS, et al. Infective endocarditis: diagnosis, antimicrobial therapy, and management of complications. *Circulation*. 2005;111:3167-3184.

Houpikian P, Raoult D. Blood culture negative endocarditis in a reference center: etiologic diagnosis of 348 cases. *Medicine*. 2005;84:162-173.

Karchmer AW. Infective endocarditis. In: Longo DL, Fauci AS, Kasper DL, et al., eds. *Harrison's Principles of Internal Medicine*. 18th ed. New York, NY: McGraw-Hill; 2012:1052-1063.

Mylonakis E, Calderwood SB. Infective endocarditis in adults. *N Engl J Med*. 2001;345:1318-1330.

A 58-year-old man presents to the emergency center (EC) complaining of severe pain in his left calf and foot that woke him from his sleep. He has a history of chronic stable angina, hypercholesterolemia, and hypertension, for which he takes aspirin, atenolol, and simvastatin. He has experienced pain in both calves and feet with walking for several years, and the pain has gradually progressed so that he can now walk only 100 ft before he has to stop because of pain. He occasionally has experienced mild pain in his feet at night, but the pain usually gets better when he sits up and hangs his feet off the bed. This time, the pain was more severe and did not improve, and he now feels like the foot is numb and he cannot move his toes.

On physical examination, he is afebrile, with heart rate 72 bpm and blood pressure 125/74 mm Hg. Head and neck examination is significant for a right carotid bruit. His chest is clear to auscultation; his heart rhythm is regular with a nondisplaced apical impulse, an S_4 gallop, and no murmurs. His abdomen is benign, with no tenderness or masses. He has bilateral femoral bruits, and palpable femoral and popliteal pulses bilaterally. His pedal pulses are diminished; they are present on the right but absent on the left. The left distal leg and foot are pale and cold to touch, with very slow capillary refill.

▶ What is the most likely diagnosis?
▶ What is your next step?

ANSWERS TO CASE 13:

Limb Ischemia (Peripheral Vascular Disease)

Summary: A 58-year-old man presents to the EC with severe pain and numbness of his left foot. He has angina and a carotid bruit suggesting systemic atherosclerotic disease. He previously had symptoms of bilateral calf claudication, but now has the sudden onset of pain, pallor, and pulselessness in the left foot.

- **Most likely diagnosis:** Acute limb ischemia, either thrombotic arterial occlusion or embolism from a more proximal source.

- **Next step:** Angiogram of the lower extremity.

ANALYSIS

Objectives

1. Understand the clinical presentation of a patient with atherosclerotic peripheral vascular disease, including acute limb ischemia.

2. Know the evaluation and medical management of peripheral vascular disease.

3. Understand the indications for extremity revascularization.

Considerations

This patient has diffuse atherosclerotic vascular disease, including coronary artery disease, carotid disease, and peripheral vascular disease. His **history of calf pain with walking, but resolution with rest, is classic for claudication.** Recently, the perfusion of his left leg likely was worsening, requiring his waking up and dangling his leg to enable blood flow and to help the pain. **Rest pain is a warning sign of possible critical limb vascular insufficiency.** The patient complains of the sudden onset of **pain, pallor, and pulselessness**, indicative of acute arterial occlusion. His limb ischemia may result from acute arterial occlusion caused by an embolus, usually arising from a dislodged thrombus from the heart, or from the aorta or a large proximal artery such as the iliac. Depending on the level of occlusion, the patient may require urgent arterial thromboembolectomy. Magnetic resonance (MR) or computed tomography (CT) angiography, or possibly a conventional arteriogram would be needed to first determine the arterial anatomy and define the best mode of revascularization.

APPROACH TO:

Peripheral Vascular Disease

DEFINITIONS

ANKLE-BRACHIAL INDEX (ABI): Ratio of ankle to brachial systolic blood pressure, determined using Doppler ultrasound flow.

CLAUDICATION: Pain, ache, or cramp in muscles that increases with walking or leg exertion in a predictable manner and resolves with rest.

CLINICAL APPROACH

Although atherosclerosis is a systemic disease, clinicians often focus on the coronary circulation and are pay less attentive to the extremities. Yet atherosclerotic peripheral arterial disease (PAD) is estimated to affect up to 16% of Americans that are 55 years and older and may exist without clinically recognized coronary or cerebrovascular disease. Furthermore, PAD confers the same risk of cardiovascular death as in persons with a prior myocardial infarction or stroke. **The most important risk factors** for PAD are **cigarette smoking and diabetes mellitus.** Hypertension, dyslipidemia, and elevated homocysteine levels also play significant roles.

Diagnosis

The most common symptom associated with chronic arterial insufficiency caused by PAD is **intermittent claudication**, characterized by pain, ache, a sense of fatigue, or other discomfort that occurs in one or both legs during exercise, such as walking, and is relieved with rest. It is ischemic pain and occurs distal to the site of the arterial stenosis, most commonly in the calves. The symptoms often are progressive and may severely limit a patient's activities and reduce the patient's functional status. An individual with proximal stenosis, such as aortoiliac disease, may complain of exertional pain in the buttocks and thighs. Severe occlusion may produce **rest pain**, which often occurs at night and may be relieved by sitting up and dangling the legs, using gravity to assist blood flow to the feet.

On physical examination, palpation of the **peripheral pulses may be diminished** or absent below the level of occlusion; **bruits** may indicate accelerated blood flow velocity and turbulence at the sites of stenosis. Bruits may be heard in the abdomen with aortoiliac stenosis and in the groin with femoral artery stenosis. **Elevation of the feet** above the level of the heart in the supine patient often induces **pallor in the soles.** If the legs are then placed in the dependent position, they frequently develop rubor as a result of reactive hyperemia. Chronic arterial insufficiency may cause **hair loss on the legs and feet**, thickened and brittle toenails, and shiny atrophic skin. Severe ischemia may produce ulcers or gangrene.

When PAD is suspected, the test most commonly used to evaluate for arterial insufficiency is **ABI**. Systolic blood pressures are measured by Doppler ultrasonography in each arm and in the dorsalis pedis and posterior tibial arteries in each ankle. Normally, blood pressures in the large arteries of the legs and arms are similar. In fact, blood pressures in the legs often are higher than in the arms because of an artifact of measurement, so the normal ratio of ankle to brachial pressures is more than 1. Patients with claudication typically have ABI values ranging from 0.41 to 0.90, and those with critical leg ischemia have ABI values less than or equal to 0.40. Further evaluation with exercise treadmill testing can clarify the diagnosis when symptoms are equivocal, can allow for assessment of functional limitations (eg, maximal walking distance), and can evaluate for concomitant coronary artery disease.

Management

The goals of therapy include reductions in cardiovascular morbidity and mortality, improvement in quality of life by decreasing symptoms of claudication and eliminating rest pain, and preservation of limb viability.

The first step in managing patients with PAD is risk factor modification. Because of the likelihood of coexisting atherosclerotic vascular disease such as coronary artery disease, patients with **symptomatic PAD** have an estimated **mortality** rate of **50% in 10 years**, most often as a consequence of cardiovascular events. **Smoking** is, by far, the **single most important risk factor** impacting both claudication symptoms and overall cardiovascular mortality. Besides slowing the progression to critical leg ischemia, **tobacco cessation reduces the risk of fatal or nonfatal myocardial infarction by as much as 50%,** more than any other medical or surgical intervention. In addition, treatment of hypercholesterolemia, control of hypertension and diabetes, and use of antiplatelet agents such as aspirin or clopidogrel all have been shown to improve cardiovascular health and may have an effect on peripheral arterial circulation. Carefully supervised exercise programs can improve muscle strength and prolong walking distance by promoting the development of collateral blood flow.

Specific medications for improving claudication symptoms have been used, with some benefit. Pentoxifylline, a substituted xanthine derivative that increases erythrocyte elasticity, has been reported to decrease blood viscosity, thus allowing improved blood flow to the microcirculation; however, results from clinical trials are conflicting, and the benefit of pentoxifylline, if present, appears small. A newer agent, cilostazol, a phosphodiesterase inhibitor with vasodilatory and antiplatelet properties, has been approved by the Food and Drug Administration (FDA) for treatment of claudication. It has been shown in randomized controlled trials to improve maximal walking distance. Figure 13–1 shows an algorithm for management of PAD.

Patients with **critical leg ischemia**, defined as **ABI** less than **0.40, severe or disabling claudication, rest pain**, or **nonhealing ulcers**, should be **evaluated for a revascularization procedure**. This can be accomplished by percutaneous angioplasty, with or without placement of intra-arterial stents, or surgical bypass grafting. Angiography (either conventional or magnetic resonance arteriography) should be performed to define the flow-limiting lesions prior to any vascular procedure. Ideal candidates for arterial revascularization are those with discrete stenosis of large vessels; diffuse atherosclerotic and small-vessel disease respond poorly.

Less common causes of chronic peripheral arterial insufficiency include thromboangiitis obliterans, or **Buerger disease**, which is an inflammatory condition of small- and medium-sized arteries that may affect the upper or lower extremities and is found almost exclusively in smokers, especially males younger than 40 years. **Fibromuscular dysplasia** is a hyperplastic disorder **affecting medium and small arteries that usually occurs in women**. Generally, the renal or carotid arteries are involved, but when the arteries to the limbs are affected, the clinical symptoms are identical to those of atherosclerotic PAD. **Takayasu arteritis** is an inflammatory condition, seen primarily in younger women, that usually affects branches of the aorta, most commonly the subclavian arteries, and causes **arm claudication and Raynaud phenomenon**, along with constitutional symptoms such as **fever** and **weight loss**.

Figure 13–1. Algorithm for management of peripheral arterial disease. (Data from Hiatt W. Medical treatment of peripheral arterial disease and claudication. *N Engl J Med.* 2001;344:1608–1621.)

Patients with chronic peripheral arterial insufficiency who present with sudden unremitting pain may have an **acute arterial occlusion**, most commonly the result of **embolism** or **in situ thrombosis. The heart is the most common source of emboli;** conditions that may cause cardiogenic emboli include atrial fibrillation, dilated cardiomyopathy, and endocarditis. Artery-to-artery embolization of atherosclerotic debris from the aorta or large vessels may occur spontaneously or, more often, after an intravascular procedure, such as arterial catheterization. Emboli tend to lodge at the bifurcation of two vessels, most often in the femoral, iliac, popliteal, or tibioperoneal arteries. Arterial thrombosis may occur in atherosclerotic vessels at the site of stenosis or in an area of aneurysmal dilation, which may also complicate atherosclerotic disease.

Patients with acute arterial occlusion may present with a number of signs, which can be remembered as **"six Ps": pain, pallor, pulselessness, paresthesias, poikilothermia (coolness), and paralysis.** The first five signs occur fairly quickly with acute ischemia; paralysis will develop if the arterial occlusion is severe and persistent.

Rapid restoration of arterial supply is mandatory in patients with an **acute arterial occlusion that threatens limb viability.** Initial management includes anticoagulation with heparin to prevent propagation of the thrombus. The affected limb should be placed below the horizontal plane without any pressure applied to it. Conventional arteriography usually is indicated to identify the location of the occlusion and to evaluate potential methods of revascularization. Surgical removal of an embolus or arterial bypass may be performed, particularly if a large proximal artery is occluded. A balloon catheter may also be attempted to remove the clot. Alternatively, a catheter can be used to deliver intra-arterial thrombolytic therapy directly into the thrombus. In comparison with systemic fibrinolytic therapy, localized infusion is associated with fewer bleeding complications.

CASE CORRELATION

- See also Case 2 (Hypercholesterolemia), Case 3 (Myocardial Infarction, Acute), and Case 6 (Hypertension).

COMPREHENSION QUESTIONS

13.1 A 49-year-old smoker with hypertension, diabetes, and hypercholesterolemia comes to the clinic complaining of pain in his calves when he walks two to three blocks. Which of the following therapies might offer him the greatest benefit in symptom reduction and in overall mortality?

A. Aspirin

B. Limb revascularization procedure

C. Cilostazol

D. Smoking cessation

E. Pravastatin

13.2 A 31-year-old male smoker presents with resting pain in his legs and a nonhealing foot ulcer. Which of the following is the most likely cause of arterial insufficiency in this patient?

A. Cholesterol embolism

B. Fibromuscular dysplasia

C. Thromboangiitis obliterans (Buerger disease)

D. Takayasu arteritis

E. Psychogenic pain

13.3 A 21-year-old woman presents with fever, fatigue, and unequal pulses and blood pressures in her arms. Which of the following is the most likely cause of arterial insufficiency in this patient?

A. Cholesterol embolism

B. Fibromuscular dysplasia

C. Thromboangiitis obliterans (Buerger disease)

D. Takayasu aortitis

E. Psychogenic pain

13.4 A 62-year-old man presents with livedo reticularis and three blue toes, including one with gangrene following cardiac catheterization. Which of the following is the most likely cause of this patient's findings?

A. Cholesterol embolism

B. Fibromuscular dysplasia

C. Thromboangiitis obliterans (Buerger disease)

D. Takayasu aortitis

E. Psychogenic pain

13.5 A 67-year-old woman is noted to have significant peripheral vascular disease. She is evaluated by the cardiovascular surgeon but not felt to be a surgical candidate. Which of the following conditions is likely to be present in this patient?

A. Diffuse atherosclerotic disease

B. Leg pain at rest

C. Symptoms that do not improve with pharmacologic management

D. Nonhealing ulcers of the ankle

ANSWERS

13.1 **D.** Tobacco cessation is the most important intervention to improve cardio-vascular morbidity and mortality in high-risk patients, such as those with PAD, and to improve claudication symptoms. Cilostazol may help with claudication symptoms but will not affect cardiovascular mortality. Aspirin, angiotensin-converting enzyme (ACE) inhibitors, and beta-hydroxy-beta-methylglutaryl coenzyme A (HMG-CoA) reductase inhibitors are important adjuncts for risk factor modification and for relief of symptoms, but their benefits pale in comparison to smoking cessation.

13.2 **C.** Thromboangiitis obliterans, or Buerger disease, is a disease of young male smokers and may cause symptoms of chronic arterial insufficiency in either legs or arms. Cholesterol embolisms are most likely to occur after a cardiac catheterization or other vascular procedure. Location of arterial insufficiency is also important for differentiation. Fibromuscular dysplasia is more likely to involve the renal arteries and extracranial cerebrovascular arteries rather than peripheral arteries of the extremities. Lastly, Takayasu arteritis is a large vessel vasculitis primarily affecting the aorta and the primary branches.

13.3 **D.** Takayasu aortitis is associated with symptoms of inflammation such as fever, and most often affects the subclavian arteries, producing stenotic lesions that may cause unequal blood pressures, diminished pulses, and ischemic pain in the affected limbs.

13.4 **A.** Embolism of cholesterol and other atherosclerotic debris from the aorta or other large vessels to small vessels of skin or digits may complicate any intra-arterial procedure.

13.5 **A.** Surgical therapy is reserved for severe symptoms after exercise and pharmacologic agents are used, and quality of life is impaired. Pain at rest, lack of symptoms for medical therapy, nonhealing ulcers, and gangrene are some of those indications. Duplex ultrasound can help to discern whether the patient is a potential surgical candidate. Arteriography may also be performed. Diffuse atherosclerotic disease is a contraindication for surgery since bypass would not help in the face of significant and widespread disease.

CLINICAL PEARLS

▶ Smoking cessation is the single most important intervention for atherosclerotic peripheral vascular disease. Other treatments include pentoxifylline or cilostazol, regular exercise, and cardiovascular risk factor modification.

▶ Revascularization by angioplasty or bypass grafting may be indicated for patients with debilitating claudication, ischemic rest pain, or tissue necrosis.

▶ Acute arterial occlusion that threatens limb viability is a medical emergency and requires immediate anticoagulation and investigation with conventional arteriography.

▶ Acute severe ischemia of an extremity causes the "six Ps": *pain, pallor, pulselessness, paresthesias, poikilothermia,* and *paralysis*. Chronic incomplete arterial occlusion may result only in exertional pain or fatigue, pallor on elevation of the extremity, and rubor on dependency.

REFERENCES

Creager M, Loscalzo J. Vascular disease of the extremities. In: Longo DL, Fauci AS, Kasper DL, et al., eds. *Harrison's Principles of Internal Medicine.* 18th ed. New York, NY: McGraw-Hill; 2012: 2066-2076.

Hankey GJ, Normal PE, Eikelboom JW, et al. Medical treatment of peripheral arterial disease. *JAMA.* 2006;295:547.

Hirsch AT, Haskal ZJ, Hertzer NR, et al. ACC/AHA 2005 practice guidelines for the management of patients with peripheral arterial disease. *Circulation.* 2006;113:e463.

Katzen BT. Clinical diagnosis and prognosis of acute limb ischemia. *Rev Cardiovasc Med.* 2002;3 (suppl 2):S2-S6.

A 48-year-old woman calls 911 and is brought to the emergency center complaining of a sudden onset of dyspnea. She reports she was standing in the kitchen making dinner, when she suddenly felt as if she could not get enough air, her heart started racing, and she became light-headed and felt as if she would faint. She denied chest pain or cough. Her medical history is significant only for gallstones, for which she underwent a cholecystectomy 2 weeks previously. The procedure was complicated by a wound infection, requiring her to stay in the hospital for 8 days. She takes no medications regularly, and only takes acetaminophen as needed for pain at her abdominal incision site.

On examination, she is tachypneic with a respiratory rate of 28 bpm, oxygen saturations 84% on room air, heart rate 124 bpm, and blood pressure 118/89 mm Hg. She appears uncomfortable, diaphoretic, and frightened. Her oral mucosa is slightly cyanotic, her jugular venous pressure is elevated, and her chest is clear to auscultation. Her heart rhythm is tachycardic but regular with a loud second sound in the pulmonic area, but no gallop or murmur. Her abdominal examination is benign, with a clean incision site without signs of infection. Her right leg is moderately swollen from mid-thigh to her feet, and her thigh and calf are mildly tender to palpation. Laboratory studies including cardiac enzymes are normal; her electrocardiogram (ECG) reveals only sinus tachycardia, and her chest x-ray is interpreted as normal.

▶ What is the most likely diagnosis?
▶ What is the most appropriate diagnostic step?

ANSWERS TO CASE 14:

Pulmonary Embolism

Summary: A 48-year-old woman is brought to the hospital for very acute onset of dyspnea and is found to be tachypneic, tachycardic, and hypoxemic. On physical examination, she has elevated jugular venous pressure and a loud pulmonic closure sound, perhaps signifying acutely elevated pulmonary pressures. All of these findings, especially the hypoxemia despite a clear chest radiograph, strongly suggest a pulmonary embolism (PE), most likely caused by a lower extremity deep venous thrombosis (DVT), a late complication of her recent hospitalization and relative immobilization.

- **Most likely diagnosis:** Pulmonary embolism.

- **Most appropriate diagnostic step:** Chest computed tomography (CT) with intravenous contrast, or other imaging study as indicated.

ANALYSIS

Objectives

1. Understand the factors that predispose patients to develop thromboembolic disease.

2. Recognize the clinical presentation of PE.

3. Know the strategies to diagnose PE.

4. Understand the goals and methods of treatment of thromboembolism.

Considerations

PE is a difficult diagnosis to establish because of the nonspecificity of presenting signs and symptoms and the probabilistic nature of the most common noninvasive diagnostic tests. In patients with suspected PE, initial treatment is supportive to maintain adequate oxygenation and hemodynamic stability, and efforts are undertaken to try to diagnose the PE or other cause of the patient's symptoms. Often, a series of diagnostic tests is necessary to determine the likely diagnosis. Specific treatment of PE may include thrombolysis or surgical embolectomy for unstable patients and initiation of anticoagulation as a long-term measure to prevent recurrence.

APPROACH TO:

Suspected Pulmonary Embolism

DEFINITION

DEEP VENOUS THROMBOSIS: Blood clot in the deep venous system that usually affects the lower extremities or pelvic veins.

PULMONARY EMBOLISM: A blot clot (usually originating from the lower extremity veins) that travels through the venous circulation and becomes lodged in the pulmonary artery. PE causes acute pulmonary hypertension and can be labeled as a "massive PE" if it causes hemodynamic instability or "submassive" or "moderate" if it causes right ventricular enlargement, strain, or dysfunction but does not cause hemodynamic instability.

CLINICAL APPROACH

Etiology and Risk Factors

Diagnosis and management of PE require a combination of clinical suspicion and appropriate use of diagnostic tools. Pulmonary emboli usually arise from deep venous thrombi and occasionally from less common sources, including air, fat, amniotic fluid, or tumor thrombus. More than 100 years ago, **Rudolf Virchow** postulated three factors that predispose to venous thrombus: **local trauma to vessel wall, a state of hypercoagulability**, and **venous stasis**. Genetic predisposition to hypercoagulability accounts for approximately 20% of PEs. **The most common inherited conditions are the factor V Leiden mutation** and the **prothrombin gene mutations.** Malignancy is also a predisposing condition for deep venous thrombosis. These neoplastic cells are thought to generate thrombin or to synthesize various procoagulants. Surgery and immobilization also increase the risk of PE as late as 1 month postoperatively.

Pathophysiology

When venous thrombi dislodge from their site of formation, they may embolize to the pulmonary arteries causing PE. The **deep proximal lower extremity veins** are the **most common sites of clot formation**, although thromboses in pelvic, calf, and upper extremity veins may also embolize. **Obstruction to the pulmonary artery causes platelets to release vasoactive agents such as serotonin, thereby elevating pulmonary vascular resistance.** The resulting increase in alveolar dead space and subsequent redistribution of blood flow create areas of ventilation/perfusion (V/Q) mismatch and impair gas exchange. Reflex bronchoconstriction causes increasing airway resistance. This cascade can result in pulmonary edema, hemorrhage, or loss of surfactant, further decreasing lung compliance. As pulmonary vascular resistance increases, right heart wall tension rises, resulting in dilation and dysfunction that ultimately may impair left heart function. **Progressive right heart failure is the usual cause of death from PE.**

Clinical and Nonimaging Evaluation

PE can often mimic other cardiopulmonary diseases, making the diagnosis challenging. Acute onset of dyspnea is the most common symptom of PE, and tachypnea is the most frequently observed sign. Severe dyspnea accompanied by syncope, hypotension, or cyanosis may indicate massive PE, whereas pleuritic pain, cough, or hemoptysis may suggest a smaller more peripheral embolus causing infarction of lung tissue. Classic findings on physical examination include tachycardia and signs of right ventricular dysfunction, including bulging neck veins, left parasternal lift, accentuated pulmonic component of the second heart sound, and systolic murmur that increases with inspiration. Findings suggestive of DVT include pain, swelling, and erythema to the lower extremity, particularly the back of the leg below the knee. Some patients complain of calf tenderness.

The most useful nonimaging diagnostic test is the serum **D-dimer** enzyme-linked immunosorbent assay (ELISA). It is elevated (>500 ng/mL) in more than 95% of patients with PE, reflecting the breakdown of fibrin and thrombolysis. Although the D-dimer ELISA has a high negative predictive value and thus is useful in excluding PE, it lacks specificity. **Elevations may be seen in patients with myocardial infarction, pneumonia, heart failure, cancer, or sepsis.** Additional laboratories can assist in risk stratification of submassive PE, including brain natriuretic peptide (BNP) and cardiac troponins. Abnormalities on the ECG are less useful in the evaluation of PE. The most common finding is sinus tachycardia. The $S_1Q_3T_3$ (S wave in lead I, a Q wave in lead III, and an inverted T wave in lead III) is often discussed but less commonly seen, but when present, is relatively specific.

Imaging Modalities

Radiologic studies are critical in the diagnosis of PE and DVT. A chest x-ray is the first study indicated in a symptomatic patient with new-onset dyspnea. A normal or near-normal chest x-ray is the most common finding in PE, sometimes with nonspecific abnormalities, such as atelectasis. In general, **acute onset** of **hypoxemia in a patient with a normal chest x-ray should be interpreted as PE until otherwise proven.** Classic abnormalities associated with PE include Westermark sign (nonspecific prominence of the central pulmonary artery with decreased pulmonary vascularity), Hampton hump (peripheral wedge-shaped density above the diaphragm), and Palla sign (enlargement of the right descending pulmonary artery). The chest radiograph probably is more important in identifying other significant pulmonary parenchymal disease (pneumonia, pulmonary edema) and cardiac disease (cardiomyopathy) as the cause of the respiratory symptoms.

For any imaging modality, the most accurate diagnosis will be achieved in combination with the clinical suspicion. The **Wells score** is a useful clinical calculator to clinically estimate pretest probability of PE. A point score less than 4 *with* a negative D-dimer assay indicates a low probability for PE. A score of 2 to 6 points indicates moderate probability, and more than 6 points is high probability (Table 14–1).

Chest CT with intravenous contrast is now the principal imaging modality to diagnose suspected pulmonary embolism. Current generation spiral CT can acquire high-resolution images in a single breath hold, and can visualize small branch artery emboli. In addition, the chest CT has the additional benefit of visualizing other abnormalities such as pneumonia, aortic abnormalities, or pulmonary masses that may not have been apparent on routine chest radiograph, and which may provide an alternative diagnosis for the patient's symptomatology. The main caveats in the use of CT are the image quality and the experience of the center in interpreting this type of scan. In general, however, CT has been shown to be at least as accurate as the previously accepted standard imaging modality, ventilation/perfusion (V/Q) lung scanning.

In patients in whom a CT with radiocontrast cannot be obtained or is contraindicated (advanced renal insufficiency, severe contrast allergy), a **V/Q scan** remains a useful tool. A normal scan or a low-probability scan with a low clinical suspicion for PE effectively excludes the diagnosis.

Table 14–1 • CLINICAL PREDICTION SCORE FOR ESTIMATING LIKELIHOOD OF PE	
Clinical Variable	Score
Symptoms of DVT	3.0
Alternative Dx less likely than PE	3.0
Heart rate >100/min	1.5
Immobilization >3 days, surgery within 4 weeks	1.5
Prior PE or DVT	1.5
Hemoptysis	1.0
Presence of malignancy	1.0

7 points or more = high probability for PE.
Less than 4 points, with negative D-dimer = low probability for PE.
(Data from Wells PS, Anderson DR, Rodger M, et. al. Derivation of a simple clinical model to categorize patients probability of pulmonary embolism: increasing the models utility with the SimpliRED D-dimer. Thromb Haemost. 2000 Mar;83(3):416-20.)

If the CT and/or V/Q scan are nondiagnostic, and yet the clinical suspicion remains high, other imaging modalities may be obtained. A **lower extremity venous ultrasound** demonstrating an acute DVT in a patient with signs and symptoms of PE would be sufficient to diagnose and treat PE (especially since the treatment with anticoagulation is the same). It should be noted, though, that a normal ultrasound does not exclude the diagnosis of PE, since most patients with PE do not have evidence of residual DVT, and in many cases because the clot has already embolized.

Other imaging studies such as **contrast-enhanced magnetic resonance imaging (MRI)** or **echocardiography** (especially transesophageal echocardiography) may be used when the clinical suspicion remains high, but other diagnostic studies are inconclusive. Figure 14–1 gives a diagnostic algorithm for suspected PE.

Treatment

Treatment options can be categorized in terms of primary and secondary therapy based on different management goals. **Primary therapy** consists of clot dissolution or **thrombolysis (with tissue plasminogen activator or tPA) or removal of clot by surgical embolectomy** and usually is reserved for patients with a high risk for adverse outcomes if the clot remains, that is, those with **right heart failure or hypotension. The main criteria for thrombolytic administration is a systolic blood pressure <90 mm Hg in the absence of absolute contraindications to tPA.** The main complications of thrombolytic administration are bleeding, **a very small percentage of which can be devastating intracerebral hemorrhages. Patients that have conventional surgical embolectomy have a higher mortality (approaching 50%) if the procedure is done emergently. Newer therapies include half-dose thrombolytics and catheter-directed thrombolysis for submassive PE. Patients with hemodynamic collapse may require mechanical circulatory support with venoarterial extracorporeal membrane oxygenation (ECMO), which provides cardiac and pulmonary support, but this should only be employed in patients that are likely to improve with a definitive therapy (ie, surgical embolectomy).**

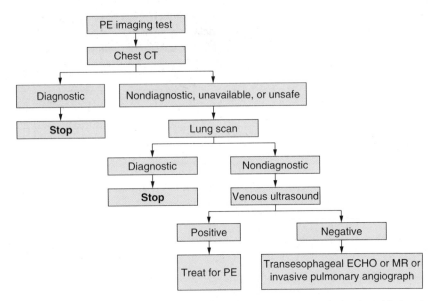

Figure 14–1. Diagnostic algorithm for patients with suspected pulmonary embolism. (Modified, with permission, from Braunwald E, Fauci AS, Kasper KL, et al, *Harrison's Principles of Internal Medicine*, 17th ed. New York: McGraw-Hill, 2008: 1655.)

For patients who are normotensive with normal right ventricle (RV) function, treatment is with **anticoagulation**, with the goal of **secondary prevention** of thrombus extension or recurrence. Anticoagulation does not dissolve existing thrombus, but allows for endothelialization and organization, which begins within days of treatment. Immediate anticoagulation should be initiated with intravenous **unfractionated heparin** (UFH), subcutaneous **low-molecular-weight heparin** (LMWH), enoxaparin or tinzaparin, or the direct factor Xa inhibitor **fondaparinux**. While UFH requires a continuous infusion and frequent laboratory monitoring every 4 to 6 hours, LMWH and fondaparinux provide rapid onset of action and predictable dose response, and no laboratory monitoring is generally required.

Patients can then be started on the oral vitamin K antagonist **warfarin**. It may cause an initial paradoxical prothrombotic state, and thus requires overlap with UFH, LMWH, or fondaparinux when beginning therapy. Because its biological effect is unpredictable, warfarin requires routine monitoring of the prothrombin time, standardized across laboratories as the international normalized ratio (**INR**). The target therapeutic INR is usually 2.5. When initiating warfarin therapy, the usual course is to use UFH, LMWH, or fondaparinux for at least 5 days while overlapping with warfarin until the INR has been therapeutic for 2 consecutive days. **The duration of treatment relates to the risk of recurrence.** One factor in assessing this risk is whether the DVT or PE was provoked (ie, occurred due to a readily identifiable and transient event such as trauma or surgery) or unprovoked. For provoked DVT of the calf or upper extremity, 3 months of anticoagulation are recommended. Six months are recommended for patients with provoked proximal leg DVT or PE. For patients with idiopathic or unprovoked DVT or PE, or with ongoing risk factors, such as malignancy or antiphospholipid syndrome, the duration of therapy is controversial, but indefinite anticoagulation may be required.

Inferior vena cava filter placement to prevent recurrent PE is recommended when there is active bleeding or other contraindication to anticoagulation, or recurrent DVT or PE despite therapeutic anticoagulation.

CASE CORRELATION

- See also Case 3 (Myocardial Infarction, Acute), Case 5 (Aortic Dissection), Case 10 (Acute Pericarditis), Case 15 (Chronic Obstructive Pulmonary Disease), and Case 16 (Asthma).

COMPREHENSION QUESTIONS

14.1 A 35-year-old woman complains of calf tenderness and acute dyspnea. The arterial blood gas reveals partial pressure of oxygen (PO_2) of 76 mm Hg. Which of the following is the most common physical examination finding of pulmonary embolism?

    A. Wheezing

    B. Increased pulmonary component of the second heart sound

    C. Tachypnea

    D. Calf swelling

    E. Pulmonary rales

14.2 A 39-year-old man is noted to have a deep venous thrombosis without any known risk factors. He notes that his brother also developed a pulmonary embolism at age 45, and his mother developed a "clot in the leg" when she was in her thirties. Which of the following is the most likely inherited disorder in this patient?

    A. Protein S deficiency

    B. Antithrombin III deficiency

    C. Factor V Leiden mutation

    D. Antiphospholipid antibody syndrome

    E. Familial malignancy syndrome

14.3 A 54-year-old woman is noted to have cervical cancer and presents with significant vaginal bleeding with a hemoglobin level of 7 g/dL. Her left leg is swollen, which on Doppler investigation reveals a deep venous thrombosis. Which of the following is the best treatment for the thrombus?

    A. Intravenous unfractionated heparin

    B. Fractionated subcutaneous heparin

    C. Subcutaneous unfractionated heparin

    D. Oral warfarin (Coumadin)

    E. Vena cava filter

ANSWERS

14.1 **C.** Tachypnea is the most common physical sign associated with pulmonary embolus. Calf or thigh pain and/or swelling occurs less frequently than tachypnea. Other common clinical manifestations of pulmonary embolus in decreasing frequency include pleuritic pain, cough, and orthopnea.

14.2 **C.** Factor V Leiden mutation is the most common hereditary thrombophilia. It is inherited in an autosomal dominant fashion and therefore will affect both men and women.

14.3 **E.** Cervical cancer with significant vaginal bleeding is a relative contraindication for anticoagulation. Thus, a vena cava filter is the most appropriate choice in this patient.

CLINICAL PEARLS

▶ Acute onset of dyspnea or hypoxemia with a normal chest x-ray should be considered a pulmonary embolism until proven otherwise.

▶ Diagnosis of pulmonary embolism is usually established using imaging tests such as chest CT considered in the light of clinical pretest probability.

▶ The primary therapy of DVT or PE is anticoagulation, with the goal of preventing recurrence.

REFERENCES

Jaff MR, McMurty MS, Archer SL, et al. Management of massive and submassive pulmonary embolism, iliofemoral deep vein thrombosis, and chronic thromboembolic pulmonary hypertension. *Circulation.* 2011;123:1788-1830.

Goldhaber SZ. Deep venous thrombosis and pulmonary thromboembolism. In: Longo DL, Fauci AS, Kasper DL, et al., eds. *Harrison's Principles of Internal Medicine.* 18th ed. New York, NY: McGraw-Hill; 2012:2170-2177.

Sharifi M, Bay C, Skrocki L, et al. Moderate pulmonary embolism treated with thrombolysis (the MOPETT Trial). *Am J Cardiol.* 2013;111:273-277.

Van Belle A, Buller HR, Huisman MV, et al. Effectiveness of managing suspected pulmonary embolism using an algorithm combining clinical probability, D-dimer testing, and computed tomography. *JAMA.* 2006;295:172-179.

Wells PS, Anderson DR, Rodger M, et al. Derivation of a simple clinical model to categorize patients' probability of pulmonary embolism: increasing the models utility with the SimpliRED D-dimer. *Thromb Haemost.* 2000;83(3):416-420.

A 58-year-old man comes to your office, because of shortness of breath. He has experienced mild dyspnea on exertion for a few years, but more recently he has noted worsening shortness of breath with minimal exercise and the onset of dyspnea at rest. He has difficulty reclining; as a result, he spends the night sitting up in a chair trying to sleep. He reports a cough with production of yellowish-brown sputum every morning throughout the year. He denies chest pain, fever, chills, or lower extremity edema. He has smoked about two packs of cigarettes per day since age 15. He does not drink alcohol. A few months ago, the patient went to an urgent care clinic for evaluation of his symptoms, and he received a prescription for some inhalers, the names of which he does not remember. He was also told to find a primary care physician for further evaluation. On physical examination, his blood pressure is 135/85 mm Hg, heart rate is 96 bpm, respiratory rate is 28 bpm, and temperature is 97.6°F. He is sitting in a chair, leaning forward, with his arms braced on his knees. He appears uncomfortable with labored respirations and cyanotic lips. He is using accessory muscles of respiration, and chest examination reveals wheezes and rhonchi bilaterally, but no crackles are noted. The anteroposterior diameter of the chest wall appears increased, and he has inward movement of the lower rib cage with inspiration. Cardiovascular examination reveals distant heart sounds but with a regular rate and rhythm, and his jugular venous pressure is normal. His extremities show no cyanosis, edema, or clubbing.

▶ What is the most likely diagnosis?
▶ What is the next best diagnostic test?
▶ What is the best initial treatment?

ANSWERS TO CASE 15:

Chronic Obstructive Pulmonary Disease

Summary: A 58-year-old smoker has noted worsening shortness of breath with minimal exercise and the onset of dyspnea at rest and difficulty reclining. He reports a productive cough with yellowish-brown sputum every morning throughout the year. He is sitting in a characteristic "tripod" position to facilitate use of accessory muscles of respiration. He appears to have airway obstruction with respiratory distress, with lower chest retractions, and bilateral wheezes and rhonchi. His perioral cyanosis suggests hypoxemia. The anteroposterior diameter of the chest wall appears increased. Cardiovascular examination reveals distant heart sounds but no signs of significant cardiac disease.

- **Most likely diagnosis:** Chronic obstructive pulmonary disease (COPD) with acute exacerbation.

- **Next diagnostic step:** Arterial blood gas to assess oxygenation and acid-base status.

- **Best initial treatment:** Oxygen by nasal cannula, followed closely by bronchodilators, and steroids for airway inflammation.

ANALYSIS

Objectives

1. Know the definition and etiologies of chronic bronchitis, COPD, and emphysema.

2. Be familiar with spirometry and flow-volume loops for diagnosis of obstructive and restrictive lung diseases.

3. Be familiar with the treatment of chronic stable COPD, as well as management of acute exacerbations, including the indications for mechanical ventilation.

Considerations

This 58-year-old long-time smoker likely has COPD. He is now in respiratory distress with labored respirations, cyanosis, and wheezing. The urgent issue is his current respiratory status. Rapid clinical assessment is critical in case this patient is headed toward respiratory failure, perhaps necessitating endotracheal intubation and mechanical ventilation. An arterial blood gas will quickly provide information regarding the adequacy of oxygenation status (PaO_2) and ventilation $(PaCO_2)$.

APPROACH TO:

Chronic Obstructive Pulmonary Disease

DEFINITIONS

PULMONARY FUNCTION TEST (PFT): Complete PFTs comprise respiratory tests of spirometry, lung volumes, and diffusion.

SPIROMETRY: Method of evaluating respiratory flow volumes and flow rates to assess pulmonary function.

FORCED VITAL CAPACITY (FVC): Total volume of air expired after full inspiration. FVC is reduced in restrictive lung disease. Patients with obstructive lung disease usually have normal FVC.

FORCED EXPIRATORY VOLUME IN ONE SECOND (FEV_1): Volume of air expired in the first second during maximal expiratory effort. FEV_1 is reduced in both obstructive lung disease (increased airway resistance) and restrictive lung disease (low vital capacity).

FEV_1/FVC: Percentage of the vital capacity that is expired during the first second of maximal effort, reduced in obstructive lung disease.

OBSTRUCTIVE LUNG DISEASE: Chronic pulmonary disorder that is characterized by a disproportional decrease in maximal airflow from the lung in relation to maximal volume that can be displaced from the lung. Typically, FEV_1 will be decreased relative to FVC and therefore the FEV_1/FVC will be decreased. Most common types of obstructive lung disease are asthma and COPD.

CHRONIC OBSTRUCTIVE PULMONARY DISEASE: Chronic airflow obstruction caused by chronic bronchitis or emphysema. COPD is a preventable and treatable disease characterized by persistent airflow limitation that is usually progressive and associated with enhanced chronic inflammatory response in the lungs to the noxious particles and gases. Diagnosis in the right clinical setting is usually supported by FEV_1/FVC ratio of less than 70?. Severity of COPD on spirometry is based on FEV_1/FEV_1 ratio vs. predicted: of >80% of predicted indicates mild disease, 50% to 80% of predicted is moderate, 30% to 50% of predicted is severe, and <30% is indicative of very severe disease.

EMPHYSEMA: COPD component that is diagnosed pathologically with abnormal, permanent enlargement of air spaces distal to the terminal bronchiole, with destruction of their walls and without obvious fibrosis.

CHRONIC BRONCHITIS: COPD component that is diagnosed clinically, and is characterized by excessive secretion of bronchial mucus and productive cough for 3 months or more in at least 2 consecutive years in the absence of any other disease that might account for this symptom.

RESTRICTIVE LUNG DISEASE: Chronic pulmonary disorder characterized by low lung volumes because of alterations of either the lung parenchyma (intrinsic), or chest wall, pleura, or respiratory muscles (extrinsic). Typically the FVC and FEV_1 are reduced, but the FEV_1/FVC is normal. The diagnosis is best made by a reduced total lung capacity (TLC).

CLINICAL APPROACH

The most common etiology for COPD is inhalation injury, specifically cigarette smoking. Another important cause is α_1-antitrypsin deficiency, which is hereditary; pulmonary disease may become evident by age 40 and often occurs without cough or smoking history. Therapy by replacement of α_1-antitrypsin enzyme is available. Characteristically, patients with COPD present with progressively worsening dyspnea (first on exertion, then with activity, then at rest). Patient may vary in appearance from a "blue bloater" (chronic bronchitis, overweight, edematous, cyanotic) to a "pink puffer" (emphysema, thin, ruddy cheeks).

Arterial blood gases (ABGs) often are normal in the early phase of the disease; however, in more advanced disease, there is evidence of hypoxemia and hypercapnia, often with a chronic compensated respiratory acidosis as a consequence of CO_2 retention. Such chronic stable patients may have a PaO_2 near 50 mm Hg and a $PaCO_2$ near 50 mm Hg, but a near-normal pH (the "50-50" club). During an acute exacerbation, more severe hypoxemia or hypercapnia, or respiratory acidosis noted on ABG may be an indication of impending respiratory failure and need for ventilatory support.

Spirometry is the most basic, inexpensive, widely valuable pulmonary function test to diagnose pulmonary diseases (Figure 15–1). Spirometric tracings of **forced expiration** (Figure 15–2) and **flow-volume loops** (Figure 15–3) help to identify the type of lung disease (obstructive vs restrictive), as well as potential reversibility of airflow obstruction. Restrictive lung diseases tend to have lower lung volumes (decreased TLC and vital capacity [VC]), whereas obstructive diseases have larger lung volumes (TLC normal or increased) with decreased expiratory flow rates (reduced FEV_1 to <80% expected, and FEV_1/FVC <0.7). Specific parameters help to classify the type and degree of lung dysfunction (Table 15–1). Reduced FEV_1/FVC with minimal response to bronchodilators is the hallmark of COPD.

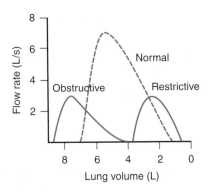

Figure 15–1. Expiratory flow-volume loops of normal, obstructive, and restrictive lung disease.

Figure 15–2. Spirographic tracing of forced expiration, comparing normal tracing (**A**) with that of patients with obstructive (**B**) and restrictive (**C**) lung disease. Calculation of FVC, FEV$_1$, and forced expiratory flow (FEF) (25%-75%) are shown for the normal tracing. The curves are positioned to show the relative starting lung volumes in each of these different conditions. Lung volumes increase to the left on the horizontal axis. VC, vital capacity. (Reproduced, with permission, from Braunwald E, Fauci AS, Kasper KL, et al, *Harrison's Principles of Internal Medicine*, 17th ed. New York: McGraw-Hill, 2008: 1586.)

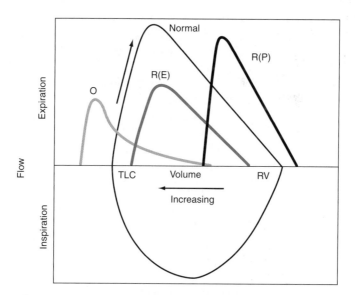

Figure 15–3. Flow-volume curves showing forced inspiratory and expiratory volumes in lung disease: O, obstructive lung disease, eg, COPD; R(P), parenchymal restrictive disease, eg, pulmonary fibrosis; R(E), extraparenchymal restrictive disease, eg, chest wall deformity, with limitation of both inspiration and expiration. Lung volumes increase to the left on the horizontal axis. TLC, total lung capacity. (Reproduced, with permission, from Braunwald E, Fauci AS, Kasper KL, et al, *Harrison's Principles of Internal Medicine*, 17th ed. New York: McGraw-Hill, 2008: 1588.)

Table 15–1 • OBSTRUCTIVE AND RESTRICTIVE LUNG DISEASE CHARACTERISTICS

	Obstructive Lung Disease	Restrictive Lung Disease	
Pulmonary function Tests	Decreased FEV_1 <80% of predicted; FEV_1/FVC <0.7; TLC usually normal or increased; diffusion capacity decreased	Decreased lung volumes: decreased VC and TLC (this is diagnostic hallmark) FEV_1/FVC is normal	
Example of diseases	**B**ronchiectasis (ie, cystic fibrosis) **A**sthma **B**ronchitis (chronic) **E**mphysema	Extrapulmonary: poor breathing mechanics **P**oliomyelitis **M**yasthenia gravis **S**coliosis	Pulmonary: poor lung expansion **P**neumonia **A**RDS **P**ulmonary edema **I**nterstitial fibrosis

Abbreviations: ARDS, acute respiratory distress syndrome; FEV_1, forced expiratory volume in first second; FVC, forced vital capacity; TLC, total lung capacity; VC, vital capacity.

Management of severe COPD exacerbations focuses simultaneously on relieving airway obstruction and correcting life-threatening abnormalities of gas exchange. Bronchodilators (beta-agonist and anticholinergic agents) are administered via handheld nebulizers; systemic glucocorticoids accelerate the rate of improvement in lung function among these patients; antibiotics should be given if there is suspicion of a respiratory infection. Controlled oxygen administration with nasal oxygen at low flows or oxygen with Venturi masks will correct hypoxemia without causing severe hypercapnia. **Caution must be exercised in patients with chronic respiratory insufficiency whose respiratory drive is dependent on "relative hypoxemia"; these individuals may become apneic if excessive oxygen is administered!**

Positive-pressure mask ventilation, such as continuous positive airway pressure (CPAP) or bilevel positive airway pressure (BiPAP), offers an alternative to intubation and mechanical ventilation in the treatment of cooperative patients with an acute exacerbation of COPD and severe hypercapnia. Signs of **acute respiratory failure** include **tachypnea** (respiratory rate >40 bpm), **inability to speak** because of dyspnea, **accessory muscle use with fatigue** despite maximal therapy, confusion, restlessness, agitation, lethargy, a rising $PaCO_2$ **level**, and extreme **hypoxemia**. Acute respiratory failure is generally treated with endotracheal intubation and mechanical ventilatory support to correct the gas-exchange disorders. Complications of mechanical ventilation include difficulty in extubation, ventilator-associated pneumonia, pneumothorax, and acute respiratory distress syndrome.

Long-term complications of COPD from hypoxemia can cause pulmonary hypertension, secondary erythrocytosis, exercise limitation, and impaired mental functioning. For patients with COPD who are stable, only **smoking cessation, supplemental oxygen therapy for patients with chronic hypoxemia, and lung volume reduction surgery** in selected patients have been shown to **alter the natural history of the disease**, and provide any **reduction in mortality**. Patients with a resting hypoxemia (PaO_2 <55 mm Hg or SaO_2 <88%) generally benefit from home oxygen therapy, which must be utilized at least 18 h/d. Other therapies such as inhaled bronchodilators (beta-agonists and/or anticholinergics) or inhaled glucocorticoids are used for symptomatic relief and to try to reduce the frequency of exacerbations.

> ## CASE CORRELATION
>
> - See also Case 14 (Pulmonary Embolism), Case 16 (Chronic Cough/Asthma), Case 17 (Pleural Effusion), and Case 19 (Pneumonia).

COMPREHENSION QUESTIONS

15.1 Which of the following is the most likely physical examination findings in a patient with COPD?

    A. Diffuse expiratory wheezing

    B. Clubbing of the fingers

    C. Bibasilar inspiratory crackles with increased jugular venous pressure (JVP)

    D. Inspiratory stridor

    E. Third heart sound

15.2 A 56-year-old woman admits to a 60-pack-year smoking history. She complains of fatigue and dyspnea with minimal exertion, and a cough that is productive each morning. Which of the following is the most likely finding in this patient?

    A. Higher diffusing capacity of lung for carbon monoxide (DLCO)

    B. Decreased residual volume

    C. Normal to slightly increased FEV_1

    D. Decreased FEV_1/FVC

    E. Decreased FVC

15.3 Which of the following therapies is most likely to provide the greatest benefit to a patient with chronic stable emphysema and a resting oxygen saturation of 86%?

    A. Inhaled tiotropium daily

    B. Inhaled albuterol as needed

    C. Oral prednisone daily

    D. Supplemental oxygen used at night

    E. Supplemental oxygen used continuously

ANSWERS

15.1 **A.** COPD is characterized by chronic airway obstruction, with most airflow resistance occurring in small airways of the lower respiratory tract, producing expiratory wheezing. Inspiratory stridor would occur with upper airway, usually extrathoracic, obstruction. Clubbing is not generally a feature of COPD and should prompt investigation for another disease process such as a bronchogenic carcinoma. Crackles, elevated JVP, and an S_3 are signs of congestive heart failure.

15.2 **D.** This patient likely has COPD, based on the smoking history and symptoms. A decrease in the FEV_1/FVC ratio is the hallmark of airflow obstruction. The FEV_1 is decreased in obstructive, as well as in restrictive, lung disease. The diffusing capacity is typically deceased in COPD as well as intrinsic restrictive lung disease. The DLCO indicates the adequacy of the alveolar-capillary membrane; the residual volume is the volume of air remaining in the lungs after a maximal expiratory effort and is usually increased in COPD due to air trapping.

15.3 **E.** For patients with chronic hypoxemia, supplemental oxygen has a significant impact on mortality, with a greater benefit with continuous usage, rather than intermittent or nocturnal-only usage. Bronchodilators such as tiotropium and albuterol improve symptoms and FEV_1, but offer no mortality benefit. Chronic use of oral corticosteroids should be avoided because of unfavorable side effects such as osteoporosis, glucose intolerance, and gastrointestinal (GI) side effects.

CLINICAL PEARLS

▶ Patients with obstructive lung disease have air flow limitation on expiration (reduced FEV_1/FVC), whereas patients with restrictive lung disease have difficulty in expanding their lung volumes in response to exercise (reduced TLC).

▶ The mainstay for treatment of chronic obstructive pulmonary disease exacerbations includes bronchodilators, oxygen, and glucocorticoids, as well as antibiotics if infection is suspected.

▶ Controlled supplemental oxygen along with positive-pressure mask ventilation (bilevel positive airway pressure) may prevent respiratory failure requiring endotracheal intubation.

▶ Smoking cessation and supplemental oxygen to treat chronic hypoxemia are the only medical therapies shown to decrease mortality among persons with chronic obstructive pulmonary disease.

▶ In both obstructive and restrictive lung disease, the FEV_1 is decreased, the FEV_1/FVC is decreased in obstructive processes and normal in restrictive processes.

▶ The hallmark of restrictive lung disease is decreased lung capacities, particularly the TLC but also the VC.

REFERENCES

Reilly JJ, Silverman EK, Shapiro SD. Chronic obstructive pulmonary disease. In: Longo DL, Fauci AS, Kasper DL, et al., eds. *Harrison's Principles of Internal Medicine*. 18th ed. New York, NY: McGraw-Hill; 2012:1380-1388.

Sutherland ER, Chemiak RM. Management of chronic obstructive pulmonary disease. *N Engl J Med.* 2004;350:2689-2697.

Weinberger SE, Rosen IM. Disturbances of respiratory function. In: Longo DL, Fauci AS, Kasper DL, et al., eds. *Harrison's Principles of Internal Medicine*. 18th ed. New York, NY: McGraw-Hill; 2012:1380-1388.

A 37-year-old man presents to your office with the complaint of cough. The cough began approximately 3 months prior to this appointment, and it has become more annoying to the patient. The cough is nonproductive and worse at night and after exercise. He has had a sedentary lifestyle but recently started an exercise program, including jogging, and says he is having a much harder time with the exertion. He runs out of breath earlier than he did to previously, and he coughs a lot. He has not had any fever, blood-tinged sputum, or weight loss. He denies nasal congestion and headaches. He does not smoke and has no significant medical history. His examination is notable for a blood pressure of 134/78 mm Hg and lung findings of occasional expiratory wheezes on forced expiration. A chest radiograph is read as normal.

▶ What is the most likely diagnosis?
▶ How would you confirm the diagnosis?

ANSWERS TO CASE 16:

Chronic Cough/Asthma

Summary: A 37-year-old nonsmoking man complains of a 3-month history of a nonproductive cough that is worse at night and with exercise. He does not have fevers or other symptoms to suggest infection. He is normotensive, and his respiratory examination reveals an occasional expiratory wheeze on forced expiration. A chest radiograph is read as normal.

- **Most likely diagnosis:** Asthma.

- **Confirmation of diagnosis:** Spirometry with testing for bronchodilator responsiveness and bronchoprovocation testing if indicated.

ANALYSIS

Objectives

1. Know the differential diagnosis of chronic cough in adult patients.

2. Understand the stepwise approach to finding the cause of cough in these patients.

3. Learn how to diagnose and treat asthma.

Considerations

This is a 37-year-old man who presents with a chronic cough of more than 8 weeks' duration. With the history of exercise intolerance, worsening cough at night, and occasional wheezes on examination, asthma is the most likely diagnosis in this patient. A chest radiograph is important to evaluate for more serious processes such as tumor, infection, or other etiologies of lung injury. A focused history should look for exposure to environmental irritants, medications such as angiotensin-converting enzyme (ACE) inhibitors, or other etiologies such as postnasal drip or gastroesophageal reflux.

APPROACH TO:

Chronic Cough

DEFINITIONS

ACUTE COUGH: Cough lasting less than 3 weeks, most commonly caused by acute upper respiratory infection, but may also be caused by congestive heart failure, pneumonia, and pulmonary embolism, allergic rhinitis, or exacerbation of existing structural lung disease.

SUBACUTE COUGH: Cough that is typically defined as lasting 3 to 8 weeks in duration and is most often infectious or postinfectious in etiology. Infectious etiologies of subacute cough include viruses, such as respiratory syncytial virus (RSV), influenza, and adenovirus, as well as bacteria. Bacterial infections causing subacute cough are usually due to pertussis, *Chlamydia*, or mycoplasma.

CHRONIC COUGH: Cough that often lasts more than 8 weeks. In a smoker, chronic cough is usually a symptom of chronic obstructive pulmonary disease (COPD), but bronchogenic carcinoma would be in the differential diagnosis in this population; in a nonsmoker with a normal chest radiograph and absence of ACE inhibitor use, it may be due to upper airway cough syndrome (UACS), gastroesophageal reflux disease (GERD), or asthma.

ASTHMA: Condition of bronchial hyperactivity and smooth muscle hypertrophy leading to a chronic inflammatory condition of the airways associated with widespread bronchospasm that has characteristically reversible obstruction on pulmonary function tests.

CLINICAL APPROACH

Chronic cough is a common complaint and accounts for a large portion of health care expenditures. Physiologically, cough is a reflexive defense mechanism to clear the upper airways. The action of cough serves two main functions: (1) to protect the lungs against aspiration and (2) to clear secretions or other material into more proximal airways to be expectorated from the tracheobronchial tree. Evaluation begins with a detailed history and physical examination, including smoking habits, complete medication list, environmental and occupational exposures, and any history of lung disease. Specific questions regarding the precipitating factors, duration and nature of the cough should be elicited. Although the physical examination or nature of the cough rarely identifies the cause, meticulous review of the ears, nose, throat, and lungs may suggest a particular diagnosis. For example, a cobblestone appearance of the oropharynx (representing lymphoid hyperplasia) or boggy erythematous nasal mucosa can be consistent with UACS. **End-expiratory wheezing suggests active bronchospasm, whereas localized wheezing may be consistent with a foreign body or a bronchogenic tumor.**

In more than 90% of cases, a normal chest radiograph in an immunocompetent nonsmoker guides the physician to one of three diagnoses: **UACS, asthma, or GERD.** Chronic cough in an immunocompromised patient is beyond the scope of this discussion. In the outpatient setting, the mainstay of diagnosis relates to the response with empiric therapy, and multiple etiologies (UACS and GERD) are often simultaneously addressed. Often, a definitive diagnosis for chronic cough depends on observing a successful response to therapy. A rational approach includes discontinuing an ACE inhibitor if patient is using one, obtaining a chest radiograph, and avoiding environmental irritants. If persistent, then UACS, asthma, and GERD should be considered. Referral to a pulmonologist is recommended when the diagnostic and empiric therapy options are exhausted. If suspicion for carcinoma is high, a high-resolution computed tomographic (CT) scan of the thorax or bronchoscopy should be pursued. A diagnosis of psychogenic cough should be one of exclusion. See Figure 16–1 for example of an algorithm.

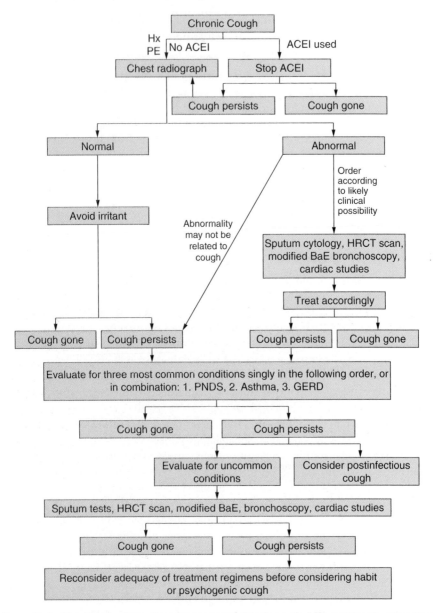

Figure 16–1. Algorithm for diagnosis and treatment of chronic cough. ACEI, angiotensin-converting enzyme inhibitor; BaE, barium esophagography; GERD, gastroesophageal reflux disease; HRCT, high-resolution computed tomography; Hx, history; PE, physical examination; PNDS, postnasal drip syndrome. (Data from Irwin RS, Boulet L-P, Cloutier MM, et al. Managing cough as a defense mechanism and as a symptom: A consensus panel report of the American College of Chest Physicians. *Chest* 1998;114[Suppl]: 133S–181S.)

Upper Airway Cough Syndrome

UACS can be attributed to sinusitis and the following types of rhinitis, alone or in combination: nonallergic, allergic, postinfectious, vasomotor, drug induced, and environmental irritant induced. Since the symptoms may be nonspecific (eg, frequent throat clearing, nasal discharge, or sensation of liquid in the throat), no definitive diagnostic criteria exist for UACS, and response to therapy confirms the diagnosis. Initial treatment for a nonallergic etiology usually includes combination treatment with a first-generation antihistamine and a decongestant for 3 weeks. For allergic rhinitis, a newer-generation antihistamine, along with a nasal corticosteroid, should be used. If the patient's symptoms do not improve, sinus radiographs may be ordered. Opacification, air-fluid levels, or mucosal thickening could suggest sinusitis, which should be treated with antibiotics.

Asthma

Asthma is a chronic inflammatory disease of the airways characterized by airway obstruction, bronchial hyperresponsiveness, and mucus hypersecretion with recurring symptoms, that is often reversible spontaneously or with treatment.

Although wheezing is considered a classic sign of asthma, **cough is often the only symptom.** Cough-variant asthma usually presents with a dry cough that occurs throughout the day and night and is worsened by airway inflammation from viral infections of the upper respiratory tract, allergies, cold air, or exercise. Although the history may be suggestive of asthma, the diagnosis should be confirmed with pulmonary function tests. Spirometry can confirm airflow obstruction with reduced forced expiratory volume in 1 second (FEV_1) and FEV_1/forced vital capacity (FVC), and demonstrate reversibility with improved FEV_1 after inhalation of a bronchodilator, typically a beta-agonist. Positive bronchodilator responsiveness is defined as reversible obstruction with an increase in FEV_1 or FVC of more than 12% and increase of 200 cc of volume after bronchodilator treatment. If the diagnosis is in doubt, bronchial hyperresponsiveness (the fundamental pathophysiologic abnormality in asthma) can be confirmed by a reduction in FEV_1 after challenge with a provocative agent such as methacholine or histamine. If methacholine is used, a positive test is defined as a 20% fall in FEV_1. Approach to asthma management is stepwise with use of asthma controllers such as inhaled corticosteroids (and if needed systemic corticosteroids) which inhibit airway inflammation and bronchodilators for rapid relief of symptoms. Current guidelines emphasize a preventative approach and a stepwise approach to therapy based on asthma severity and control (Table 16–1).

Gastroesophageal Reflux Disease

Gastroesophageal reflux disease often can be clinically inapparent, and it may be the primary or coexisting cause of the cough, as a result of aspiration and vagal stimulation. Initial treatment includes lifestyle modification along with medical therapy. Recommendations include a low-fat diet, elevation of the head of the bed, avoidance of offending foods (caffeine, alcohol, chocolate), smoking cessation, and weight reduction. If the cough does not resolve with lifestyle changes,

Table 16–1 • GUIDELINES FOR DIAGNOSIS AND MANAGEMENT OF ASTHMA					
Classification	Step	Days With Symptoms	Nights With Symptoms	Daily Medication	Quick Relief Medication
Severe persistent	4	Continual	Frequent	High-dose inhaled steroids and long-acting inhaled β_2-agonist; if needed, add oral steroids	Short-acting inhaled β_2-agonist, as needed; oral steroids may be required
Moderate persistent	3	Daily	>1/wk	Low-to-medium–dose inhaled steroids and long-acting β_2-agonist (preferred) or medium-dose inhaled steroids or low-to-medium–dose inhaled steroids and either leukotriene modifier or theophylline	Short-acting inhaled β_2-agonist, as needed; oral steroids may be required
Mild persistent	2	>2/wk, but <1 time/d	>2/mo	Low-dose inhaled steroids (preferred) or cromolyn, leukotriene modifier, or nedocromil, or sustained-release theophylline to serum concentration of 5-15 µg/mL	Short-acting inhaled β_2-agonist, as needed; oral steroids may be required
Mild intermittent	1	<2/wk	<2/mo	No daily medications	Short-acting inhaled β_2-agonist, as needed; oral steroids may be required

daily treatment with an H_2 receptor antagonist such as famotidine, or a proton pump inhibitor such as omeprazole, should be initiated. If acid suppression does not resolve the symptoms and if there are other symptoms of dyspepsia, a gastric motility stimulant such as metoclopramide may be considered.

Patients who remain symptomatic after maximal medical treatment may benefit from 24-hour esophageal pH monitoring to confirm the diagnosis. An esophago-gastroduodenoscopy showing esophagitis or an upper gastrointestinal radiographic series demonstrating reflux further supports the diagnosis. Of note, gastrointestinal symptoms may resolve prior to resolution of the cough, and full resolution may require 2 to 3 months of intensive medical therapy.

> **CASE CORRELATION**
>
> • See also Case 14 (Pulmonary Embolism), Case 15 (Chronic Obstructive Pulmonary Disease), Case 17 (Pleural Effusion), and Case 19 (Pneumonia).

COMPREHENSION QUESTIONS

16.1 A patient with known asthma undergoing therapy with inhaled corticosteroids and intermittent (short-acting) β_2-agonist presents with complaints of nocturnal awakenings secondary to cough and occasional wheezing. This episode occurs three to four times per week. Pulmonary function tests in the past have shown mild obstructive lung disease. Which of the following is the best next step?

A. Oral steroids

B. Leukotriene inhibitors

C. Long-acting β_2-agonists

D. Theophylline

E. Antireflux therapy

16.2 Which of the following is most accurate?

A. Cough caused by captopril may resolve with switching to enalapril.

B. Initial treatment of a chronic cough should include codeine or a similar opiate derivative to suppress the cough.

C. Cough caused by reflux can be effectively ruled out by a negative history of heartburn or dyspepsia.

D. More than one condition is often responsible for causing chronic cough in a given patient.

16.3 A 22-year-old African-American woman presents with fatigue, arthralgias, and a nagging dry cough for the past 6 weeks, but no shortness of breath. On physical examination, her lungs are clear to auscultation, and she has bilateral pretibial tender erythematous raised nodules. Which of the following is your best next step?

A. Chest radiograph

B. High-resolution CT

C. Empiric treatment for postnasal drip

D. Antinuclear antibody

E. Initiation of antituberculosis therapy

16.4 An obese 50-year-old man with a history of asthma returns with complaints of occasional dyspepsia and nocturnal cough. He wakes up in the morning with a sour taste in his mouth. His current medications include inhaled corticosteroid and a short-acting β_2-agonist. Which of the following should be your next step?

A. 24-Hour esophageal pH monitoring

B. Chest radiograph

C. Initiation of omeprazole

D. Short course of oral corticosteroids

E. Initiation of allergy desensitization

ANSWERS

16.1 **C.** Long-acting β_2-agonists are indicated in this situation. The asthma would be classified as moderate persistent, and the recommended treatment is addition of long-acting β_2-agonists (such as salmeterol) to the inhaled corticosteroids, which are particularly helpful with nocturnal symptoms.

16.2 **D.** Often more than one condition is responsible for causing chronic cough in a given patient. Cough from ACE inhibitors is class dependent, and change to another class of antihypertensives is more appropriate. The etiology of chronic cough should be determined prior to suppression of the cough because treatment of the underlying condition is the most effective approach. A patient with GERD may present with the sole manifestation of cough, or it may present "silently."

16.3 **A.** The patient has clinical features suggestive of sarcoidosis given the new cough, arthralgias, and description of erythema nodosum. The initial, most cost-effective study is a chest radiograph. Hilar lymphadenopathy with or without interstitial infiltrates would solidify a diagnosis of sarcoidosis. A high-resolution CT may be ordered if the patient has interstitial lung disease, but it is not the first study of choice. Postnasal drip does not explain the patient's other symptoms. An antinuclear antibody would not necessarily identify the cause of the cough or provide a diagnosis.

16.4 **C.** The dyspepsia and the sour taste suggest GERD. Aside from acid suppression, other recommendations include dietary modifications and weight reduction. 24-Hour esophageal pH monitoring is indicated only if there is no response to treatment.

CLINICAL PEARLS

▶ A normal chest radiograph excludes most, **but not all**, of the serious and uncommon causes of chronic cough.

▶ The three most common causes of chronic cough in immunocompetent nonsmokers who are not taking ACE inhibitors are upper airway cough syndrome, asthma, and gastroesophageal reflux disease.

▶ Cough caused by ACE inhibitors can be triggered after the first dose or may occur after months of therapy.

▶ Treatment of asthma is a stepwise process based on frequency of symptoms and response to prescribed medications.

▶ Asthma can be the cause of cough in a patient with normal examination and pulmonary function tests. If suspicion is high, a positive methacholine challenge has a high predictive value.

▶ Definitive diagnosis of the etiology of chronic cough is not always necessary for successful treatment.

REFERENCES

Barnes PJ. Asthma. In: Longo DL, Fauci AS, Kasper DL, et al., eds. *Harrison's Principles of Internal Medicine*. 18th ed. New York, NY: McGraw-Hill; 2012:2102-2115.

Guidelines for the Diagnosis and Management of Asthma, National Asthma Education and Prevention Program. National Heart, Lung and Blood Institute; August 2007.

Irwin RS, Bauman MH, Bolser DC, et al. Diagnosis and management of cough executive summary: ACCP evidence-based clinical practice guidelines. *Chest*. 2006;129(suppl 1):S1-S23.

Irwin RS, Madison JM. The diagnosis and treatment of cough. *N Engl J Med*. 2000;343:1715-1721.

Morice AH, Kastelik JA. Chronic cough in adults. *Thorax*. 2003;58:901-907.

Williams SG, Schmidt DK, Redd SC, et al. National Asthma Education and Prevention Program. Key clinical activities for quality asthma care. Recommendations of the National Asthma Education and Prevention Program. *MMWR Recomm Rep*. 2003;52(RR-6):1-8.

A 32-year-old woman presents to the emergency center complaining of productive cough, fever, and chest pain for 4 days. She was seen 2 days ago in her primary care physician's clinic with the same complaints, was diagnosed clinically with pneumonia, and was sent home with oral azithromycin. Since then, her cough has diminished in quantity. However, the fever has not abated, and she still experiences left-sided chest pain, which is worse when she coughs or takes a deep breath. In addition, she has started to feel short of breath when she walks around the house. She has no other medical history. She does not smoke and has no history of occupational exposure. She has not traveled outside of the United States and has no sick contacts.

On physical examination, her temperature is 103.4°F, heart rate is 116 bpm, blood pressure is 128/69 mm Hg, respiratory rate is 24 bpm and is shallow. Her pulse oximetry is 94% saturation on room air. Physical examination is significant for decreased breath sounds in the lower half of the left lung fields posteriorly, with dullness to percussion about halfway up. There are a few inspiratory crackles in the mid-lung fields, and her right side is clear to auscultation. Her heart is tachycardic but regular with no murmurs. She has no cyanosis. Figure 17–1 shows her chest x-ray films.

► What is your most likely diagnosis?
► What is your next step?

Figure 17–1. (**A**) Posteroanterior film of the chest. (**B**) Lateral chest film of the same patient. (Courtesy of Dr. Jorge Albin.)

ANSWERS TO CASE 17:
Pleural Effusion, Parapneumonic

Summary: A 32-year-old previously healthy woman comes in with a clinical diagnosis of community-acquired pneumonia that has not improved with outpatient treatment. She has diminished breath sounds and dullness to percussion on the left side of her chest, suggesting a large left-sided pleural effusion, which is confirmed by chest radiography. The effusion likely is caused by infection in the adjacent lung parenchyma and may be the cause of her failure to improve on antibiotics.

- **Most likely diagnosis:** Parapneumonic effusion as a complication of pneumonia.

- **Next step:** Diagnostic thoracentesis to help diagnose the cause of the pleural effusion and to determine the necessity for fluid drainage.

ANALYSIS
Objectives

1. Understand the use of Light criteria to distinguish transudative effusions from exudative effusions, as a guide to the etiology of the effusion.

2. Learn what pleural fluid characteristics suggest a complicated parapneumonic effusion or empyema, and the need for drainage.

3. Know the treatment of a complicated parapneumonic effusion that does not improve after thoracentesis.

Considerations

In this patient, the pleural effusion is large, and if it is free-flowing, which would be evaluated with a lateral decubitus film, then diagnostic thoracentesis can easily be accomplished. It is important to determine if the effusion is, in fact, caused by the pneumonia, and, if so, whether it is likely to resolve with antibiotics alone or will require drainage with tube thoracostomy.

APPROACH TO:
Pleural Effusion

DEFINITIONS

PLEURAL EFFUSION: Accumulation of fluid in the pleural space.

TRANSUDATE: Effusion caused by alteration of oncotic forces, usually with low protein and low lactate dehydrogenase (LDH) levels.

EXUDATE: Effusion caused by inflammatory or malignant causes, usually with high protein or high LDH levels.

CLINICAL APPROACH

Diagnostic thoracentesis should be considered for every patient who presents with a pleural effusion for which the cause is unknown. Possibly the only exception to this rule is if the patient is known to have congestive heart failure (CHF) with equal bilateral effusions or if the effusion is too small, that is, less than 10 mm on lateral decubitus film. If the pleural effusion of CHF does not significantly improve after a trial of diuresis, however, a diagnostic thoracentesis should be performed. Table 17–1 gives the correlations of pleural fluid appearance. As little as 5 to 10 mL can be visualized on a lateral decubitus film (more reliable in detecting smaller effusions), and fluid volume more than 500 mL usually obscures the whole hemidiaphragm.

Indications for thoracentesis:

All new pleural effusions must be investigated, except in the setting of CHF where a trial of diuretics is attempted, or fluid overload states such as end-stage renal disease or nephrotic syndrome where dialysis will help with clearing of effusions. A simple "diagnostic" thoracentesis can be performed, but if the effusion is significant in size and the patient is dyspneic, especially at rest, a "therapeutic" thoracentesis may also be performed, with safe removal until the patient develops a vague chest discomfort. With removal of more fluid, the patient is at risk for developing reexpansion pulmonary edema.

Transudate Versus Exudate

To appreciate the pathophysiology of the formation of a transudate versus an exudate is to understand the causes under each category. Approximately 10 mL of pleural fluid is formed every day by the visceral pleura and absorbed by the parietal pleura (capillaries and lymphatics). Processes that disturb this "equilibrium" lead to fluid accumulation. Clinical settings in which the hydrostatic pressure is increased, for example, CHF and constrictive pericarditis; the oncotic pressure is decreased, for example, nephrotic syndrome and cirrhosis; or the intrapleural pressure is reduced, for example, atelectasis, lead to the formation of a "transudate." In contrast, "exudates" are more a result of local inflammation, for example, infection, malignancy, and connective tissue diseases, which cause a protein leak into the pleural space. Less commonly, impaired lymphatic drainage, as occurs in chylothorax,

Table 17–1 • PLEURAL FLUID APPEARANCE	
Clear yellow	Transudative, eg, secondary to CHF, cirrhosis, nephrotic syndrome
Frank pus	Infectious process, empyema
Bloody	If hematocrit (Hct) of pleural fluid is >1/2 of Hct in peripheral blood: *Hemothorax*, mostly due to trauma, but also rupture of blood vessel, or seen in malignancy—would require tube thoracostomy. If Hct <50% of peripheral blood: cancer, pulmonary embolism, tuberculosis
Milky, turbid	Chylothorax triglycerides >110 mg/dL resulting from disruption of thoracic duct, cholesterol effusion
Dark green	Biliothorax

Table 17–2 • CAUSES OF TRANSUDATIVE PLEURAL EFFUSIONS	
Transudate	Clinical Correlates or Radiographic Features
Congestive heart failure	Most commonly bilateral and symmetric, at times isolated right-sided effusion
Nephrotic syndrome	Bilateral and subpulmonic effusion
Cirrhosis with ascites	Patients usually have significant ascites
Myxedema	Uncommon, usually occurs along with ascites, signs of heart failure in advanced hypothyroidism
Pulmonary embolism	May also be exudative or bloody; rarely large
Nephrotic syndrome	Due to hypoalbuminemia, third-spacing

or lymphangitic spread of a malignancy may cause an exudative fluid. Pulmonary emboli can cause both exudative and transudative effusions. Tables 17–2 and 17–3 list the etiologies of transudative and exudative pleural effusions, respectively.

Pleural Fluid—Light Criteria: The most widely used criteria to distinguish between a transudative and exudative fluid are the Light criteria first described in 1997. For a fluid to be labeled an **exudate**, it must meet **at least one of the following criteria** (transudates meet none of these criteria):

1. Pleural fluid protein/serum protein ratio >0.5

2. Pleural fluid LDH/serum LDH ratio >0.6

3. Pleural fluid LDH >2/3 the upper limit of normal for serum LDH

Table 17–3 • CAUSES OF EXUDATIVE PLEURAL EFFUSIONS	
Exudate	Comment
Infection	Bacterial pneumonia, viral etiology, fungal infection, parasitic (eosinophilic) involvement; subdiaphragmatic abscesses
Tuberculosis	One-third have parenchymal involvement; lymphocytes >80%; adenosine deaminase >43 U/L; total protein >4.0 g/dL; diagnostic yield of fluid for acid-fast bacilli <10%; pleural biopsy increases yield to between 80% and 90%
Malignancy	Lymphocytic predominant and occasionally bloody; cytologic examination positive in >50% of cases; usually indicative of dismal prognosis
Connective tissue disease	Rheumatoid pleurisy: very low glucose, rheumatoid factor >1:320 and > serum titer and LDH >1000 IU/L; more common in men
	Lupus pleuritis: positive lupus erythematosus cells; pleural fluid/serum antinuclear antibody >1.0; usually responsive to steroid treatment
Pancreatitis	Elevated pancreatic amylase isoenzyme; salivary isoenzyme seen in esophageal rupture with associated low pH
Chylothorax	Triglycerides >110 mg/dL
Asbestos exposure	Spectrum of disease ranges from pleural plaques to effusion and malignancy; also usually eosinophilic

Pleural LDH correlates with the degree of **pleural inflammation** and, along with **fluid protein**, should always be sent in the initial evaluation.

Parapneumonic Effusions and Empyemas

Pleural effusions occur in 40% of patients with an underlying bacterial pneumonia. Most of these effusions should resolve with appropriate antibiotic treatment, but if the fluid characteristics predict a **"complicated"** parapneumonic effusion, urgent tube drainage is indicated to prevent formation of fibrous peels, which may need surgical decortication.

The following fluid characteristics suggest the need for chest tube drainage:

- Empyema (frank pus in the pleural space)
- Positive Gram stain or culture of fluid
- Presence of loculations
- pH less than 7.20 (pleural fluid pH is normally alkaline with pH of 7.6)
- Glucose less than 60 mg/dL
- LDH more than 1000 U/L

If the patient does not meet the criteria for immediate drainage, a 1-week trial of antibiotics is indicated, with close reevaluation of those patients who do not respond or who clinically deteriorate.

If tube thoracostomy drainage is required, a chest tube is placed until the drainage rate has decreased to less than 50 mL/d. Postdrainage imaging must be obtained to confirm complete drainage of fluid and to assess the need for placement of a second tube if the fluid has not been adequately drained (as is often seen if the effusion is loculated). Complete sterilization of the cavity is desirable when treating an empyema with 4 to 6 weeks of antibiotics, as is complete obliteration of the space by lung expansion. Multiloculated empyemas are treated further by administering a combination of fibrinolytic agents such as tissue plasminogen activator (t-PA) and deoxyribonuclease (DNAase) through the chest tube. Video-assisted thoracoscopic surgery (VATS) with debridement and drainage is the next option if the combination of t-PA and DNAse fail in clearing the loculations.

CASE CORRELATION

- See also Case 14 (Pulmonary Embolism), Case 15 (Chronic Obstructive Pulmonary Disease), and Case 16 (Chronic Cough/Asthma).

COMPREHENSION QUESTIONS

17.1 A 55-year-old man with congestive heart failure develops bilateral pleural effusions. Which of the following is the most likely pleural fluid characteristic if thoracentesis is performed?

A. Pleural fluid LDH 39, LDH ratio 0.2, protein ratio 0.7

B. Pleural fluid LDH 39, LDH ratio 0.2, protein ratio 0.1

C. Pleural fluid LDH 599, LDH ratio 0.9, protein ratio 0.1

D. Pleural fluid LDH 599, LDH ratio 0.9, protein ratio 0.7

17.2 A 39-year-old man develops a moderate free-flowing pleural effusion following a left lower lobe pneumonia. Thoracentesis reveals straw-colored fluid with gram-positive diplococci on Gram stain, pH 6.9, glucose 32 mg/dL, and LDH 1890. Which of the following is the best next step?

A. Send the fluid for culture.

B. Continue treatment with antibiotics for pneumococcal infection.

C. Tube thoracostomy to drain the effusion.

D. Schedule a follow-up chest x-ray in 2 weeks to document resolution of the effusion.

17.3 A 69-year-old man complains of gradually worsening dyspnea and a nagging cough over the past 3 months but no fevers. He is found to have a right-sided pleural effusion, which is tapped and is grossly bloody. Which of the following is the most likely diagnosis?

A. Parapneumonic effusion

B. Malignancy in the pleural space

C. Rupture of aortic dissection into the pleural space

D. Pulmonary embolism with pulmonary infarction

ANSWERS

17.1 **B.** Congestive heart failure is commonly associated with bilateral pleural effusions, which are transudative, as a consequence of alteration of Starling forces. The effusions of heart failure are best managed by treating the heart failure, for example, with diuretics, and typically do not require thoracentesis. Per Light Criteria, all other options would be classified as an exudative pleural effusion.

17.2 **C.** The positive Gram stain, low pH, low glucose, and markedly elevated LDH all suggest that this parapneumonic effusion is "complicated," that is, it is unlikely to resolve with antibiotic therapy and is likely to produce loculated pockets of pus, which will require drainage with tube thoracostomy.

17.3 **B.** The most common causes of hemorrhagic pleural effusion are trauma, malignancy, and pulmonary embolism. Pulmonary embolism would be suggested by acute onset of dyspnea and pleuritic chest pain rather than this subacute presentation. Similarly, aortic rupture can produce a hemothorax but would have an acute presentation with pain and hemodynamic compromise.

CLINICAL PEARLS

▶ Transudative effusions meet none of the following criteria (exudative effusions meet at least one): (a) Pleural fluid protein/serum protein ratio more than 0.5. (b) Pleural fluid LDH/serum LDH ratio more than 0.6. (c) Pleural fluid LDH greater than two-thirds normal serum LDH.

▶ Tube thoracostomy or more aggressive drainage of parapneumonic effusion usually is required with gross pus (empyema), positive Gram stain or culture, glucose less than 60 mg/dL, pH less than 7.20, and loculations.

▶ The most common cause of pleural effusion is congestive heart failure, which typically gives bilateral symmetric transudative effusions and is best treated with diuresis.

▶ The most common causes of bloody pleural effusion (in the absence of trauma) are malignancy and pulmonary embolism with infarction.

REFERENCES

Colice GL, Curtis A, Deslauriers J, et al. Medical and surgical treatment of parapneumonic effusions: an evidence-based guideline. *Chest.* 2000;118:1158-1171.

Light RW. Disorders of the pleura and mediastinum. In: Longo DL, Fauci AS, Kasper DL, et al., eds. *Harrison's Principles of Internal Medicine.* 18th ed. New York, NY: McGraw-Hill; 2012:2178-2182.

Light RW. Pleural effusion. *N Engl J Med.* 2002;346:1971-1977.

CASE 18

A 68-year-old woman is brought to the emergency center after coughing up several tablespoons of bright red blood. For the previous 3 to 4 months, she has had a chronic nonproductive cough but no fevers. More recently, she has noticed some scant blood-streaked sputum. On review of her symptoms, she reports increased fatigue, decreased appetite, and a 25-lb weight loss in the past 3 months. She denies chest pain, fever, chills, or night sweats. The patient has smoked one pack of cigarettes per day for the past 35 years. She drinks two martinis every day and has not had any significant medical illness. She worked in a library for 35 years and has no history of occupational exposures. She does not take any medication except for one aspirin per day.

The patient is a thin woman who is mildly anxious, alert, and oriented. Her blood pressure is 150/90 mm Hg, heart rate is 88 bpm, respiratory rate is 16 bpm, and temperature is 99.2°F. Neck examination reveals no lymphadenopathy, thyromegaly, or carotid bruit. The chest has scattered rhonchi bilaterally, but there are no wheezes or crackles. Cardiovascular examination reveals a regular rate and rhythm, without rubs, gallops, or murmurs. The abdomen is benign with no hepatosplenomegaly. Examination of her extremities reveals no cyanosis; there is finger clubbing. Neurologic examination is normal.

▶ What is your next step?
▶ What is the most likely diagnosis?

ANSWERS TO CASE 18:

Hemoptysis, Lung Cancer

Summary: A 68-year-old female smoker has expectorated bright red blood. She has had a chronic nonproductive cough and, more recently, some blood-streaked sputum. She reports increased fatigability, reduced appetite, and unintentional weight loss. She has no fever, chills, or night sweats to suggest infection. On examination, her chest reveals scattered rhonchi bilaterally without wheezes or crackles. She has clubbing of the fingers.

- **Next step:** Chest imaging, either x-ray or computed tomography (CT) scan.

- **Most likely diagnosis:** Lung cancer.

ANALYSIS

Objectives

1. Know the differential diagnosis for hemoptysis.

2. Be familiar with the risk factors for and the clinical presentation of lung cancer (including superior vena cava [SVC] syndrome and Horner syndrome).

3. Know the workup of the solitary pulmonary nodule.

4. Be familiar with the general principles of the treatment of lung cancer.

Considerations

The most likely diagnosis in this case is lung cancer. On physical examination, there was finger clubbing, an enlargement of the terminal digital phalanges with loss of the nail bed angle. In pulmonary disease, clubbing of fingers is most commonly seen in patients with lung cancer or with chronic septic conditions, such as bronchiectasis or lung abscess. She will require imaging studies such as a chest x-ray and likely CT of the chest, and if abnormalities are seen, a biopsy procedure to establish a tissue diagnosis. In the meantime, she will benefit from rest and cough suppression to minimize her hemoptysis, which may be acutely life threatening if massive bleeding occurs.

APPROACH TO:

Hemoptysis

DEFINITIONS

MASSIVE HEMOPTYSIS: A consensus definition has not been established but typically is defined as at least 250 mL or more of fresh blood coughed up in 24 hours.

HORNER SYNDROME: Symptoms are ptosis, loss of pupillary dilation (miosis), and loss of sweating on the ipsilateral side (anhidrosis) caused by compression of the superior cervical ganglion and resultant loss of sympathetic innervation. This is usually related to a superior sulcus tumor.

SUPERIOR VENA CAVA SYNDROME: Obstruction of venous drainage, usually by extrinsic compression of the SVC, leading to edema of the face, neck, and upper part of the torso often with formation of collateral veins on the upper chest.

CLINICAL APPROACH

Hemoptysis is defined as an expectoration of blood from the respiratory tract. It is an alarming symptom, both because it may be a manifestation of a serious underlying diagnosis, such as malignancy, and because massive hemoptysis can fill up alveolar air spaces and cause asphyxiation. Hemoptysis, particularly if in large amounts or recurrent, is a potentially fatal event requiring an immediate search for the cause and precise location of the bleeding. Hemoptysis must be differentiated from hematemesis and epistaxis. **Currently, the most common causes of hemoptysis in the United States are bronchitis and lung cancer.** In prior eras, the most common causes have been tuberculosis, lung abscess, and bronchiectasis. History is an important diagnostic step: blood-streaked purulent sputum suggests bronchitis; **chronic copious sputum production suggests bronchiectasis. Hemoptysis with an acute onset of pleuritic chest pain and dyspnea** suggests a **pulmonary embolism.** Every patient with hemoptysis should undergo a chest x-ray or CT to look for a mass lesion, evidence of bronchiectasis, or parenchymal lung disease. If the chest imaging reveals a lung mass, the patient should undergo fiberoptic bronchoscopy to localize the site of bleeding and to visualize and attempt to biopsy any endobronchial lesion. Patients with massive hemoptysis require measures to maintain their airway and to prevent spilling blood into unaffected areas of the lungs. These patients should be kept at rest with suppression of cough. If the bleeding is localized to one lung, the affected side should be placed in a dependent position so that bleeding does not flow into the contralateral side. They may also require endotracheal intubation and rigid bronchoscopy for better airway control and suction capacity. Urgent referral to interventional radiology for bronchial artery embolization or thoracic surgery for resection may also be required if bleeding is not amenable to bronchoscopic intervention.

Risk Factors for Lung Cancer

Primary lung cancer, or bronchogenic carcinoma, is the leading cause of cancer deaths in both men and women. Approximately 85% of lung cancers of all cell types are linked to smoking. Of the 15% of lung cancers that are not related to smoking, the majority are found in women for reasons that are unknown. Thoracic radiation exposure as well as exposure to occupational or environmental toxins such as asbestos or radon are also associated with increased risk of developing lung cancer.

Clinical Presentation of Lung Cancer

Only 5% to 15% of patients with lung cancer are asymptomatic when diagnosed. In these cases, a lung nodule usually is found incidentally on chest x-ray or CT.

Endobronchial tumors may present with cough or with hemoptysis. Chest pain is also a possible symptom of lung cancer and suggests pleural involvement or neoplastic invasion of the chest wall. Symptoms of weight loss, malaise, and fatigue usually develop later in the disease course. Malignant pleural effusion is common. **Horner syndrome** is caused by the invasion of the cervicothoracic sympathetic nerves and occurs with apical tumors (**Pancoast tumor**). Phrenic nerve invasion may cause diaphragmatic paralysis. SVC obstruction is produced by direct extension of the tumor or by compression from the neighboring lymph nodes. **SVC syndrome** has a dramatic clinical presentation and requires urgent care.

Once a patient presents with symptoms or radiographic findings suggestive of lung cancer, the next steps are as follows:

1. Tissue diagnosis to establish malignant diagnosis and histologic type

2. Staging to determine resectability or curative potential

3. Cancer treatment: surgery, radiotherapy, traditional chemotherapy, or targeted therapies

Lung Cancer Classification

Histologically, primary lung cancer can be divided into two major categories with important therapeutic implications: **small cell lung cancer** (SCLC) and **non-small cell lung cancer** (NSCLC). NSCLC accounts for approximately 86% or all primary lung cancers compared with only 14% for SCLC. NSCLC is further classified into three or more major histologic types including squamous cell carcinoma, adenocarcinoma, large cell carcinoma, and other.

Squamous cell carcinoma usually does not metastasize early. It usually is a central/hilar lesion with local extension that may present with symptoms caused by bronchial obstruction, such as atelectasis and pneumonia. It may present on chest x-ray as a cavitary lesion; **squamous cell cancer is by far the most likely to cavitate.** It may also produce parathyroid hormone (PTH)-like hormone and present with hypercalcemia. **Adenocarcinoma** and large cell cancer are peripheral lesions. Adenocarcinoma metastasizes early, especially to the central nervous system (CNS), bones, and adrenal glands. **Adenocarcinoma has the least association with smoking** and a stronger association with pulmonary scars/fibrosis. **Large cell cancer** usually is a peripheral lesion and tends to metastasize to the CNS and mediastinum, **causing SVC syndrome or hoarseness as a consequence of laryngeal nerve paralysis.** Individually, the other NSCLC subtypes represent only a fraction of total lung cancer cases and have a varied presentation.

Small cell carcinoma is made up of poorly differentiated cells of neuroendocrine origin. It is extremely aggressive but is more likely to respond to chemotherapy than NSCLC. The primary lesion is usually central. Eighty percent of patients have metastasis at the time of diagnosis, so its treatment usually is different from that of other lung cancers. Contrary to other lung cancers, cavitation never occurs in small

Table 18-1 • LUNG CANCER CHARACTERISTICS				
	Small Cell	Squamous Cell	Adenocarcinoma	Large Cell
Location	Central	Central	Peripheral	Peripheral
Associated with smoking	Yes	Yes	Often not associated	Yes
Cavitation	Never	Most likely		
Metastases	Early	Late	Early	Late
Extrapulmonary manifestations	SIADH, ectopic ACTH, Eaton-Lambert, Cushing, peripheral neuropathy	Hypercalcemia	Thrombophlebitis	SVC syndrome or hoarseness

Abbreviations: ACTH, adrenocorticotropic hormone; SIADH, syndrome of inappropriate secretion of antidiuretic hormone; SVC, superior vena cava.

cell cancer. SCLC can cause the syndrome of inappropriate secretion of antidiuretic hormone (SIADH), ectopic adrenocorticotropic hormone (ACTH) production, and Eaton-Lambert syndrome. Table 18–1 lists typical characteristics of various cell types.

SCLC is initially very responsive to chemotherapy and radiation therapy, but unfortunately, most SCLC relapse. Additionally, SCLC has almost always spread at time of diagnosis, so surgical treatment with curative intent is not possible. In contrast, NSCLC is much less responsive to chemotherapy or to radiation, but tumors that are localized at time of diagnosis may be treated with curative surgery, or with radiation therapy. The majority of NSCLC subtypes has similar prognoses at similar stages and is treated similarly.

General Principles of Treatment

Treatment of lung cancer consists of surgical resection, chemotherapy, and/or radiation therapy in different combinations, depending on the tissue type and extent of the disease, and may be performed with either curative or palliative intent. Targeted therapies against mutations prevalent in adenocarcinoma subtypes are increasingly being used with variable success.

SCLC is nearly always metastatic at time of diagnosis and, therefore, not eligible for surgical resection. It is staged as either **limited-stage** disease, that is, disease confined to one hemithorax that can be treated within a radiotherapy port, or **extensive-stage** disease, that is, contralateral lung involvement or distant metastases. Patients with untreated SCLC have a poor prognosis, with survival measured in weeks. With treatment, survival can be prolonged, and approximately 20% to 30% of patients with limited-stage disease can be cured with radiotherapy and chemotherapy. The prognosis for relapsed patients is poor.

Once the diagnosis of NSCLC is made, the next step is to stage the disease to decide whether the cancer is resectable and, thus, potentially curable. In general, patients are candidates for resection if the cancer is localized to one hemithorax which may include ipsilateral, but not contralateral, hilar and mediastinal lymph nodes, and there are no major anatomic barriers to successful resection.

Because most lung cancer occurs in older patients who have been smokers, they frequently have underlying cardiopulmonary disease and require preoperative evaluation, including pulmonary function testing, to predict whether they have sufficient pulmonary reserve to tolerate a lobectomy or pneumonectomy.

Solitary Pulmonary Nodule

The solitary pulmonary nodule is defined as a nodule surrounded by normal parenchyma. The majority of incidentally discovered nodules are benign, but differentiation between benign etiologies and early-stage malignancy can be challenging. Proper management of a solitary nodule in an individual patient depends on a variety of elements: age, risk factors, presence of calcifications, and size of the nodule. Of these factors, size is highly predictive. Larger lesions are more likely to be malignant than smaller lesions. In one study, the likelihood of malignancy was 0.2% for nodules smaller than 3 mm, 0.9% for nodules 4 to 7 mm, 18% for nodules 8 to 20 mm, and 50% for nodules larger than 20 mm. Put another way, greater than 99% of nodules measuring less than 8 mm are benign.

The presence and type of calcification on a solitary pulmonary nodule can be helpful. "Popcorn" and "bull's-eye" calcifications suggest a benign process, whereas absence of calcification increases the likelihood of malignancy.

Professional organizations such as the Fleischner Society offer a widely accepted algorithm for follow-up imaging of solitary pulmonary nodules. Generally speaking, for lesions 8 mm or less, serial CT imaging is an acceptable strategy to monitor for growth. Radiographic stability for 2 years or longer is strong evidence of benign etiology. For lesions 1 cm or greater, additional studies such as positron emission tomography (PET) scan or transthoracic needle biopsy or bronchoscopic evaluation may be indicated.

Screening

Data from the National Lung Screening Trial (NLST) demonstrated a reduction in lung cancer mortality in select high-risk patient who undergo an annual low-dose CT scan of the chest. These findings have been endorsed by a variety of professional and government organization and routine lung cancer screening is now entering clinical practice. Concern over cost-benefit, the cumulative effects of regular CT scans, and the increase rate of invasive diagnostic procedures remains controversial.

CASE CORRELATION

- See also Case 15 (Chronic Obstructive Pulmonary Disease), Case 16 (Chronic Cough/Asthma), Case 17 (Pleural Effusion), and Case 19 (Pneumonia).

COMPREHENSION QUESTIONS

18.1 A 67-year-old long-time smoker with chronic obstructive pulmonary disease presents with 3 days of headaches and plethoric swelling of his face and right arm. Which of the following is the most likely diagnosis?

A. Angioedema

B. Hypothyroidism

C. Superior vena cava syndrome

D. Trichinosis

18.2 A 64-year-old woman comes to your office complaining of hoarse voice for 4 months. She has not had fever, sore throat, or a cough. On examination, she has expiratory wheezes in her left mid-lung fields. Which of the following is the best next step?

A. Prescribe antibiotics for bronchitis.

B. Order a chest x-ray.

C. Advise gargling with saltwater solution.

D. Prescribe an albuterol inhaler.

18.3 A 33-year-old woman who is a nonsmoker has lost 30 lb and has a cough. She is noted to have a lung mass on chest radiograph. Which of the following lung cancers is the most likely cell type?

A. Squamous cell

B. Adenocarcinoma

C. Small cell

D. Large cell

18.4 A 52-year-old man presents with dyspnea, and chest x-ray shows a hilar mass with ipsilateral pleural effusion. Which of the following is the best next step?

A. CT scan of the chest, head, and abdomen for cancer staging.

B. Pulmonary function testing to evaluate pulmonary reserve to evaluate for pulmonectomy.

C. Obtain a specific tissue diagnosis by biopsy of the hilar mass.

D. Initiate palliative radiation because the patient is not a candidate for curative resection.

ANSWERS

18.1 **C.** The patient has features of SVC syndrome, caused by compression of the SVC, almost always by a thoracic malignancy. Urgent diagnosis and treatment are mandatory because of impaired cerebral venous drainage and resultant increased intracranial pressure or possibly fatal intracranial venous thrombosis. Angioedema, hypothyroidism, and trichinosis all may cause facial swelling, but not the plethora or swelling of the arm.

18.2 **B.** This patient has chronic hoarseness and unilateral wheezing. This suggests an intrathoracic mass causing bronchial obstruction and impairment of the recurrent laryngeal nerve, causing vocal cord paralysis. Thus, an imaging study of the chest is essential.

18.3 **B.** Eighty-five percent of patients with lung cancer of *all* histologic types have a smoking history. The most common form of lung cancer found in nonsmokers, young patients, and women is adenocarcinoma.

18.4 **C.** Tissue diagnosis is essential for proper treatment of any malignancy and should always be the first step. Once a specific tissue diagnosis is obtained, the cancer is staged for prognosis and to guide therapy, whether that is surgical resection, chemotherapy, or radiotherapy. Questions for this patient include the tissue type, location of spread, and whether the pleural effusion is caused by malignancy.

CLINICAL PEARLS

▶ Most patients with hemoptysis require evaluation with bronchoscopy. Massive hemoptysis may result in death by asphyxiation.

▶ Lung cancer is the leading cause of cancer deaths in men and women.

▶ A solitary pulmonary nodule measuring 8 mm or less can be followed radiographically. For larger lesions, a biopsy, whether bronchoscopic, percutaneous, or surgical, should be considered.

▶ Steps in management of a patient with suspected lung cancer include tissue diagnosis, staging, preoperative evaluation, and treatment with surgery, radiotherapy, or chemotherapy.

▶ Small cell lung cancer usually is metastatic at the time of diagnosis and not resectable. Non-small cell lung cancer may be curable by resection if it is early stage, and the patient has sufficient pulmonary reserve.

REFERENCES

Eddy JB. Clinical assessment and management of massive hemoptysis. *Crit Care Med*. 2000;28(5):1642-1647.

Horn L, Pao W, Johnson DH. Neoplasms of the lung. In: Longo DL, Fauci AS, Kasper DL, et al., eds. *Harrison's Principles of Internal Medicine*. 18th ed. New York, NY: McGraw-Hill; 2012:737-753.

Kritek P, Fanta C. Cough and hemoptysis. In: Longo DL, Fauci AS, Kasper DL, et al., eds. *Harrison's Principles of Internal Medicine*. 18th ed. New York, NY: McGraw-Hill; 2012:2170-2177.

Libby DM, Smith JP, Altorki NK, et al. Managing the small pulmonary nodule discovered by CT. *Chest*. 2004;125:1522-1529.

Aberle DR, Adams AM, Berg CD, et al. Reduced lung-cancer mortality with low-dose computed tomographic screening. *N Engl J Med*. 2011;365(5):395-409.

A 44-year-old man presents with sudden onset of shaking chills, fever, and productive cough. He was in his usual state of good health until 1 week ago, when he developed mild nasal congestion and achiness. He otherwise felt well until last night, when he became fatigued and feverish, and developed a cough associated with right-sided pleuritic chest pain. His medical history is remarkable only for his 15-pack per year smoking habit. In your office, his vital signs are normal except for a temperature of 102°F. His oxygen saturation on room air is 100%. He is comfortable, except when he coughs. His physical examination is unremarkable except for bronchial breath sounds and end-inspiratory crackles in the right lower lung field.

► What is your diagnosis?
► What is your next step?

ANSWERS TO CASE 19:

Community-Acquired Pneumonia

Summary: A 44-year-old healthy man presents with sudden onset of shaking chills, fever, and productive cough. He also complains of right-sided pleuritic chest pain. He is febrile to 102°F, but not tachypneic, and is normotensive with good oxygenation. His physical examination is unremarkable except for bronchial breath sounds and end-inspiratory crackles in the right lower lung field, and there is a right lower lobe consolidation on chest x-ray.

- **Most likely diagnosis:** Community-acquired pneumonia (CAP).

- **Next step:** Oral antibiotic therapy, pain relievers, antipyretics, and cough suppressants for relief of symptoms. Close outpatient follow-up (in 1-2 weeks).

ANALYSIS

Objectives

1. Know the causative organisms in CAP and the appropriate therapeutic regimens.

2. Understand the clinical criteria indicating inpatient versus outpatient therapy.

3. Discuss the role of radiologic and laboratory evaluation in the diagnosis of pneumonia.

4. Understand the difference between aspiration pneumonitis and aspiration pneumonia.

Considerations

This previously healthy 44-year-old man has clinical and radiographic evidence of a focal consolidation of the lungs, which is consistent with a bacterial process, such as infection with *Streptococcus pneumoniae*. The specific causative organism is usually not definitively established, so you will need to initiate empiric antimicrobial therapy and risk stratify the patient to determine whether he can safely be treated as an outpatient or requires hospitalization.

APPROACH TO:

Suspected Pneumonia

DEFINITIONS

PNEUMONIA: An infection of the lung parenchyma, which may be caused by bacteria, viruses, fungi, or rarely protozoa.

COMMUNITY-ACQUIRED PNEUMONIA: An infection of the alveoli, distal airways, and interstitium of the lungs that occurs outside the hospital setting, affecting individuals of all ages.

HEALTH CARE-ASSOCIATED PNEUMONIA (HCAP): Pneumonia occurring in a nonhospitalized patient but with extensive health care contact, including one of the following: intravenous therapy, wound care, or intravenous chemotherapy within the prior 30 days, residence in a nursing home or other long-term care facility, hospitalization in an acute care hospital for 2 or more days within the prior 90 days, or attendance at a hospital or hemodialysis clinic within the prior 30 days.

CLINICAL APPROACH

Pneumonia is an infection of the lung parenchyma. Patients may present with any of a combination of cough, fever, pleuritic chest pain, sputum production, shortness of breath, hypoxia, and respiratory distress. Certain clinical presentations are associated with particular infectious agents. For example, the "typical" pneumonia is often described as having a sudden onset of fever, cough with productive sputum, often associated with pleuritic chest pain, and possibly **rust-colored sputum**. This is the classic description of pneumococcal pneumonia. The **"atypical"** pneumonia is characterized as having a **more insidious onset, with a dry cough**, prominent extra-pulmonary symptoms such as **headache, myalgias, sore throat**, and a chest radiograph that appears much worse than the clinical or auscultatory findings. This type of presentation usually is attributed to *Mycoplasma pneumoniae*. Although these characterizations are of some diagnostic value, it is very difficult to reliably distinguish between typical and atypical organisms based on clinical history and physical examination as the cause of a specific patient's pneumonia. Therefore, pneumonias are typically classified according to the immune status of the host, the radiographic findings, and the setting in which the infection was acquired, in an attempt to identify the most likely causative organisms and to guide initial empiric therapy.

Community-acquired pneumonia, as opposed to nosocomial or hospital-acquired pneumonia, is most commonly caused by *S pneumoniae, M pneumoniae, Haemophilus influenzae, Chlamydophila pneumoniae*, or respiratory viruses, such as influenza and adenovirus. Despite careful history and physical and routine laboratory and radiographic investigation, it is difficult to determine a specific pathogen in most cases. Epidemiology and risk factors may provide some clues: *Chlamydia psittaci* (bird exposure), coccidioidomycosis (travel to the American southwest), or histoplasmosis (endemic to the Mississippi Valley) may be the cause. In a patient with acquired immunodeficiency syndrome (AIDS) or immunosuppression, *Pneumocystis jirovecii* should be added to the differential diagnosis. Tuberculosis is a possibility in patients with a history suggestive of exposure or predisposition (eg, those with AIDS) to this disease.

Pathogens in HCAP include methicillin-resistant *Staphylococcus aureus* (MRSA), *Pseudomonas aeruginosa, Acinetobacter* spp, and multidrug-resistant *Enterobacteriaceae*. Empiric antibiotic therapy should be directed accordingly.

Once the clinical diagnosis of pneumonia has been made, the next step is to try to **risk stratify** the patients, to decide which patients can be treated safely as outpatients with oral antibiotics, and which require hospitalization. Two major risk stratification tools are currently employed. The **Pneumonia Severity Index (PSI)** uses 20 variables to identify patients at low risk for death. Those in the lowest two classes have a predicted mortality less than 0.6% and are suitable for outpatient treatment. The **CURB-65** is a severity of illness score using five variables:

Confusion (1 point)

Urea greater than 20 mg/dL (1 point)

Respiratory rate greater than 30 bpm (1 point)

Blood pressure, systolic less than 90 mm Hg (1 point)

Age greater than **65** (1 point)

Patients with a score of 0 have a 30-day mortality of 1.5% and usually can be safely treated as outpatients with oral antibiotics. With a score of 2, the mortality is 9.2%, and the patient should be admitted to the hospital. In addition to these scores, patient's ability to take oral medication and the availability of outpatient support resources should be considered.

Although outpatients usually are diagnosed and empiric treatment is begun based on clinical findings, further diagnostic evaluation is important in hospitalized patients. Chest radiography is not only required for the diagnosis of CAP, but is also important to try to define the cause and extent of the pneumonia and to look for complications, such as parapneumonic effusion or lung abscess. Unless the patient cannot mount an immune response, as in severe neutropenia, or the process is very early, **every patient with pneumonia will have a visible pulmonary opacity.**

The pattern of infiltration can yield diagnostic clues. Infection with *S pneumoniae* classically presents with a dense lobar consolidation, often with an associated parapneumonic effusion. Diffuse interstitial opacities are common in *Pneumocystis* pneumonia and viral processes. Conversely, pleural effusions are almost never seen in *Pneumocystis* pneumonia. Bilateral apical alveolar opacities suggest tuberculosis. Appearance of **cavitation** suggests a necrotizing infection such as *S aureus*, tuberculosis, or gram-negative organisms such as *P aeruginosa* or *Klebsiella pneumoniae*. Serial chest radiography of inpatients usually is unnecessary, because many weeks are required for the infiltrate to resolve; serial chest radiography typically is performed if the patient does not show clinical improvement, has a pleural effusion, or has a necrotizing infection. A repeat radiograph to show complete resolution of the opacities may be prudent in patients at high risk for a postobstructive pneumonia from a potential undiagnosed lung malignancy.

Microbiologic studies, such as sputum Gram stain and culture, and blood cultures are important to try to identify the specific etiologic agent causing the illness. However, use of sputum Gram stain and culture is limited by the frequent contamination by upper respiratory flora as the specimen is expectorated. However, if the sputum appears purulent and it is minimally contaminated (>25 polymorphonuclear cells and <10 epithelial cells per low-power field), the diagnostic yield is good. Additionally, blood cultures can be helpful, because 30% to 40% of patients with pneumococcal pneumonias are bacteremic. Serologic studies can be performed to diagnose patients who are infected with organisms not easily cultured, for example, *Legionella, Mycoplasma,* or *C pneumoniae.*

Finally, fiberoptic bronchoscopy with bronchoalveolar lavage often is performed in seriously ill or immunocompromised patients, or in those patients who are not responding to therapy, to try to obtain a specimen from the lower respiratory tract for routine Gram stain and culture, as well as more sophisticated testing, such as direct fluorescent antibody testing for various organisms, for example, *Legionella.*

Initially, empiric treatment is based on the most common organisms given the clinical scenario. For outpatient therapy of **community-acquired pneumonia,** macrolide antibiotics, such as **azithromycin,** doxycycline, or antipneumococcal **quinolones,** such as moxifloxacin or levofloxacin, are good choices for treatment of *S pneumoniae, Mycoplasma,* and other common organisms. Recent use of antibiotics and known community resistance patterns to common organisms should be considered in making this choice. Duration of therapy for community-acquired pneumonia should be minimum of 5 days. **Hospitalized patients** with community-acquired pneumonia usually are treated with an **intravenous third-generation cephalosporin plus a macrolide** or with an antipneumococcal quinolone. For immunocompetent patients with hospital-acquired or ventilator-associated pneumonias, the causes include any of the organisms that can cause community-acquired pneumonia, *P aeruginosa* or *S aureus,* as well as more gram-negative enteric bacteria and oral anaerobes. Accordingly, the initial antibiotic coverage is broader and includes an antipseudomonal *beta*-lactam, such as piperacillin or cefepime, plus an aminoglycoside. If MRSA is a consideration, linezolid is often used. Vaccination for influenza and pneumococcus should be considered for all who meet criteria, and smoking cessation is an integral part of postrecovery care.

Two other commonly confused pulmonary syndromes deserve mention at this point. **Aspiration pneumonitis** is a chemical injury to the lungs caused by aspiration of acidic gastric contents into the lungs. Because of the high acidity, gastric contents are normally sterile, so this is not an infectious process but rather a chemical burn that causes a severe inflammatory response, which is proportional to the volume of the aspirate and the degree of acidity. This inflammatory response can be profound and produce respiratory distress and a pulmonary infiltrate that is apparent within 4 to 6 hours and typically resolves within 48 hours. Aspiration of gastric contents is most likely to occur in patients with a depressed level of consciousness, such as those under anesthesia or suffering from a drug overdose, intoxication, or after a seizure.

Aspiration pneumonia, by contrast, is an infectious process caused by inhalation of oropharyngeal secretions that are colonized by bacterial pathogens. It should be noted that many healthy adults frequently aspirate small volumes of oropharyngeal secretions while sleeping (this is the primary way that bacteria gain entry to the lungs), but usually the material is cleared by coughing, ciliary transport, or normal immune defenses so that no clinical infection results. However, any process that increases the volume or bacterial organism burden of the secretion or impairs the normal defense mechanisms can produce clinically apparent pneumonia. This is most commonly seen in elderly patients with dysphagia, such as stroke victims, who may aspirate significant volumes of oral secretions, and those with poor dental care. The affected lobe of the lung depends on the patient's position: in recumbent

186 CASE FILES: INTERNAL MEDICINE

patients, the posterior segments of the upper lobes and superior segments of the lower lobes are most common. In contrast to aspiration pneumonitis, where aspiration of vomitus may be witnessed, the aspiration of oral secretions typically is silent and should be suspected when any institutionalized patient with dysphagia presents with respiratory symptoms and pulmonary infiltrate in a dependent segment of the lung.

Antibiotic therapy for aspiration pneumonia is similar to that of other pneumonias, that is, it should cover typical respiratory pathogens such as *S pneumoniae* and *H influenzae*, as well as gram-negative organisms and oral anaerobes. Treatment for aspiration pneumonitis, because it usually is not infectious, is mainly supportive. Antibiotics are often added if secondary bacterial infection is suspected because of failure to improve within 48 hours, or if the gastric contents are suspected to be colonized because of acid suppression or bowel obstruction.

> ## CASE CORRELATION
>
> - See also Case 14 (Pulmonary Embolism), Case 15 (Chronic Obstructive Pulmonary Disease), Case 16 (Chronic Cough/Asthma), Case 17 (Pleural Effusion), and Case 18 (Hemoptysis/Lung Cancer)

COMPREHENSION QUESTIONS

19.1 A 65-year-old cigarette smoker with a history of hypertension and mild congestive heart failure presents to the emergency room with worsening cough, fever, and dyspnea at rest. The illness began 1 week ago with fever, muscle aches, abdominal pain, and diarrhea, with nonproductive cough developing later that week and rapidly becoming worse. Therapy for which of the following atypical organisms must be considered in this case?

A. *C pneumoniae*

B. *M pneumoniae*

C. *Legionella pneumophila*

D. Coccidioidomycosis

E. *Aspergillus fumigatus*

19.2 An 85-year-old nursing home resident with a history of congestive heart failure has dementia such that she requires assistance in all activities of daily life. She has a 3-day history of fever and productive cough. Chest x-ray reveals a right middle lobe consolidation. Which of the following is the most appropriate initial antibiotic choice?

A. Oral amoxicillin

B. Intravenous linezolid

C. Intravenous cefepime

D. Oral azithromycin

19.3 A 56-year-old man is brought into the emergency room intoxicated with alcohol. He has repeated bouts of emesis and is found choking. Lung examination reveals some crackles in the right lung base. Which of the following is the most appropriate management?

A. Initiate azithromycin.

B. Initiate corticosteroid therapy.

C. Initiate haloperidol therapy.

D. Observation with follow-up chest radiograph.

ANSWERS

19.1 **C.** *Legionella* typically presents with myalgias, abdominal pain, diarrhea, and severe pneumonia. This patient is also more susceptible to Legionella given his smoking status. C. pneumoniae would be more likely in an older patient with a more gradual onset of symptoms and associated pharyngitis, hoarseness and/or sinus involvement. M. pneumonia are more common in a young adults and a common tested association is with bullous myringitis (blisters seen on the tympanic membrane). Coccidioidomycosis is endemic to the southwest United States and often causes a subclinical infection often after dust exposure. Aspergillus is more common in immunocompromised individuals and can present with hemoptysis and lung infarction.

19.2 **C.** This nursing home resident would be considered to have a nosocomial rather than community-acquired infection, with a higher incidence of gram-negative infection. Her age and comorbid medical conditions place her at high risk, requiring hospitalization for intravenous antibiotics such as a third-generation cephalosporin.

19.3 **D.** Antibiotic therapy is generally not indicated for aspiration pneumonitis, but patients need to be observed for clinical deterioration. Azithromycin would be appropriate to treat an atypical pneumonia such as Mycoplasma. If this was an aspiration pneumonia as evidenced by fever, purulent sputum production and a patient known to aspirate antibiotic treatment with clindamycin would be appropriate.

CLINICAL PEARLS

▶ It is difficult to reliably distinguish clinically between typical and atypical causes of pneumonia. Therefore, diagnosis and empiric treatment of pneumonia are based on the setting in which it was acquired (community acquired or health care associated) and the immune status of the host.

▶ Clinical criteria, such as patient's age, vital signs, mental status, and renal function, can be used to risk stratify patients with pneumonia to decide who can be treated as an outpatient and who requires hospitalization.

▶ Although initial antibiotic therapy is empiric, the etiologic agent frequently can be identified based on chest radiography, blood cultures, or sputum Gram stain and culture.

▶ Aspiration pneumonitis is a noninfectious chemical burn caused by inhalation of acidic gastric contents in patients with a decreased level of consciousness, such as seizure or overdose.

▶ Aspiration pneumonia is pulmonary infection caused by aspiration of colonized oropharyngeal secretions and is seen in patients with impaired swallowing, such as stroke victims.

REFERENCES

Halm EA, Teirstein AS. Management of community-acquired pneumonia. *N Engl J Med*. 2002;347: 2039-2045.

Mandell LA, Wunderink R. Pneumonia. In: Longo DL, Fauci AS, Kasper DL, et al., eds. *Harrison's Principles of Internal Medicine*. 18th ed. New York, NY: McGraw-Hill; 2012:2130-2141.

Mandell LA, Wunderink RG, Anzueto A, et al. Infectious Diseases Society of America/American Thoracic Society consensus guidelines on the management of community-acquired pneumonia in adults. Clin Infect Dis. 2007;44(suppl 2):S27-S72.

Marik P. Aspiration pneumonitis and aspiration pneumonia. *N Engl J Med*. 2001;344:665-671.

A 37-year-old executive returns to your clinic for follow-up of recurrent upper abdominal pain. He initially presented 3 weeks ago, complaining of an increase in frequency and severity of burning epigastric pain, which he has experienced occasionally for more than 2 years. Now the pain occurs three or four times per week, usually when he has an empty stomach, and it often awakens him at night. The pain usually is relieved within minutes by food or over-the-counter antacids, but then recurs within 2 to 3 hours. He admitted that stress at work had recently increased and that because of long working hours, he was drinking more caffeine and eating a lot of take-out foods. His medical history and review of systems were otherwise unremarkable, and, other than the antacids, he takes no medications. His physical examination was normal, including stool guaiac that was negative for occult blood. You advised a change in diet and started him on a proton pump inhibitor. His symptoms resolved completely with the diet changes and daily use of the medication. Results of laboratory tests performed at his first visit show no anemia, but his serum *Helicobacter pylori* antibody test was positive.

► What is your diagnosis?
► What is your next step?

ANSWERS TO CASE 20:
Peptic Ulcer Disease

Summary: A 37-year-old man presents with complaints of chronic and recurrent upper abdominal pain with characteristics suggestive of duodenal ulcer: the pain is burning, occurs when the stomach is empty, and is relieved within minutes by food or antacids. He does not have evidence of gastrointestinal (GI) bleeding or anemia. He does not take nonsteroidal anti-inflammatory drugs, which might cause ulcer formation, but he does have serologic evidence of *H pylori* (Hp) infection.

- **Most likely diagnosis:** Peptic ulcer disease (PUD).

- **Next step:** Triple antibiotic therapy for *H pylori* infection, and acid suppression.

ANALYSIS

Objectives

1. Know how to differentiate common causes of abdominal pain by historical clues.

2. Recognize clinical features of duodenal ulcer, gastric ulcer, and features that increase concern for gastric cancer.

3. Understand the role of *H pylori* infection and use of nonsteroidal anti-inflammatory drugs (NSAIDs) in the etiology of PUD.

4. Understand the use and interpretation of tests for *H pylori*.

Considerations

This is a 37 year old man, whose symptoms are suggestive of duodenal ulcer. He does not have "alarm symptoms," such as weight loss, bleeding, or anemia, and his young age and chronicity of complaints make gastric malignancy an unlikely cause for his symptoms. *H pylori* is commonly associated with PUD and requires eradication to promote ulcer healing and prevent recurrence. This patient's symptoms might also represent nonulcer dyspepsia.

APPROACH TO:
Peptic Ulcer Disease

DEFINITIONS

DYSPEPSIA: Pain or discomfort centered in the upper abdomen (mainly in or around the midline), which can be associated with fullness, early satiety, bloating, or nausea. Dyspepsia can be intermittent or continuous, and it may or may not be related to meals.

FUNCTIONAL (NONULCER) DYSPEPSIA: Symptoms as described for dyspepsia, persisting for at least 12 weeks but without evidence of ulcer on endoscopy.

HELICOBACTER PYLORI: A gram-negative microaerophilic bacillus that resides within the mucus layer of the gastric mucosa and causes persistent gastric infection and chronic inflammation. It produces a urease enzyme that splits urea, raising local pH and allowing it to survive in the acidic environment. *H pylori* is associated with 30% to 60% of gastric ulcers and with 50% to 70% of duodenal ulcers.

PEPTIC ULCER DISEASE: Presence of gastric or duodenal mucosal ulceration as demonstrated by endoscopy or by upper gastrointestinal barium study.

CLINICAL APPROACH

Upper abdominal pain is one of the most common complaints encountered in primary care practice. Many patients have benign functional disorders (ie, no specific pathology can be identified after diagnostic testing), but others have potentially more serious conditions such as PUD or gastric cancer. Historical clues, knowledge of the epidemiology of diseases, and some simple laboratory assessments can help to separate benign from serious causes of pain. However, endoscopy is often necessary to confirm the diagnosis.

Dyspepsia refers to upper abdominal pain or discomfort that can be caused by PUD, but it also can be produced by a number of other gastrointestinal disorders. **Gastroesophageal reflux** typically produces "heartburn," or burning epigastric or mid chest pain, usually occurring after meals and worsening with recumbency. **Biliary colic** caused by gallstones typically has acute onset of severe pain located in the right upper quadrant or epigastrium, usually is precipitated by meals, especially fatty foods, lasts 30 to 60 minutes with spontaneous resolution, and is more common in women. **Irritable bowel syndrome** is a diagnosis of exclusion but is suggested by chronic dysmotility symptoms (bloating, cramping) often relieved with defecation, sometimes alternating constipation and diarrhea, without weight loss or GI bleeding. If these causes are excluded by history or other investigations, it is still difficult to clinically distinguish the patients with PUD from those without ulcers, termed *nonulcer dyspepsia.*

The classic findings of **duodenal ulcers** are caused by the presence of acid without food or other buffers. Symptoms are typically produced after the stomach is emptied but food-stimulated acid production still persists, typically 2 to 5 hours after a meal. They may awaken patients at night, when circadian rhythms increase acid production. The pain is typically relieved within minutes by neutralization of acid by food or antacids (eg, calcium carbonate, aluminum-magnesium hydroxide).

Gastric ulcers, by contrast, are more variable in their presentation. Food may actually worsen symptoms in patients with gastric ulcer, or pain might not be relieved by antacids. In fact, many patients with gastric ulcers have no symptoms at all. Five percent to 10% of gastric ulcers are malignant, and so should be investigated endoscopically and biopsied to exclude malignancy.

Gastric cancers may present with pain symptoms, with dysphagia if they are located in the cardiac region of the stomach, with persistent vomiting if they block the pyloric channel, or with early satiety by their mass effect or infiltration of the stomach wall. Because the incidence of gastric cancer increases with age, patients **older than 45 years** who present with **new-onset dyspepsia** should generally undergo endoscopy. In addition, patients with **alarm symptoms** (eg, weight loss, recurrent vomiting, dysphagia, evidence of GI bleeding, or iron deficiency anemia) should be referred for prompt endoscopy. Finally, endoscopy should be recommended for patients whose symptoms have **failed to respond** to empiric therapy. When endoscopy is undertaken, besides visualization of the ulcer, biopsy samples can be taken to exclude the possibility of malignancy, and specimens can be obtained for urease testing or microscopic examination to document active *H pylori* infection.

In **younger patients with no alarm features**, an acceptable strategy is to perform a **noninvasive test** to detect *H pylori*, such as serology, urea breath test, or fecal *H pylori* antigen test. The two most commonly used tests are the **urea breath test**, which provides evidence of current active infection, and **H *pylori* antibody** tests, which provide evidence of prior infection, but will remain positive for life, even after successful treatment. Because chronic infection with *H pylori* is found in the large majority of duodenal and gastric ulcers, the standard of care is to test for infection and, if present, to treat it with a combination antibiotic regimen for 14 days and acid suppression with a proton pump inhibitor. Several different regimens are used, such as omeprazole twice daily, plus clarithromycin, plus metronidazole or amoxicillin. A bismuth compound such as bismuth subsalicylate along with metronidazole plus tetracycline may be used in patients who are penicillin allergic, or who fail an initial treatment regimen. Successful treatment depends on a high level of patient compliance with the course of treatment, and selection of a drug regimen based on local resistance patterns.

Aside from its association with PUD, *H pylori* is associated with the development of gastric carcinoma and gastric mucosa-associated lymphoid tissue (MALT) lymphoma. Whether treatment of *H pylori* infection reduces or eliminates dyspeptic symptoms in the absence of ulcers (nonulcer dyspepsia) is uncertain. Similarly, whether treatment of asymptomatic patients found to be *H pylori* positive is beneficial is unclear. In *H pylori*-positive patients with dyspepsia, antibiotic treatment may be considered, but a follow-up visit is recommended within 4 to 8 weeks. If symptoms persist or alarm features develop, then prompt upper endoscopy is indicated.

In addition to *H pylori*, the other major cause of duodenal and gastric ulcers is the use of **NSAIDs**. They promote ulcer formation by inhibiting gastroduodenal prostaglandin synthesis, resulting in reduced secretion of mucus and bicarbonate and decreased mucosal blood flow. In other words, they impair local defenses against acid damage. The risk of ulcer formation caused by NSAID use is dose dependent and can occur within days after treatment is initiated. If ulceration occurs, the NSAID should be discontinued if possible, and acid-suppression therapy with a proton pump inhibitor should be initiated.

A rare cause of ulcer is the **Zollinger-Ellison syndrome** (ZES), a condition in which a gastrin-producing tumor (usually pancreatic) causes acid hypersecretion, peptic ulceration, and often diarrhea. This condition should be suspected if patients have ulcers refractory to standard medical therapy, ulcers in unusual locations (beyond the duodenal bulb), or ulcers without a history of NSAID use or *H pylori* infection. About 25% of gastrinomas occur in patients with multiple endocrine neoplasia I (MEN I) syndrome, an autosomal dominant genetic disorder characterized by parathyroid, pancreatic, and pituitary neoplasms. To diagnose Zollinger-Ellison syndrome, the first step is to measure a fasting gastrin level, which may be markedly elevated (>1000 pg/mL), and then try to localize the tumor with an imaging study.

Hemorrhage is the most common severe complication of PUD and can present with hematemesis or melena. **Free perforation** into the abdominal cavity may occur in association with hemorrhage, with sudden onset of pain and development of peritonitis. If the perforation occurs adjacent to the pancreas, it may induce pancreatitis. Some patients with chronic ulcers later develop gastric outlet obstruction, with persistent vomiting and weight loss but no abdominal distention. Perforation and obstruction are indications for the patient to undergo surgery.

CASE CORRELATION

- For a differential diagnosis of chest/abdominal pain, see also Case 3 (Myocardial Infarction, Acute), Case 5 (Aortic Dissection), Case 10 (Acute Pericarditis), Case 22 (Diverticulitis), and Case 25 (Pancreatitis).

COMPREHENSION QUESTIONS

20.1 A 42-year-old overweight but otherwise healthy woman presents with sudden onset of right upper abdominal colicky pain 45 minutes after a meal of fried chicken. The pain is associated with nausea and vomiting, and any attempt to eat since then has caused increased pain. Which of the following is the most likely cause?

    A. Gastric ulcer

    B. Cholelithiasis

    C. Duodenal ulcer

    D. Acute hepatitis

20.2 Which of the following is the most accurate statement regarding *H pylori* infection?

    A. It is more common in North America than in the developing world.

    B. It is associated with the development of colon cancer.

    C. Eradication of *H pylori* eliminates most cases of nonulcer dyspepsia.

    D. The route of transmission is believed to be sexually transmitted.

    E. It is a cause of both duodenal and gastric ulcers.

20.3 A 45-year-old man was brought to the emergency room (ER) after vomiting bright red blood. He has a blood pressure of 88/46 mm Hg and heart rate of 120 bpm. Which of the following is the best next step?

A. Intravenous fluid resuscitation and preparation for a transfusion

B. Administration of a proton pump inhibitor

C. Guaiac test of the stool

D. Treatment for H pylori

20.4 Which one of the following patients should be promptly referred for endoscopy?

A. A 65-year-old man with new onset of epigastric pain and weight loss

B. A 32-year-old patient whose symptoms are not relieved with ranitidine

C. A 29-year-old H pylori-positive patient with dyspeptic symptoms

D. A 49-year-old woman with intermittent right upper quadrant pain following meals

ANSWERS

20.1 **B.** Right upper abdominal pain of acute onset that occurs after ingestion of a fatty meal and is associated with nausea and vomiting is most suggestive of biliary colic as a result of gallstones. Duodenal ulcer pain is likely to be diminished with food, and gastric ulcer pain is not likely to have acute severe onset. Acute hepatitis is more likely to produce dull ache and tenderness.

20.2 **E.** Although H pylori is clearly linked to gastric and duodenal ulcers and probably to gastric carcinoma and lymphoma, whether it is more common in patients with nonulcer dyspepsia is unclear. Less than 10% of patients with nonulcer dyspepsia improve after H pylori treatment. H pylori infection is more common in developing countries.

20.3 **A.** This patient is hemodynamically unstable with hypotension and tachycardia as a consequence of the acute blood loss. Volume resuscitation, immediately with crystalloid or colloid solution, followed by blood transfusion, if necessary, is the initial step to prevent irreversible shock and death. Later, after stabilization, acid suppression and H pylori treatment might be useful to heal an ulcer, if one is present.

20.4 **A.** Patient in answer A has "red flag" symptoms: he is older than 45 years and has new-onset symptoms. Patient in answer B may benefit from the reassurance of a negative endoscopic examination. Patient in answer C, however, may benefit from treatment of H pylori first. Some studies indicate this approach may be cost-saving overall. This patient could be sent for an endoscopic examination if she does not improve following the therapy.

CLINICAL PEARLS

▶ The most common causes of duodenal and gastric ulcers are *H pylori* infection and use of nonsteroidal anti-inflammatory drugs.

▶ *H pylori* is associated with duodenal and gastric ulcers, chronic active gastritis, gastric adenocarcinoma, and gastric MALT lymphoma.

▶ Treatment of peptic ulcers requires acid suppression with a proton pump inhibitor to heal the ulcer, as well as antibiotic therapy of *H pylori* infection, if present, to prevent recurrence.

▶ Patients with dyspepsia who have "red flag" symptoms (new dyspepsia after the age of 45, weight loss, dysphagia, evidence of bleeding, or anemia) should be referred for an early endoscopic examination.

▶ Other patients (patients with dyspepsia who do not have "red flag" symptoms) may be tested for *H pylori* and treated first. Antibody tests show evidence of infection but remain positive for life, even after successful treatment. Urea breath tests are evidence of current infection.

▶ Common treatment regimens for *H pylori* infection include a 14-day course of a proton pump inhibitor in high doses along with antibiotic therapy, which may include clarithromycin and amoxicillin, or metronidazole and tetracycline, along with a bismuth compound.

REFERENCES

Atherton JC, Blaser MJ. Helicobacter pylori infections. In: Kasper DL, Fauci AS, Hauser SL, et al., eds. *Harrison's Principles of Internal Medicine*. 19th ed. New York, NY: McGraw-Hill Education; 2015:1038-1042.

Del Valle J. Peptic ulcer disease and related disorders. In: Kasper DL, Fauci AS, Hauser SL, et al., eds. *Harrison's Principles of Internal Medicine*. 19th ed. New York, NY: McGraw-Hill Education; 2015:1911-1932.

Talley NJ, Vakil N; Practice Parameters Committee of the American College of Gastroenterology. Guidelines for the management of dyspepsia. *Am J Gastroenterol*. 2005;100:2324-2337.

A 28-year-old man comes to the emergency center complaining of 2 days of abdominal pain and diarrhea. He describes his stools as frequent, with 10 to 12 per day, small volume, sometimes with visible blood and mucus, and preceded by the sudden urge to defecate. The abdominal pain is crampy, diffuse, and moderately severe, and it is not relieved with defecation. In the past 6 to 8 months, he has experienced similar episodes of abdominal pain and loose mucoid stools with some bleeding, but the episodes were milder and resolved within 24 to 48 hours. He has no other medical history and takes no medications. He has neither traveled out of the United States nor had contact with anyone with similar symptoms. He works as an accountant and does not smoke or drink alcohol. No member of his family has gastrointestinal (GI) problems.

On examination, his temperature is 99°F, heart rate is 98 bpm, and blood pressure is 118/74 mm Hg. He appears uncomfortable and is lying still on the stretcher. His sclerae are anicteric, and his oral mucosa is pink and clear without ulceration. His chest is clear, and his heart rhythm is regular, without murmurs. His abdomen is soft and mildly distended, with hypoactive bowel sounds and minimal diffuse tenderness but no guarding or rebound tenderness.

Laboratory studies are significant for a white blood cell (WBC) count of 15,800/mm^3 with 82% polymorphonuclear leukocytes, hemoglobin 10.3 g/dL, and platelet count 754,000/mm^3. The human immunodeficiency virus (HIV) assay is negative. Renal function and liver function tests are normal. A plain film radiograph of the abdomen shows a mildly dilated air-filled colon with a 4.5-cm diameter and no pneumoperitoneum or air/fluid levels.

▶ What is the most likely diagnosis?
▶ What is your next step?

ANSWERS TO CASE 21:
Ulcerative Colitis

Summary: A 28-year-old man comes in with a moderate to severe presentation of colitis, as manifested by crampy abdominal pain with tenesmus, low-volume bloody mucoid stool, and colonic dilation on x-ray. He has no travel or exposure history to suggest infection. He reports a history of previous similar episodes, which suggests a chronic inflammatory rather than acute infectious process.

- **Most likely diagnosis:** Colitis, probably ulcerative colitis.

- **Next step:** Admit to the hospital, obtain stool samples to exclude infection, and begin therapy with corticosteroids.

ANALYSIS

Objectives

1. Know the typical presentation of inflammatory bowel disease (IBD).

2. Know the differences between Crohn disease and ulcerative colitis.

3. Know the treatment of IBD.

Considerations

Although the likelihood is low, infection must be excluded, and it is necessary to check for infections with organisms such as *Entamoeba histolytica*, *Salmonella*, *Shigella*, *Entamoeba coli*, and *Campylobacter*, as well as *Clostridium difficile*, which can occur in the absence of prior antibiotic exposure. The main consideration in this case would be IBD versus infectious colitis. The absence of travel history, sick contacts, and the chronicity of the illness all point away from infection.

At the moment, the patient does not appear to have any life-threatening complication of colitis, such as perforation or toxic megacolon, but he must be monitored closely, and surgical consultation may be helpful. The combination of abdominal pain, bloody diarrhea, and the abdominal x-ray localizing the disease to the colon points to a "colitis."

APPROACH TO:
Colitis

DEFINITIONS

COLITIS: Inflammation of the colon, which may be due to infectious, autoimmune, ischemic, or idiopathic causes.

INFLAMMATORY BOWEL DISEASE: Autoimmune-mediated intestinal inflammation primarily due to either Crohn disease or ulcerative colitis.

CLINICAL APPROACH

The differential diagnosis for colitis includes ischemic colitis, infectious colitis (*C difficile, E coli, Salmonella, Shigella, Campylobacter*), radiation colitis, and IBD (Crohn disease vs. ulcerative colitis). Mesenteric ischemia usually is encountered in people older than 50 years with known atherosclerotic vascular disease or other cause of hypoperfusion. The pain usually is acute in onset following a meal ("intestinal angina") and not associated with fevers. Infectious colitis is usually characterized by an acute onset of symptoms, often in patients with a recent history of foreign travel, or recent use of antibiotics.

Inflammatory bowel disease (IBD) is most commonly diagnosed in young patients between the ages of 15 and 35. There is a second peak in the incidence of IBD between the ages of 60 and 70. IBD may present with a low-grade fever. The chronic nature of this patient's disease (several months) is typical of IBD. Anemia may be present due to either iron deficiency from chronic GI blood loss or anemia of chronic disease. Patients with IBD may also report fatigue and weight loss.

Ulcerative colitis usually presents with grossly bloody stool, whereas symptoms of Crohn disease are much more variable, mainly chronic abdominal pain, diarrhea, and weight loss. Ulcerative colitis involves only the large bowel, whereas Crohn disease may affect any portion of the GI tract, typically the colon and terminal ileum. **Ulcerative colitis always begins in the rectum** and proceeds proximally in a **continuous** pattern; disease is **limited to the colon.** Crohn disease classically involves the terminal ileum but may occur anywhere in the GI tract from the mouth to the anus. Anal fissures and nonhealing ulcers are often seen in Crohn disease. Additionally, the pattern of **Crohn disease** is **not contiguous** in the GI tract; classically, it has a patchy distribution that is often referred to as "skip lesions." Patients with Crohn disease may develop strictures caused by fibrosis from repeated inflammation which can lead to bowel obstruction, with crampy abdominal pain and nausea/vomiting. **Ulcerative colitis** is characterized by diarrhea and bleeding, but usually not severe pain. The diagnosis usually is confirmed after colonoscopy with biopsy of the affected segments of bowel and histologic examination. In ulcerative colitis, inflammation will be limited to the **mucosa and submucosa,** whereas in **Crohn disease,** the inflammation will be **transmural** (throughout all layers of the bowel). Tables 21–1 and 21–2 list further clinical features. Surgery is indicated for complications of Crohn disease, such as obstruction, fistulas, or perforation, but recurrent disease is common.

Crohn Disease Versus Ulcerative Colitis

The treatment of ulcerative colitis can be complex because the pathophysiology of the disease is incompletely understood. Management is aimed at reducing the inflammation. Most commonly, **sulfasalazine** and other 5-aminosalicylic acid (ASA) compounds such as **mesalamine** are used and are available in oral and rectal preparations. They are used in mild to moderate ulcerative colitis to induce remission. **Corticosteroids** such as prednisone or budesonide may be used (PO, PR, or IV) to treat patients with moderate to severe disease. Once remission is achieved, the steroids should be tapered over a period of weeks and then discontinued if possible to minimize their side effects. Immune modulators are used for more severe,

Table 21–1 • COMPARISON OF CROHN DISEASE VS ULCERATIVE COLITIS		
	Crohn Disease	Ulcerative Colitis
Site of origin	Terminal ileum (most common)	Rectum
Pattern of progression	"Skip" lesions/irregular	Proximally contiguous
Thickness of inflammation	Transmural	Submucosa or mucosa
Symptoms	Crampy abdominal pain	Bloody diarrhea
Complications	Fistulas, abscess, obstruction	Hemorrhage, toxic megacolon, cancer
Radiographic findings	String sign on barium x-ray	Lead pipe colon on barium x-ray
Surgery	For complications such as stricture	Curative

refractory disease. Such medications include 6-mercaptopurine, azathioprine, methotrexate, and the tumor necrosis factor (TNF) antibody infliximab. Anti-TNF therapy, such as **infliximab**, has been an important treatment of patients with Crohn disease who are refractory to steroids, and more recently has shown efficacy in ulcerative colitis. Patients receiving the potent anti-TNF therapies are at increased risk of infection, including reactivation of latent tuberculosis.

Surgery is indicated for complications of ulcerative colitis. **Total colectomy** is performed in patients with **carcinoma or dysplasia, toxic megacolon, perforation, and uncontrollable bleeding.** Surgery is curative for ulcerative colitis if symptoms persist despite medical therapy. Two very important and potentially life-threatening complications of ulcerative colitis are toxic megacolon and colon cancer. **Toxic megacolon** occurs when the colon dilates to a diameter more than 6 cm. It usually is accompanied by **fever, leukocytosis, tachycardia, and evidence of serious toxicity, such as hypotension or altered mental status.** Therapy is designed to reduce the chance of perforation and includes IV fluids, nasogastric suction, and placing the patient

Table 21–2 • EXTRAINTESTINAL MANIFESTATIONS OF INFLAMMATORY BOWEL DISEASE		
	Crohn Disease	Ulcerative Colitis
Skin manifestations	Erythema nodosum: 15% pyoderma gangrenosum: rare	Erythema nodosum: 10% Pyoderma gangrenosum: 1%-12%
Rheumatologic	Arthritis (polyarticular, asymmetric): common Ankylosing spondylitis: 10%	Arthritis: less common Ankylosing spondylitis: less common
Ocular	Uveitis: more common (photophobia, blurred vision, headache)	Uveitis: 3%-4% (photophobia, blurred vision, headache)
Hepatobiliary	Cholelithiasis fatty liver: common Primary sclerosing cholangitis: rare	**Fatty liver: common** **Primary sclerosing cholangitis: 5%**
Urologic	Nephrolithiasis (10%-20%) after small bowel resection or ileostomy	

NPO, broad-spectrum IV antibiotics, and IV steroids are given to reduce inflammation. The most severe consequence of toxic megacolon is colonic perforation complicated by peritonitis or hemorrhage.

Patients with **ulcerative colitis** have a marked **increase in the incidence of colon cancer** compared to the general population. The risk of cancer increases over time and is related to disease duration and extent. It is seen both in patients with active disease and in those whose disease has been in remission. **Annual or biennial colonoscopy is advised in patients with ulcerative colitis, beginning 8 years after diagnosis of pancolitis,** and random biopsies should be sent for evaluation. If colon cancer or dysplasia is found, a colectomy is recommended.

CASE CORRELATION

- For a differential diagnosis of chronic diarrhea and abdominal pain, see also Case 22 (Diverticulitis) and Case 23 (Diarrhea).

COMPREHENSION QUESTIONS

21.1 A 32-year-old woman has a history of chronic diarrhea and gallstones and now has rectovaginal fistula. Which of the following is the most likely diagnosis?

A. Crohn disease

B. Ulcerative colitis

C. Systemic lupus erythematosus

D. Laxative abuse

21.2 A 45-year-old man with a history of ulcerative colitis is admitted to the hospital with 2 to 3 weeks of right upper quadrant abdominal pain, jaundice, and pruritus. He has no fever and a normal WBC count. Endoscopic retrograde cholangiopancreatography (ERCP) shows multifocal strictures of both the intrahepatic and extrahepatic bile ducts with intervening segments of normal and dilated ducts. Which of the following is the most likely diagnosis?

A. Acute suppurative cholangitis

B. Cholangiocarcinoma

C. Primary sclerosing cholangitis (PSC)

D. Choledocholithiasis with resultant biliary strictures

21.3 A 25-year-old man is hospitalized for ulcerative colitis. He has now developed abdominal distention, fever, and transverse colonic dilation of 7 cm on x-ray. Which of the following is the best next step?

A. 5-ASA

B. Oral steroids

C. IV antibiotics and prompt surgical consultation

D. Infliximab

21.4 A 35-year-old woman has chronic crampy abdominal pain and intermittent constipation and diarrhea, but no weight loss or gastrointestinal bleeding. Her abdominal pain is usually relieved with defection. Colonoscopy and upper endoscopy with biopsies are normal, and stool cultures are negative. Which of the following is the most likely diagnosis?

A. Infectious colitis

B. Irritable bowel syndrome

C. Crohn disease

D. Ulcerative colitis

ANSWERS

21.1 **A.** Fistulas are common with Crohn disease because of its transmural nature but are uncommon in ulcerative colitis. Gallstones are common in patients with Crohn disease due to ileal bile salt malabsorption and depletion, causing the formation of more cholesterol-rich lithogenic bile.

21.2 **C.** The ERCP shows the typical appearance for PSC, which is associated with IBD in 75% of cases. Stone-induced strictures should be extrahepatic and unifocal. Cholangiocarcinoma is less common but may develop in 10% of patients with PSC.

21.3 **C.** Colonic dilation greater than or equal to 6 cm with signs of systemic toxicity (i.e. fever) makes the diagnosis of toxic megacolon more likely. With toxic megacolon, antibiotics and surgical intervention are often necessary and lifesaving. Medical therapy includes bowel rest with total parenteral nutrition (TPN), IV steroids, and antibiotics, but there is no role for sulfasalazine and 5-ASA compounds.

21.4 **B.** Irritable bowel syndrome is characterized by intermittent diarrhea and crampy abdominal pain often relieved with defecation, but no weight loss or abnormal blood in the stool. It is a diagnosis of exclusion once other conditions, such as inflammatory bowel disease and parasitic infection (eg, giardiasis), have been excluded.

CLINICAL PEARLS

▶ Ulcerative colitis always involves the rectum and may extend proximally in a continuous distribution.

▶ Crohn disease most commonly involves the distal ileum, but it may involve any portion of the gastrointestinal tract and has "skip lesions."

▶ Because of transmural inflammation, Crohn disease often is complicated by fistula formation.

▶ Toxic megacolon is characterized by dilation of the colon along with systemic toxicity; failure to improve with medical therapy may require surgical intervention.

▶ Ulcerative colitis is associated with increased risk of colon cancer; the risk increases with duration and extent of disease.

▶ Both ulcerative colitis and Crohn disease can be associated with extraintestinal manifestations, such as uveitis, erythema nodosum, pyoderma gangrenosum, arthritis, and primary sclerosing cholangitis.

REFERENCES

Banerjee S, Peppercorn MA. Inflammatory bowel disease. Medical therapy of specific clinical presentations. *Gastroenterol Clin North Am.* 2002;341:147-166.

Danese S, Fiocchi C. Medical progress: ulcerative colitis. *N Engl J Med.* 2011;365:1713-1725.

Friedman S, Blumberg RS. Inflammatory bowel disease. In: Kasper DL, Fauci AS, Hauser SL, et al., eds. *Harrison's Principles of Internal Medicine.* 19th ed. New York, NY: McGraw-Hill; 2015:1947-1965.

CASE 22

A 61-year-old man comes to the emergency center complaining of 3 days of worsening abdominal pain. The pain is localized to the left lower quadrant of his abdomen. It began as an intermittent crampy pain and now has become steady and moderately severe. He feels nauseated, but he has not vomited. He had a small loose stool at the beginning of this illness, but he has not had any bowel movements since. He has never had symptoms like this before, nor any gastrointestinal (GI) illnesses.

On examination, his temperature is 100.2°F, heart rate is 98 bpm, and blood pressure is 110/72 mm Hg. He has no pallor or jaundice. His chest is clear, and his heart rhythm is regular without murmurs. His abdomen is mildly distended with hypoactive bowel sounds and marked left lower quadrant tenderness with voluntary guarding. Rectal examination reveals tenderness, and his stool is negative for occult blood.

Laboratory studies are significant for a white blood cell (WBC) count of 12,800/mm³ with 74% polymorphonuclear leukocytes, 22% lymphocytes, and a normal hemoglobin and hematocrit. A plain film of the abdomen shows no pneumoperitoneum and a nonspecific bowel gas pattern.

▶ What is the most likely diagnosis?
▶ What is the most appropriate next step?

ANSWERS TO CASE 22:

Acute Sigmoid Diverticulitis

Summary: A 61-year-old man has 3 days of new-onset, worsening, left lower quadrant abdominal pain, with slight nausea but no diarrhea. He has a low-grade fever and is hemodynamically stable. His abdomen is mildly distended with hypoactive bowel sounds and marked left lower quadrant tenderness, with voluntary guarding. He has leukocytosis and normal hemoglobin with no occult blood in his stool. A plain film of the abdomen shows no acute changes.

- **Most likely diagnosis:** Acute sigmoid diverticulitis.

- **Most appropriate next step:** Admit to the hospital for intravenous antibiotics and monitoring. Computed tomographic (CT) scan of the abdomen will be very useful to confirm the diagnosis and to exclude pericolic abscess or other complications, such as fistula formation.

ANALYSIS

Objectives

1. Understand the complications of diverticular disease.

2. Understand the appropriate therapy of acute diverticulitis, which is dependent on the age of the patient and the severity of the disease presentation.

3. Learn the complications of diverticulitis and the indications for surgical intervention.

Considerations

This is an older patient with new-onset, progressively severe, lower abdominal pain on the left side, suggesting diverticulitis as a diagnosis. The abdominal film reveals no pneumoperitoneum, making perforation less likely. **Diverticulosis,** that is, non-inflammatory diverticuli, may present with bright red bleeding per rectum. Ischemic colitis is another diagnostic consideration in an older patient, but it usually is associated with signs of bleeding, whereas diverticulitis is not. Because the clinical presentation may be similar, it is important to evaluate the patient for colon cancer with perforation, once all signs of inflammation have subsided.

APPROACH TO:

Suspected Diverticulitis

DEFINITIONS

COLONIC DIVERTICULUM: Herniation of the mucosa and submucosa through a weakness of the muscle lining of the colon.

DIVERTICULITIS: Inflammation of a colonic diverticulum, typically on the left colon, such as the sigmoid.

DIVERTICULOSIS: Presence of diverticular disease in the colon without inflammation, and is often asymptomatic, or may present with painless bright red rectal bleeding.

CLINICAL APPROACH

Diverticulosis is extremely common, affecting 50% to 80% of people older than 80 years. Colonic diverticula are, in fact, *pseudodiverticula* through weakness in the muscle lining, typically at areas of vascular penetration to the smooth muscle. Therefore, their walls do not contain the muscle layers surrounding the colon. They are typically 5 to 10 mm in diameter and occur mainly in the distal colon in Western societies. The development of diverticula has been linked to insufficient dietary fiber leading to alteration in colonic transit time and increased resting colonic intraluminal pressure. The majority of patients will remain asymptomatic. However, some patients will have chronic symptoms resembling those of irritable bowel syndrome (nonspecific lower abdominal pain aggravated by eating with relief upon defecation, bloating, and constipation or diarrhea). They may even present with acute symptoms that could be confused with acute diverticulitis, but without evidence of inflammation upon further workup. This entity has been named "painful diverticular disease without diverticulitis." **Complications of diverticulosis** include **acute diverticulitis, hemorrhage, and obstruction.**

Diverticular hemorrhage is the most common cause of hematochezia in patients older than 60 years, and typically presents as **painless passage of bright red blood.** Only 20% of patients with diverticulosis will experience GI bleeding. Generally, the hemorrhage is **abrupt in onset and abrupt in resolution.** The diagnosis may be established by finding diverticula on endoscopy without other pathology. Most diverticular hemorrhages are self-limited, and treatment is supportive, with intravenous fluid or blood replacement as needed. Treatment of diverticulosis consists of dietary measures with increased fiber. Avoidance of nuts or foods with small seeds (eg, strawberries) is traditionally advised, although data supporting this recommendation are lacking. For patients with recurrent or chronic bleeding, resection of the affected colonic segment may be indicated.

Acute diverticulitis is another common complication of diverticulosis, developing in approximately 20% of all patients with diverticula. Patients often present with acute abdominal pain and signs of peritoneal irritation localizing to the left lower quadrant, often **presenting like "left-sided appendicitis."** Inspissated stool particles (fecaliths) appear to obstruct the diverticular neck, setting up for more inflammation and diminished venous outflow, as well as bacterial overgrowth, which ultimately leads to abrasion and perforation of the thin diverticular wall. Most cases are uncomplicated and may be managed medically, but 25% of cases develop complications that may require surgical intervention (Table 22–1).

Table 22–1 • PRESENTATION OF DIVERTICULITIS	
Uncomplicated (75%)	Abdominal pain, fever, leukocytosis, anorexia, constipation/obstipation
Complicated (25%)	Abscess (15%) Perforation (10%) Stricture (5%) Fistula (1%)

Diagnosis

Patients usually present with visceral pain that localizes later to the **left lower quadrant** and is associated with fever, nausea, vomiting, or constipation. A right lower quadrant presentation would not exclude this diagnosis because ascending colon or cecal diverticulitis can occur. On examination, the patient may have localized left lower quadrant tenderness or more diffuse abdominal tenderness with peritoneal irritation signs, such as guarding or rebound tenderness.

Plain film radiographs, including abdominal erect and supine films with a chest x-ray, are routinely performed but usually are not diagnostic. They help in identifying patients with pneumoperitoneum and assessing their cardiopulmonary status, especially in patients with other comorbid conditions. Barium enemas are contraindicated for fear of perforation and spillage of contrast into the abdominal cavity, a catastrophic complication. Endoscopy is also relatively contraindicated in the acute phase and usually is reserved for use at least 6 weeks after resolution of the attack and then is performed primarily to exclude colonic neoplasia, which may have similar findings on imaging.

CT scan typically is the **preferred modality of choice for diagnosing diverticulitis.** Findings consistent with diverticulitis include sigmoid diverticula, thickening of the bowel wall to more than 4 mm, pericolic fat stranding signifying inflammation, or the finding of a diverticular abscess.

Therapy

Patients with **uncomplicated diverticulitis** can usually be managed conservatively (with **bowel rest and antibiotics**). Selected patients may be managed as outpatients (less severe presentation, ability to tolerate oral intake, no significant comorbid conditions). Oral antibiotics may include a quinolone plus metronidazole, or amoxicillin-clavulanate for 10 to 14 days. Patients should be instructed to take clear liquids only, and advance their diet slowly only if clinical improvement is evident after 2 to 3 days.

Factors that advocate for **inpatient** therapy include elderly or immunosuppressed patients, those with significant comorbidities, and those with high fever or significant leukocytosis, or the need for narcotics to control pain. Patients requiring hospitalization can be treated with clear liquids or NPO with intravenous hydration, depending on the severity of symptoms. Intravenous empiric antibiotics with broad-spectrum activity against gram-negative rods and anaerobic organisms (eg, piperacillin/tazobactam or ceftriaxone plus metronidazole) should

Table 22–2 • COMPLICATIONS OF DIVERTICULITIS		
Complication	**Characteristics**	**Treatment**
Abscess	Suspected in patients with a tender mass on examination, persistent fever and leukocytosis in spite of adequate therapy, or a suggestive finding on imaging studies.	Conservative management for small pericolic abscesses. A CT-guided percutaneous drainage or surgical drainage for other abscesses depending on the size, content, location, and peritoneal contamination.
Fistulas	Majority is colovesical with male predominance (because of bladder protection by the uterus in females). Others include colovaginal, coloenteric, colouterine, and colouretral. Colocutaneous fistulas are extremely rare.	Single-stage surgery with fistula closure and primary anastomosis.
Obstruction	Either acutely or chronically. Ileus or pseudo-obstruction is more likely than complete mechanical obstruction. Small bowel obstruction may occur if a small bowel loop was incorporated in the inflamed mass.	Usually amenable to medical management (NPO, gastric decompression). If not, prompt surgical intervention is required.
Strictures	Occur as a result of recurrent attacks of diverticulitis. Insidious-onset colonic obstruction is likely. Colonoscopy is important for an accurate diagnosis and to exclude a stenosing neoplasm as the cause of the stricture.	A trial of endoscopic therapy (bougienage, balloon, laser, electrocautery, or a blunt dilating endoscope) reasonably can be attempted. Surgery is indicated if neoplasm could not be excluded or if such trial has failed.

be started. Pain, fever, and leukocytosis are expected to diminish with appropriate management in the first few days of treatment, at which point the dietary intake can be advanced gradually. CT imaging is indicated to identify complications (Table 22–2) such as abscess, stricture, or obstruction in the patient with persistent fever or pain.

Surgical management such as sigmoid resection is indicated for **low surgical risk** patients with **complicated diverticulitis.** Patients who have suffered two or more episodes of uncomplicated diverticulitis are often treated surgically, but medical management may also be continued without increased risk of perforation. Indications for **emergent surgical intervention** include **generalized peritonitis, uncontrolled sepsis, perforation, and clinical deterioration.**

Once the acute phase has resolved, medical management to prevent symptoms includes use of high-fiber diet, anti-inflammatory medications such as mesalazine for chronic low-grade inflammation, and probiotics. Colonoscopy is commonly performed 6 weeks after an attack of diverticulitis to evaluate for colorectal carcinoma, which may mimic the clinical presentation of diverticulitis.

> **CASE CORRELATION**
>
> • For a differential diagnosis of abdominal pain and diarrhea, see also Case 20 (Peptic Ulcer Disease), Case 21 (Ulcerative Colitis), Case 23 (Diarrhea), and Case 25 (Pancreatitis).

COMPREHENSION QUESTIONS

22.1 A 48-year-old woman is admitted to the hospital with left lower quadrant abdominal pain, leukocytosis, and a CT showing sigmoid wall thickening consistent with a pericolic abscess. Her only significant medical history is a similar hospitalization with the same diagnosis less than 1 year previously. Which of the following is the most appropriate treatment?

A. Surgical consultation for exploratory laparotomy and sigmoid resection

B. Intravenous antibiotics with follow-up colonoscopy after hospital discharge

C. Intravenous antibiotics and barium enema to evaluate for possible colonic malignancy

D. Intravenous antibiotics and recommendations for postdischarge diet high in fiber with whole grains and nuts to minimize the risk of diverticular progression

22.2 A 78-year-old is noted to have fever and chills, decreased mentation, tachycardia, and right lower quadrant abdominal tenderness and guarding. Which of the following is the most likely diagnosis?

A. Ruptured diverticulitis

B. Meningitis

C. Ruptured appendicitis

D. Ischemic bowel

E. Urosepsis

22.3 A 58-year-old man presents to the emergency room with a temperature of 102°F, abdominal pain localizing to the left lower quadrant, and mild rebound tenderness. Which of the following diagnostic tests is the best next step?

A. Barium enema

B. Flexible sigmoidoscopy

C. CT imaging of the abdomen

D. Laparoscopic examination

ANSWERS

22.1 **A.** This patient has complicated diverticulitis, with recurrent disease (as defined by > or equal to 2 complicated episodes), and is a low surgical risk, and thus should be evaluated for resection. Barium enema is contraindicated due to risk of perforation, and dietary recommendations regarding nuts and seeds are unsupported by data.

22.2 **C.** The most common cause of an acute abdomen at any age is appendicitis.

22.3 **C.** CT imaging is the modality of choice in evaluating diverticulitis. Barium enema and endoscopy tend to increase intraluminal pressure and can worsen diverticulitis or lead to colonic rupture. Colonoscopy is also contraindicated in the acute setting and should be delayed to 6 weeks after to rule out a neoplasm.

CLINICAL PEARLS

▶ Acute diverticulitis usually presents with left lower quadrant pain, fever, leukocytosis, and constipation, and often with signs of peritoneal inflammation.

▶ Uncomplicated diverticulitis can be treated medically with antibiotics and bowel rest. Complicated diverticulitis is usually treated surgically.

▶ Diverticulitis can be complicated by perforation with peritonitis, pericolic abscess, fistula formation, often to the bladder, and strictures with colonic obstruction.

▶ Enemas and endoscopy are usually avoided in acute diverticulitis because of the risk of perforation.

REFERENCES

Ahmed R, Gearhart SL. Diverticular disease and common anorectal disorders. In: Kasper DL, Fauci AS, Hauser SL, et al., eds. *Harrison's Principles of Internal Medicine*. 19th ed. New York, NY: McGraw-Hill Education; 2015:1971-1978.

Ferzoco LB, Raptopoulos V, Silen W. Acute diverticulitis. *N Engl J Med*. 1998;338:1521-1526.

Stollman N, Raskin J. Diverticular disease of the colon. *J Clin Gastroenterol*. 1999;29:241-252.

CASE 23

A 38-year-old man without a significant medical history presents for an office evaluation. He reports a 9- to 12-month history of intermittent diarrhea, associated with some mild cramping. He says the stools are usually large in volume, are nonbloody, and sometimes look greasy. He has lost more than 20 lb during this period without trying, but says that his appetite and oral intake have been good. He has tried taking a proton pump inhibitor daily for the last several months, but it has not improved his symptoms. He also tried refraining from any intake of dairy products, but that did not affect the diarrhea, either. He has not experienced fever or any other constitutional symptoms. He does not smoke and drinks an occasional beer on the weekends, but not regularly. He is married and monogamous, and he was adopted and does not know his family medical history.

On examination, he is afebrile and normotensive and comfortable appearing. He has some glossitis, but no other oral lesions. His chest is clear to auscultation, and his heart is regular in rate and rhythm. On abdominal examination, his bowel sounds are active and there is no tenderness, and no masses or organomegaly. Rectal examination is negative for occult blood. He has a few papulovesicular lesions on his elbows and knees with some excoriations.

▶ What is the most likely diagnosis?
▶ What is the best diagnostic test?

ANSWERS TO CASE 23:

Chronic Diarrhea

Summary: A 38-year-old man presents with chronic diarrhea, which he describes as nonbloody, but sometimes greasy, suggestive of fat malabsorption. He has experienced unintentional weight loss. There has been no fever or other systemic symptoms to suggest an infectious or inflammatory process. He has glossitis on examination, which is concerning for deficiencies of iron, vitamin B_{12}, or other vitamin B. The rash on his extensor surfaces is consistent with dermatitis herpetiformis, which is strongly associated with celiac disease.

- **Most likely diagnosis:** Chronic diarrhea due to celiac disease.

- **Best diagnostic test:** Endoscopic examination with small bowel biopsy.

ANALYSIS

Objectives

1. Understand the initial evaluation and management of acute infectious diarrhea.

2. Know the indications for antibiotic treatment of acute diarrhea.

3. Be able to evaluate patients with chronic diarrhea and understand pathophysiologic mechanisms.

4. Understand the diagnosis, management, and complications of celiac disease.

Considerations

This patient complains of chronic diarrhea with worrisome features (weight loss, probable malabsorption with nutritional deficiency). It is important to distinguish between functional causes of chronic diarrhea, such as irritable bowel syndrome (IBS), and more significant causes of diarrhea (inflammatory diseases, malabsorption from whatever cause, or underlying systemic disease) that may lead to complications or adverse long-term sequelae. Celiac disease is an important diagnosis to consider, as the clinical manifestations may be subtle, but once a diagnosis is established, most patients can be managed with dietary modification to improve symptoms and prevent complications.

APPROACH TO:

Diarrhea

DEFINITIONS

DIARRHEA: Passage of abnormally liquid or unformed stool at increased frequency.

ACUTE DIARRHEA: Diarrhea of less than 14-day duration.

CHRONIC DIARRHEA: Diarrhea of more than 4-week duration (may be termed persistent diarrhea if symptoms continue for 2-4 weeks).

CELIAC DISEASE: Small bowel disorder characterized by symptoms of malabsorption, and an abnormal small bowel biopsy, which occurs with exposure to dietary gluten and improves after elimination of gluten from the diet.

CLINICAL APPROACH

Acute Diarrhea

Diarrheal illnesses are extremely common, affecting nearly one in three people in the United States each year. In developing countries, acute infectious diarrhea is one of the leading causes of mortality. In the developed world, **90% of cases of acute diarrhea are infectious,** but the large majority of those illnesses are mild and self-limited. High-risk groups include travelers, immunocompromised patients, and patients who are hospitalized or institutionalized, but those groups are outside the scope of this discussion.

Most patients with mild to moderate illness do not require specific evaluation, and their symptoms can be managed with an oral sugar-electrolyte solution, or with antimotility agents such as loperamide. Bismuth subsalicylate can also reduce symptoms of nausea and diarrhea.

A more severe illness is suggested by any of the following findings: profuse watery diarrhea with signs of hypovolemia, grossly bloody stools, fever, symptoms >48 hours, severe abdominal pain, age >70, or hospitalized patients or recent use of antibiotics.

For these patients, an evaluation should be performed to **distinguish between inflammatory and noninflammatory** causes of diarrhea. Routine evaluation includes the following:

- Testing for **fecal leukocytes** or **fecal lactoferrin** (a more sensitive marker of fecal leukocytes)
- **Routine stool culture** (performed for *Salmonella, Shigella,* and *Campylobacter*).

Additional testing might include the following:

- Examination of **stool for ova and parasites**, which may be considered in cases of persistent diarrhea, especially if patient has exposure to infants in a day care setting (*Giardia, Cryptosporidium*), or if there is a known community waterborne outbreak of these infections.
- Nonroutine cultures, such as for *Escherichia coli* **O157:H7**, may be performed in cases of acute bloody diarrhea, especially when there is a known local outbreak, or if the patient develops hemolytic uremic syndrome (HUS).
- Stool may also be tested for the ***Clostridium difficile* toxin** in patients with recent antibiotic use.

If testing suggests a **noninflammatory diarrhea,** most cases are due to viral infection (Norwalk, rotavirus), food poisoning (*Staphylococcus aureus, Bacillus cereus,*

Clostridium perfringens), or giardiasis. Viral infections and food poisoning are generally self-limited and are treated with **supportive care.** Giardiasis is treated with metronidazole or tinidazole.

If testing suggests an **inflammatory diarrhea, empiric therapy** is usually instituted, often with **quinolone antibiotics** such as ciprofloxacin or norfloxacin. An exception to this strategy is in patients with suspected **enterohemorrhagic *E coli*** **(EHEC)** infection. There is no evidence of benefit from antibiotics for EHEC infections such as the O157:H7 strain, and there is concern about increased risk of hemolytic uremic syndrome due to an increase in the production of Shiga toxin when antibiotics are administered, so **antibiotics are not recommended.**

Chronic Diarrhea

Unlike acute diarrhea, most cases of chronic diarrhea are not infectious. To evaluate and manage patients with chronic diarrhea, it is useful to classify them into their pathophysiologic mechanism (Table 23–1).

Table 23–1 • CAUSES OF CHRONIC DIARRHEA

Secretory
    Bacterial or parasitic infections, eg, *Giardia*, microsporidia
    Hormone-producing tumors (carcinoid, VIPoma, medullary cancer of thyroid, gastrinoma)
    Exogenous stimulant laxatives
    Idiopathic secretory diarrhea
    Bowel resection, disease, or fistula (inadequate absorptive surface)
    Congenital electrolyte absorption defects
    Cholerrheic diarrhea (excess bile acid entering colon stimulates secretion, eg, postcholecystectomy)

Osmotic
    Osmotic laxatives (magnesium, phosphate, sulfate)
    Lactase deficiencies
    Nonabsorbable carbohydrates (sorbitol, lactulose, polyethylene glycol)

Steatorrhea
    Chronic pancreatitis (exocrine insufficiency)
    Cystic fibrosis
    Bacterial overgrowth
    Celiac disease
    Whipple disease
    Tropical sprue
    Mycobacterium avium-intracellulare (AIDS patients)
    Amyloidosis
    First- or second-degree lymphatic obstruction

Inflammatory causes
    Inflammatory bowel disease (Crohn, ulcerative colitis)
    Lymphocytic and collagenous colitis
    Eosinophilic gastroenteritis
    Graft-vs-host disease
    Infections (invasive bacteria, viruses, and parasites, Brainerd diarrhea)
    Radiation enteritis

Dysmotility
    Irritable bowel syndrome
    Visceral neuromyopathies (diabetic diarrhea)
    Hyperthyroidism
    Drugs (prokinetic agents such as metoclopramide or erythromycin)

1. **Secretory diarrhea** is caused by a disruption of the water and electrolyte transport across the intestinal epithelium. The diarrhea is typically described as large volume, watery, without significant abdominal pain, and with no evidence of stool fat or fecal leukocytes.

   Hormone-producing tumors are less common but important causes of secretory diarrhea. **Carcinoid** tumors typically arise in the small bowel, and may present with diarrhea, episodic flushing, and wheezing. Diagnosis is established by demonstration of elevated serotonin levels, usually through finding high concentrations of its metabolite 5-hydroxyindoleacetic acid (5-HIAA) in a 24-hour urine collection. **Gastrinomas** are uncommon neuroendocrine tumors, usually located in the pancreas that secrete gastrin, causing high gastric acid levels and most often present with recurrent peptic ulcers, but also commonly causing diarrhea. The chronic diarrhea may be the presenting feature in 10% of cases. Initial diagnostic testing includes finding a markedly elevated fasting gastrin level. **VIPoma** is a rare pancreatic neuroendocrine tumor that secretes vasoactive intestinal peptide (VIP) as well as other peptide hormones that cause profuse, sometimes massive, watery diarrhea with profound dehydration and hypokalemia.

2. **Osmotic diarrhea** occurs with ingestion of large amounts of poorly absorbed, osmotically active solute that draws water into the intestinal lumen. Common solutes include unabsorbed carbohydrates (sorbitol, lactulose, or lactose in patients with lactase deficiency) or divalent ions (magnesium or sulfate, often used in laxatives). The fecal water output is proportional to the solute load, so the diarrhea can be large or small volume. An important clinical clue to distinguish between osmotic and secretory diarrhea is that **secretory diarrhea will persist during a 24- to 28-hour fast**, whereas **osmotic diarrhea should abate with fasting**, or when the patient stops ingesting the poorly absorbed solute.

   By far, the most common cause of osmotic diarrhea is **lactose intolerance**, which affects the large majority of the world's nonwhite population, and approximately 20% to 30% of the US population. Most people lose the brush border lactase enzyme with age, and by adulthood, can no longer digest lactose. Diagnosis is made clinically, by history, and with a trial of lactose avoidance. Symptoms are managed by avoiding dairy products or supplementation with oral lactase enzyme.

3. **Inflammatory diarrhea** is characterized by systemic symptoms such as fever, and may have abdominal pain, with presence of blood in the stool. Stool studies will typically show fecal leukocytes. The most common and important causes are the inflammatory bowel diseases, ulcerative colitis, and Crohn disease, which are discussed more fully in Case 21.

4. **Dysmotility** is most often due to altered bowel motility due to a secondary cause (hyperthyroidism, prokinetic medications), or due to visceral autonomic dysregulation, as in diabetic diarrhea. An extremely common but poorly understood dysmotility disorder is **IBS**. It is characterized by chronic abdominal pain and altered bowel habits without a clear organic cause. Pain is typically relieved with defecation, and there is often mucus discharge

with stools and a sensation of incomplete voiding. Presence of any of the following findings is **not characteristic of IBS** and should prompt investigation for an organic cause of diarrhea: large-volume diarrhea, bloody stools, greasy stools, significant weight loss, anemia, occult or overt gastrointestinal bleeding, or nocturnal awakening with pain or diarrhea.

5. **Malabsorption/steatorrhea.** Malabsorption, or impaired absorption of nutrients, can be caused by either intraluminal maldigestion or mucosal epithelial defects. In conditions causing malabsorption, steatorrhea is commonly assessed as an indicator of global malabsorption primarily because the process of fat absorption is complex and is sensitive to interference from absorptive disease processes. Significant fat malabsorption produces greasy, foul-smelling diarrhea. Hydroxylation by gut bacteria leads to increased concentration of intraluminal fatty acids, causing an osmotic effect and increased stool output.

The **most common cause of intraluminal maldigestion** is pancreatic exocrine insufficiency due to **chronic pancreatitis**, most often due to alcohol abuse. Patients present with chronic abdominal pain, steatorrhea, and pancreatic calcifications on imaging, and may often have diabetes due to pancreatic endocrine dysfunction and insulin deficiency. Treatment of malabsorption is with oral pancreatic enzyme supplementation.

The **most common and important cause of mucosal malabsorption** is **celiac disease**. Originally described in pediatric patients with severe diarrhea and failure to thrive, it is now understood that it is much more common than previously recognized, **affecting approximately 1% of the population,** with highest incidence in white people of northern European ancestry. Patients with severe disease may present with classic manifestations of malabsorption: greasy, voluminous, foul-smelling stools, weight loss, severe anemia, neurologic disorders from deficiencies of B vitamins, and osteopenia from deficiency of vitamin D and calcium. However, this spectrum of findings is relatively uncommon, even in generalized mucosal disease. **Adult patients with undiagnosed celiac disease rarely present with profuse diarrhea and severe metabolic disturbances.** The majority of patients have relatively mild gastrointestinal (GI) symptoms, which often mimic more common disorders such as IBS, and may present solely with symptoms that are attributable to a nutritional deficiency. For example, patients with **unexplained iron deficiency anemia, especially if it fails to correct adequately with iron supplementation, should be suspected to have celiac disease.**

The exact pathophysiology of celiac disease is uncertain, but current understanding is that **genetically predisposed** individuals develop an **immune disorder** that is triggered by exposure to the **gliadin component of gluten** (a protein composite found in foods processed from wheat and related grain species, including barley and rye). Characteristic mucosal changes include villous atrophy and crypt hyperplasia in the proximal small bowel.

In patients for whom there is a **high clinical suspicion of disease,** one should proceed to **endoscopic evaluation with small bowel biopsy, and a serologic evaluation. IgA antiendomysial antibodies** and **antitissue transglutaminase (tTG) antibodies** are highly specific and reasonably sensitive tests for celiac disease. For patients with a low (<5%) clinical suspicion (no family history, no clinical or laboratory evidence of malabsorption), one can screen with serologic evaluation only. Negative serology adequately excludes the diagnosis in such patients. Note that **all testing should be done with patients on a gluten-rich diet** for at least several weeks, as the mucosal abnormalities may disappear and serologic titers fall after gluten withdrawal from the diet.

The mainstay of treatment of celiac disease is **adherence to a gluten-free diet.** Referral to a nutritionist may be appropriate, and there are a number of gluten-free foods that are commercially available. In addition, nutritional deficiencies should be repleted, and patients should be evaluated for bone loss using a dual x-ray absorptiometry (DEXA) scan. Patients with celiac disease may also have a higher risk of malignancy (GI tract malignancies and lymphoma), so one should maintain a higher index of suspicion.

CASE CORRELATION

- See also Case 21 (Ulcerative Colitis) and Case 22 (Acute Diverticulitis).

COMPREHENSION QUESTIONS

23.1 Which of the following features is *not* consistent with the diagnosis of irritable bowel syndrome?

A. Abdominal pain relieved with defecation

B. Sensation of incomplete evacuation

C. Passage of mucus

D. Nocturnal awakening with pain or diarrhea

E. Normal bowel habits alternating with either diarrhea or constipation

23.2 Which of the following findings is more consistent with an osmotic, rather than a secretory, diarrhea?

A. The diarrhea persists despite a 48-hour fast.

B. Stool osmolality = 290 mOsm, stool Na = 95 mOsm, stool K = 15 mOsm.

C. Diarrhea is large volume and watery, and is accompanied by paroxysms of flushing and wheezing.

D. Profuse, painless "rice-water" stool in a patient in a cholera-endemic area.

23.3 Which of the following patients is not a good candidate for evaluation for celiac disease, with either endoscopy or serologic testing?

A. A 26-year-old woman who experiences with intermittent abdominal bloating but no diarrhea and is found to have osteopenia and vitamin D deficiency.

B. A 19-year-old college freshman with bulky, foul-smelling, floating stools and excessive flatulence, who has lost 20 lb unintentionally.

C. A thin, 39-year-old man with a family history of celiac disease, who has been adhering to a gluten-free vegetarian diet for the last 3 years, and now complains of gassiness and reflux.

D. A 42-year-old man who was found to have iron deficiency anemia, but has no gastrointestinal symptoms, and recently had a negative colonoscopy.

ANSWERS

23.1 **D.** Nocturnal diarrhea is not typically associated with IBS, and should prompt further investigation, for example, with imaging or colonoscopy. The other symptoms listed are included in commonly used diagnostic criteria for IBS. It should be remembered that IBS is essentially a diagnosis of exclusion, and is established when patients have typical symptoms, but other conditions with similar clinical presentations have been excluded in a cost-effective manner.

23.2 **B.** Normal stool osmolality is equal to plasma, about 290 mOsm. In secretory diarrhea, most of the osmotically active particles are electrolytes, and can be calculated as $2 \times [Na + K]$. The size of osmotic gap (the difference between calculated and directly measured osmolality) is equivalent to the concentration of the poorly absorbed unmeasured solute in the fecal water. This patient has a stool osmotic gap of 70 (gap >50 is indicative of osmotic diarrhea). Answer A is incorrect given that an osmotic diarrhea will often decrease with fasting. Answers C and D are suggestive of carcinoid syndrome and cholera infection, respectively, both are causes of secretory diarrhea.

23.3 **C.** While GI symptoms in a patient with a family history of celiac disease are reasonable to investigate, the fact that he has been on a gluten-free diet for a prolonged period greatly diminishes the sensitivity of both endoscopic and serologic testing. Unexplained osteopenia and vitamin D deficiency in a young woman, unexplained iron deficiency anemia in any patient, and the classic presentation with steatorrhea and weight loss should all be investigated.

CLINICAL PEARLS

▶ Most cases of acute infectious diarrhea in the United States cause mild to moderate illness that is self-limited, and can be managed with oral rehydration solution or with antimotility agents such as loperamide.

▶ Empiric treatment with quinolone antibiotics is usually indicated for acute inflammatory diarrhea. An exception is for EHEC infection, where antibiotics may increase the risk of HUS.

▶ Symptoms of malabsorption include greasy, voluminous stools, weight loss, anemia, neurologic disorders from deficiencies of B vitamins, and osteopenia from deficiency of vitamin D and calcium.

▶ Adults with undiagnosed celiac disease often present with relatively mild gastrointestinal symptoms, and may only present with unexplained nutritional deficiency (eg, refractory iron deficiency anemia).

▶ If there is a high clinical suspicion for celiac disease, patients should undergo endoscopic evaluation with small bowel biopsy and serologies for IgA antiendomysial antibodies and tTG antibodies.

REFERENCES

AGA Institute. AGA Institute Medical Position Statement on the Diagnosis and Management of Celiac Disease. *Gastroenterology.* 2006;131(6):1977.

Binder HJ. Disorders of absorption. In: Kasper DL, Fauci AS, Hauser SL, et al., eds. *Harrison's Principles of Internal Medicine.* 19th ed. New York, NY: McGraw-Hill Education; 2015:1932-1946.

Camilleri M, Murray JA. Diarrhea and constipation. In: Kasper DL, Fauci AS, Hauser SL, et al., eds. *Harrison's Principles of Internal Medicine.* 19th ed. New York, NY: McGraw-Hill Education; 2015:264-274.

A 49-year-old woman presents to the emergency department (ED) complaining of a 4-week history of progressive abdominal swelling and discomfort. She has no other gastrointestinal symptoms, and has a normal appetite and normal bowel habits. Her medical history is significant only for three pregnancies, one of which was complicated by excessive blood loss, requiring a blood transfusion. She has been married and monogamous for 20 years, exercises, does not smoke, and drinks only occasionally. On pointed questioning, however, she does admit that she was "wild" in her youth, and she had snorted cocaine once or twice at parties many years ago. She does not use drugs now. She was HIV negative at the time of the birth of her last child.

On examination, her temperature is 100.3°F, heart rate is 88 bpm, and blood pressure is 94/60 mm Hg. She is thin, her complexion is sallow, her sclerae are icteric, her chest is clear, and her heart rhythm is regular with no murmur. Her abdomen is distended, with mild diffuse tenderness, hypoactive bowel sounds, shifting dullness to percussion, and a fluid wave. She has no peripheral edema. Laboratory studies are normal except for Na 129 mEq/L (normal 135-145), albumin 2.8 g/dL (normal 3.5-5 g/dL), total bilirubin 4 mg/dL, prothrombin time 15 seconds (normal 11-13.5), hemoglobin 12 g/dL with mean cell volume (MCV) 102 fL (normal 78-95), and platelet count 78,000/mm^3 (normal 150,000-500,000).

▸ What is the most likely diagnosis?
▸ What is your next step?

ANSWERS TO CASE 24:
Cirrhosis, Probable Hepatitis C–Related

Summary: A 49-year-old woman presents with new-onset abdominal swelling. Her history reveals a blood transfusion and remote history of drug use. On examination, her temperature is 100.3°F, heart rate is 88 bpm, and blood pressure is 94/60 mm Hg. Her sclerae are icteric. Her abdomen is distended, with mild diffuse tenderness, shifting dullness to percussion, and a fluid wave, consistent with ascites. She has no peripheral edema. Laboratory studies show the following levels: Na 129 mmol/L, albumin 2.8 g/dL, prothrombin time 15 seconds, hemoglobin 12 g/dL with MCV 102 fL, and platelet count 78,000/mm^3.

- **Most likely diagnosis:** Ascites caused by portal hypertension as a complication of hepatic cirrhosis.

- **Next step:** Perform a paracentesis to evaluate the ascitic fluid to try to determine its likely etiology as well as evaluate for the complication of spontaneous bacterial peritonitis (SBP).

ANALYSIS

Objectives

1. Know the causes of chronic hepatitis, especially hepatitis C virus (HCV).

2. Learn the complications of chronic hepatitis, such as cirrhosis and portal hypertension.

3. Understand the utility of the serum ascites-albumin gradient (SAAG) to differentiate causes of ascites.

4. Know how to diagnose spontaneous bacterial peritonitis.

Considerations

This 49-year-old woman had been in good health until recently, when she noted increasing abdominal swelling and discomfort. The physical examination is consistent with ascites with the fluid wave and shifting dullness. Her icterus suggests liver disease as the etiology of the ascites. Her laboratory studies are significant for hypoalbuminemia and coagulopathy (prolonged prothrombin time), indicating probable impaired hepatic synthetic function and advanced liver disease. She does have prior exposures, most notably a blood transfusion, which put her at risk for hepatitis viruses, especially hepatitis C. Currently, she also has a low-grade fever and mild abdominal tenderness, both signs of infection. Bacterial infection of the ascitic fluid must be considered, because untreated cases have a high mortality.

Although the large majority of patients with ascites and jaundice have cirrhosis, other etiologies of the ascites must be considered, including malignancy. Diagnostic paracentesis can be used to assess for infection as well as to seek an etiology of the ascites.

APPROACH TO:
Chronic Hepatitis

DEFINITIONS

ASCITES: Abnormal accumulation (>25 mL) of fluid within the peritoneal cavity.

CHRONIC HEPATITIS: Evidence of hepatic inflammation and necrosis for at least 6 months.

CIRRHOSIS: Histologic diagnosis reflecting irreversible chronic hepatic injury, which includes extensive fibrosis and formation of regenerative nodules.

PORTAL HYPERTENSION: Increased pressure gradient (>10 mm Hg) in the portal vein, usually resulting from resistance to portal flow and most commonly caused by cirrhosis.

SPONTANEOUS BACTERIAL PERITONITIS: Bacterial infection of ascitic fluid without any intra-abdominal source of infection. Occurs in 10% to 20% of cirrhotic patients with ascites.

CLINICAL APPROACH

Chronic hepatitis is diagnosed when patients have evidence of hepatic inflammation and necrosis (usually found by elevated transaminases) for at least 6 months. The **most common causes of chronic hepatitis are viral infections**, such as **hepatitis B and C, alcohol use, chronic exposure to other drugs or toxins, and autoimmune hepatitis.** Less common causes are inherited metabolic disorders, such as hemochromatosis, Wilson disease, or α_1-antitrypsin deficiency. Table 24–1 lists the diagnostic markers for these disorders.

Hepatitis C infection is most commonly acquired through percutaneous exposure to blood. Risk factors for acquisition of hepatitis C include intravenous drug use, sharing of straws to snort cocaine, hemodialysis, blood transfusion, tattooing, and piercing. In contrast to hepatitis B, **sexual transmission is rare.** Vertical transmission from mother to child is uncommon but occurs more often when the mother has high viral titers or is HIV positive.

Table 24–1 • CAUSES OF CHRONIC HEPATITIS	
Cause	Test
Hepatitis C	Anti-HCV Ab, presence of HCV RNA
Hepatitis B	Persistent HBsAg, presence of HBeAg
Autoimmune	ANA, anti-LKM (liver kidney microsomal)
Hemochromatosis	High transferrin saturation (>45%), high ferritin
Wilson disease	Low serum ceruloplasmin
α_1-antitrypsin deficiency	Low α_1-antitrypsin enzyme activity

Abbreviations: ANA, antinuclear antibody; HBeAg, hepatitis B e antigen; HBsAg, hepatitis B surface antigen.

Most patients diagnosed with hepatitis C are asymptomatic and report no prior history of acute hepatitis. The clinician must have a high index of suspicion and offer screening to those individuals with risk factors for infection. To date, the best methods for detecting infection include the enzyme-linked immunosorbent assay (ELISA) test, which detects anti-HCV antibody (Ab), or the polymerase chain reaction (PCR) to detect HCV RNA. Approximately 70% to 80% of all patients infected with hepatitis C will develop chronic hepatitis in the 10 years following infection. Within 20 years, 20% of those will develop cirrhosis. Among those with cirrhosis, 1% to 4% annually may develop hepatocellular carcinoma. The goal of treatment is to eradicate HCV RNA and achieved a sustained virologic response (no measurable HCV RNA 6 months after treatment) to prevent the sequelae of end-stage cirrhosis, liver failure, and hepatocellular carcinoma. Previously, the treatment of choice for chronic hepatitis C was combination therapy with pegylated alpha-interferon and ribavirin. Trials have demonstrated a sustained virologic response in up to 75% to 80% of those with favorable HCV genotypes (types 2 and 3). Genotype 1 is the most common type of HCV genotype in the United States and has been the most difficult to treat.

Interferon-based therapy has many side effects, such as influenza-like symptoms and depression, and hemolysis with ribavirin. New agents, such as ledipasvir/sofosbuvir and daclatasvir, have the advantages of being all oral, interferon-free regimens with very favorable side effect profile, and very high rates of cure (sustained virologic response), but the regimens are very costly, which may limit their use. Treatment is rapidly evolving, and guidelines for hepatitis C are frequently updated (www.hcvguidelines.org).

Cirrhosis is the end result of chronic hepatocellular injury that leads to both fibrosis and nodular regeneration. With ongoing hepatocyte destruction and collagen deposition, the liver shrinks in size and becomes nodular and hard. Alcoholic cirrhosis is one of the most common forms of cirrhosis encountered in the United States. It is related to chronic alcohol use, but there appears to be some hereditary predisposition to the development of fibrosis, and the process is enhanced by concomitant infection with hepatitis C. Clinical symptoms are produced by the hepatic dysfunction, as well as by portal hypertension (Table 24–2).

Loss of functioning hepatic mass leads to jaundice as well as impaired synthesis of albumin (leading to edema) and clotting factors (leading to coagulopathy). Decreased liver production of steroid hormone-binding globulin (SHBG) leads to an increase in unbound estrogen manifested by spider angiomata, palmar erythema, and testicular atrophy and gynecomastia in men.

Fibrosis and increased sinusoidal resistance lead to portal hypertension and its complications. Esophageal and gastric varices are prone to bleeding, which may produce massive hemorrhage, or more subtle bleeding that can trigger encephalopathy. Treatment may include infusion of octreotide to cause splanchnic vasoconstriction and reduce portal pressure. Esophageal varices can also be treated endoscopically with ligation or banding to treat or prevent bleeding, or with sclerotherapy for active bleeding. Transjugular intrahepatic portal-systemic shunt (TIPS) may also be placed to decompress portal pressure and reduce bleeding risk, but this carries a risk of causing hepatic encephalopathy. Hepatic encephalopathy is characterized

Table 24–2 • COMPLICATIONS OF CIRRHOSIS

Disorder	Diagnosis	Clinical Presentation	Treatment
Portal hypertension	Development of clinical features, visualization of varices and splenomegaly on imaging, and evaluation of portal blood flow using Doppler ultrasonography	Ascites, splenomegaly, hypersplenism, encephalopathy, and bleeding varices	Nonselective beta-blockers such as propranolol lower portal pressure; for acute variceal bleed, IV octreotide causes splanchnic vasoconstriction
Ascites	Finding free peritoneal fluid on physical examination or on an imaging study	Abdominal distention, sometimes with peripheral edema	Sodium restriction, spironolactone; loop diuretics; large-volume paracentesis
Spontaneous bacterial peritonitis	Ascitic fluid contains >250 neutrophils/mm³ and confirmed with a positive culture; most common organisms are *Escherichia coli, Klebsiella*, other enteric flora, enterococci	Abdominal pain, distention, fever, decreased bowel sounds, or sometimes few abdominal symptoms but worsening encephalopathy	IV antibiotics, such as cefotaxime or ampicillin/sulbactam

by mental status changes, asterixis, and elevated ammonia levels. It may be precipitated by numerous factors including electrolyte disturbance, increased dietary protein load (including digestion of blood), or infection. Treatment is aimed at correcting underlying causes, as well as administration of lactulose, a nonabsorbable disaccharide that causes colonic acidification and elimination of nitrogenous waste. Poorly absorbed **antibiotics** such as neomycin may also be administered orally as adjunctive treatment.

The most common cause of ascites is portal hypertension as a consequence of cirrhosis. Ascites may be a result of exudative causes such as infection (eg, tuberculous peritonitis) or malignancy. It is important to try to determine the cause of ascites in order to look for reversible causes and for serious causes, such as malignancy, and to guide therapy. Ascitic fluid is obtained by paracentesis and examined for protein, albumin, cell count with differential, and culture. The first step in trying to determine the cause of ascites (Table 24–3) is to determine whether it is caused by portal hypertension or by an exudative process by calculating the SAAG:

Serum ascites-albumin gradient = serum albumin − ascitic albumin

The **treatment of ascites usually consists of dietary sodium restriction coupled with diuretics.** Loop diuretics are often combined with spironolactone to provide effective diuresis and to maintain normal potassium levels. **Spontaneous bacterial peritonitis** is a relatively common complication of ascites, thought to be caused by translocation of gut flora into the peritoneal fluid. Symptoms include fever and abdominal pain, but often there is paucity of signs and symptoms. Diagnosis is established by paracentesis and finding more than 250 neutrophils/mm³ or by a

Table 24-3 • DIFFERENTIAL DIAGNOSIS OF ASCITES BASED ON SAAG[a]
High gradient >1.1 g/dL: Portal hypertension
• Cirrhosis
• Portal vein thrombosis
• Budd-Chiari syndrome
• Congestive heart failure
• Constrictive pericarditis
Low gradient <1.1 g/dL: Nonportal hypertension
• Peritoneal carcinomatosis
• Tuberculous peritonitis
• Pancreatic ascites
• Bowel obstruction or infarction
• Serositis, eg, as in lupus
• Nephrotic syndrome

[a]SAAG: Serum ascites-albumin gradient = serum albumin − ascitic albumin.

positive culture. Culture of ascitic fluid often fails to yield the organism. However, fluid cultures, when positive, usually reveal a single organism, most often gram-negative enteric flora but occasionally enterococci or pneumococci. This is in contrast to secondary peritonitis, for example, as a consequence of intestinal perforation, which usually is polymicrobial. Empiric therapy includes coverage for gram-positive cocci and gram-negative rods, such as intravenous ampicillin/sulbactam, or a third-generation cephalosporin such as cefotaxime. Oral fluoroquinolones may also be used for uncomplicated SBP, but should be avoided in patients who were taking quinolones for SBP prophylaxis, as their organisms may be resistant.

Other complications of advanced cirrhosis include **hepatorenal syndrome**, which typically presents as progressive decline in renal function in patients with significant ascites. The pathogenesis is poorly understood, but appears to involve multifactorial renal vasoconstriction. Treatment is difficult, and prognosis is often poor, unless patients proceed for liver transplant.

Patients being considered for **transplant** are stratified according to scoring systems to estimate disease severity and survival. The Model for End-stage Liver Disease (**MELD**) score uses a patient's laboratory values for serum bilirubin, serum creatinine, and the international normalized ratio (INR) for prothrombin time to predict survival. An older scoring system, the **Child-Pugh system**, also classifies severity of disease, with class A having the best prognosis and class C the worst.

CASE CORRELATION

• See also Case 26 (Acute Viral Hepatitis) and Case 27 (Painless Jaundice).

COMPREHENSION QUESTIONS

24.1 A 15-year-old adolescent girl has elevated liver enzymes and a positive anti-nuclear antibody (ANA). Choose the one cause (A-G) that is probably responsible for the patient's presentation.

A. Wilson disease
B. Hematochromatosis
C. Primary biliary cirrhosis
D. Sclerosing cholangitis
E. Autoimmune hepatitis
F. Alcohol-induced hepatitis
G. Viral hepatitis

24.2 A 56-year-old man has brittle diabetes (difficult to control with widely fluctuating blood sugars), tan skin, and a family history of cirrhosis. Select the cause (A-G) that is probably responsible for the patient's presentation.

A. Wilson disease
B. Hematochromatosis
C. Primary biliary cirrhosis
D. Sclerosing cholangitis
E. Autoimmune hepatitis
F. Alcohol-induced hepatitis
G. Viral hepatitis

24.3 A 35-year-old man presents to your clinic with progressive jaundice, pruritis, and fatigue. He has ulcerative colitis. Choose the cause that is probably responsible for the patient's presentation.

A. Wilson disease
B. Hematochromatosis
C. Primary biliary cirrhosis
D. Sclerosing cholangitis
E. Autoimmune hepatitis
F. Alcohol-induced hepatitis
G. Viral hepatitis

24.4   A 56-year-old woman who presented with complaints of pruritus and fatigue
       has elevated alkaline phosphatase. Select the cause that is probably respon-
       sible for the patient's presentation.

       A. Wilson disease

       B. Hematochromatosis

       C. Primary biliary cirrhosis

       D. Sclerosing cholangitis

       E. Autoimmune hepatitis

       F. Alcohol-induced hepatitis

       G. Viral hepatitis

24.5   A 32-year-old man presents to your clinic with Kayser-Fleischer rings, dys-
       arthria, and spasticity. Pick the cause from the following that is probably
       responsible for the patient's presentation.

       A. Wilson disease

       B. Hematochromatosis

       C. Primary biliary cirrhosis

       D. Sclerosing cholangitis

       E. Autoimmune hepatitis

       F. Alcohol-induced hepatitis

       G. Viral hepatitis

ANSWERS

24.1   **E.** Idiopathic or autoimmune hepatitis is a less-well-understood cause of
       hepatitis that seems to be caused by autoimmune cell-mediated damage to
       hepatocytes. A subgroup of these patients includes young women with posi-
       tive ANAs and hypergammaglobulinemia who may have other symptoms
       and signs of systemic lupus erythematosus.

24.2   **B.** Hemochromatosis is a genetic disorder of iron metabolism. Progressive
       iron overload leads to organ destruction. Diabetes mellitus, cirrhosis of the
       liver, hypogonadotropic hypogonadism, arthropathy, and cardiomyopathy
       are among the more common end-stage developments. Skin deposition of
       iron leads to "bronzing" of the skin, which could be mistaken for a tan. Diag-
       nosis is made early in the course of disease by demonstrating elevated iron
       stores but can be made through liver biopsy with iron stains. Genetic testing
       is available. Therapy involves phlebotomy to remove excess iron stores.

24.3   **D.** Sclerosing cholangitis is an autoimmune destruction of both the intrahe-
       patic and extrahepatic bile ducts and often is associated with inflammatory
       bowel disease, most commonly ulcerative colitis. Patients present with jaun-
       dice or symptoms of biliary obstruction; cholangiography reveals the charac-
       teristic beading of the bile ducts.

24.4 **C.** Primary biliary cirrhosis is thought to be an autoimmune disease leading to destruction of small- to medium-size bile ducts. Most patients are women between the ages of 35 and 60, who usually present with symptoms of pruritus and fatigue. Alkaline phosphatase elevated two to five times above the baseline should raise suspicion; diagnosis is confirmed with antimitochondrial Ab.

24.5 **A.** Wilson disease is an inherited disorder of copper metabolism. The inability to excrete excess copper leads to deposition of the mineral in the liver, brain, and other organs. Patients can present with fulminant hepatitis, acute nonfulminant hepatitis, or cirrhosis, or with bizarre behavioral changes as a result of neurologic damage. Kayser-Fleischer rings develop when copper is released from the liver and deposits in Descemet membrane of the cornea. Patients will often have high copper levels in their urine and low serum ceruloplasmin. Treatment is chelation with penicillamine and pyridoxine supplementation.

CLINICAL PEARLS

▶ The most common causes of cirrhosis are alcohol use, hepatitis B and C, and autoimmune disorders.

▶ Hepatitis C is most commonly contracted through blood exposure and rarely through sexual contact. Most patients are asymptomatic until they develop complications of chronic liver disease.

▶ A serum ascites-albumin gradient more than 1.1 g/dL suggests that ascites is caused by portal hypertension, as occurs in cirrhosis.

▶ Treatment of cirrhotic ascites requires sodium restriction and, usually, diuretics, such as spironolactone and furosemide.

▶ Spontaneous bacterial peritonitis is infection of the ascitic fluid characterized by more than 250 polymorphonuclear cells/mm³, sometimes with a positive monomicrobial culture.

REFERENCES

Bacon BR. Cirrhosis and its complications. In: Kasper DL, Fauci AS, Hauser SL, et al., eds. *Harrison's Principles of Internal Medicine*. 19th ed. New York, NY: McGraw-Hill Education; 2015:2058-2067.

Dienstag JL. Chronic hepatitis. In: Kasper DL, Fauci AS, Hauser SL, et al., eds. *Harrison's Principles of Internal Medicine*. 19th ed. New York, NY: McGraw-Hill Education; 2015:2031-2052.

Recommendations for Testing, Managing, and Treating Hepatitis C. Joint panel from the American Association of the Study of Liver Diseases and the Infectious Diseases Society of America. http://www.hcvguidelines.org. Accessed August, 2015.

A 42-year-old Hispanic woman presents to the emergency department (ED) complaining of 24 hours of severe, steady epigastric abdominal pain, radiating to her back, with several episodes of nausea and vomiting. She has experienced similar painful episodes in the past, usually in the evening following heavy meals, but the episodes always resolved spontaneously within an hour or two. This time the pain did not improve, so she sought medical attention. She has no medical history and takes no medications. She is married, has three children, and does not drink alcohol or smoke cigarettes.

On examination, she is afebrile, tachycardic with a heart rate of 104 bpm, blood pressure of 115/74 mm Hg, and shallow respirations of 22 bpm. She is moving uncomfortably on the stretcher, her skin is warm and diaphoretic, and she has scleral icterus. Her abdomen is soft, mildly distended with marked right upper quadrant and epigastric tenderness to palpation, hypoactive bowel sounds, and no masses or organomegaly appreciated. Her stool is negative for occult blood. Laboratory studies are significant for a total bilirubin (9.2 g/dL) with a direct fraction of 4.8 g/dL, alkaline phosphatase 285 IU/L, aspartate aminotransferase (AST) 78 IU/L, alanine aminotransferase (ALT) 92 IU/L, and elevated amylase level 1249 IU/L. Her leukocyte count is 16,500/mm^3 with 82% polymorphonuclear cells and 16% lymphocytes. Serum electrolytes, blood urea nitrogen (BUN), and creatinine are normal. A plain film of the abdomen shows a nonspecific gas pattern and no pneumoperitoneum, and chest x-ray is normal.

▶ What is the most likely diagnosis?
▶ What is the most likely underlying etiology?
▶ What is your next diagnostic step?

ANSWERS TO CASE 25:

Pancreatitis, Gallstones

Summary: A 42-year-old woman with a prior history consistent with symptomatic cholelithiasis now presents with epigastric pain and nausea for 24 hours, much longer than would be expected with uncomplicated biliary colic. Her symptoms are consistent with acute pancreatitis. She also has hyperbilirubinemia and an elevated alkaline phosphatase level, suggesting obstruction of the common bile duct caused by a gallstone, which is the likely cause of her pancreatitis.

- **Most likely diagnosis:** Acute pancreatitis.

- **Most likely etiology:** Choledocholithiasis (common bile duct stone).

- **Next diagnostic step:** Right upper quadrant abdominal ultrasonography.

ANALYSIS

Objectives

1. Know the causes, clinical features, and prognostic factors in acute pancreatitis.

2. Learn the principles of treatment and complications of acute pancreatitis.

3. Know the complications of gallstones.

4. Understand the medical treatment of a patient with biliary sepsis and the indications for endoscopic retrograde cholangiopancreatography (ERCP) or surgical intervention.

Considerations

This 42-year-old woman complained of episodes of mild right upper quadrant abdominal pain with heavy meals in the past. These prior episodes were short lived. This is very consistent with biliary colic. However, this episode is different in severity and location of pain (now radiating straight to her back and accompanied by nausea and vomiting). The elevated amylase level confirms the clinical impression of acute pancreatitis. She likely has acute pancreatitis caused by a stone in the common bile duct. Biliary obstruction is suggested by the elevated bilirubin level. She is moderately ill but is hemodynamically stable and has only one prognostic feature to predict mortality. She meets criteria for systemic inflammatory response syndrome (SIRS), and should be monitored closely for signs of clinical deterioration (Table 25–1).

Table 25–1 • SIRS CRITERIA	
Temperature	≤36°C or ≥ 38°C
Heart rate	≥90 bpm
Respiratory rate	≥20 breaths/min **or** $PaCO_2$ <32 mm Hg
White blood cell count	≥12,000 or ≤4000 cells/mm³ **or** >10% bands

Data from Ranson JH. Etiological and prognostic factors in human acute pancreatitis: A review. Am J Gastroenterol 1982;77:633.

APPROACH TO:
Acute Pancreatitis

DEFINITIONS

ACUTE PANCREATITIS: An inflammatory process in which pancreatic enzymes are activated and cause autodigestion of the gland.

PANCREATIC PSEUDOCYST: Cystic space within the pancreas **not lined by epithelial cells**, often associated with chronic pancreatitis.

CLINICAL APPROACH

Acute pancreatitis can be caused by many conditions, but in most clinical investigations, **gallstones are the most common cause** (30%-60% of cases), usually due to passage of a gallstone into the common bile duct. **Alcohol use** is next most common cause (15%-30% of cases in the United States) with episodes often precipitated by binge drinking. **Hypertriglyceridemia** is another common cause (1%-4% of cases) and occurs when serum triglyceride levels are more than 1000 mg/dL, as is seen in patients with familial dyslipidemias or diabetes (etiologies are given in Table 25–2). Acute pancreatitis can be induced by **ERCP**, occurring after 5%-10% of such procedures. When patients appear to have "idiopathic" pancreatitis, that is, no gallstones are seen on ultrasonography and no other predisposing factor can be found, biliary tract disease is still the most likely cause—either biliary sludge (microlithiasis) or sphincter of Oddi dysfunction.

    Abdominal pain is the cardinal symptom of pancreatitis and often is severe, typically in the **upper abdomen with radiation to the back.** The pain often is relieved by

Table 25–2 • CAUSES OF ACUTE PANCREATITIS
Biliary tract disease (eg, gallstones)
Alcohol use
Drugs (eg, the antiretroviral didanosine [DDI], pentamidine, thiazides, furosemide, sulfonamides, azathioprine, L-asparaginase)
Surgical manipulation of the gland, or ERCP
Hypertriglyceridemia/hypercalcemia
Infections such as mumps or cytomegalovirus
Trauma such as blunt abdominal trauma

sitting up and bending forward, and is exacerbated by food. Patients **commonly experience nausea and vomiting** that is precipitated by oral intake. They **may have low-grade fever** (if temperature is >101°F, one should suspect infection) and often are volume depleted because of the vomiting and inability to tolerate oral intake, and because the inflammatory process may cause third spacing with sequestration of large volumes of fluid in the peritoneal cavity. Hemorrhagic pancreatitis with blood tracking along fascial planes would be suspected if periumbilical ecchymosis (**Cullen sign**) or flank ecchymosis (**Grey Turner sign**) is present.

The most common test used to diagnose pancreatitis is an **elevated serum amylase level**. It is released from the inflamed pancreas within hours of the attack and remains elevated for 3 to 4 days. Amylase undergoes renal clearance, and after serum levels decline, its level remains elevated in the urine. **Amylase is not specific to the pancreas**, however, and can be elevated as a consequence of many other abdominal processes, such as **gastrointestinal ischemia with infarction or perforation; even just the vomiting** associated with pancreatitis can cause elevated amylase of **salivary origin**. Elevated **serum lipase level**, also seen in acute pancreatitis, is **more specific than is amylase to pancreatic origin and remains elevated longer than does amylase**. When the diagnosis is uncertain or when complications of pancreatitis are suspected, computed tomographic (**CT) imaging of the abdomen is highly sensitive** for showing the inflammatory changes in patients with moderate to severe pancreatitis.

Treatment of pancreatitis is mainly supportive and includes "pancreatic rest," that is, **withholding food or liquids by mouth until symptoms subside**, and adequate **narcotic analgesia. Intravenous fluids** are necessary for maintenance and to replace any deficits. In patients with severe pancreatitis who sequester large volumes of fluid in their abdomen as pancreatic ascites, sometimes prodigious amounts of parenteral fluid replacement are necessary to maintain intravascular volume. ERCP with papillotomy to remove bile duct stones may lessen the severity of gallstone pancreatitis, and is usually done within 24-48 hours. When pain has largely subsided and the patient has bowel sounds, oral clear liquids can be started and the diet advanced as tolerated.

The large majority of patients with acute pancreatitis will recover spontaneously and have a relatively uncomplicated course. Several scoring systems have been developed in an attempt to identify the 15%-25% of patients who will have a more complicated course, including the BISAP score and APACHE II score. Patients with severe acute pancreatitis, or SIRS >48 hours may require management in a monitored or intensive care unit. **The most common cause of early death in patients with pancreatitis is hypovolemic shock**, which is multifactorial: third spacing and sequestration of large fluid volumes in the abdomen, as well as increased capillary permeability. Others develop pulmonary edema, which may be noncardiogenic due to acute respiratory distress syndrome (ARDS), or cardiogenic as a consequence of myocardial dysfunction.

Pancreatic complications include a **phlegmon**, which is a solid mass of inflamed pancreas, often with patchy areas of necrosis. Sometimes, extensive areas of **pancreatic necrosis** develop within a phlegmon. Either necrosis or a phlegmon can become secondarily infected, resulting in **pancreatic abscess**. Abscesses typically develop 2-3 weeks after the onset of illness and should be suspected if there is fever or leukocytosis. If pancreatic abscesses are not drained, mortality approaches 100%.

Pancreatic necrosis and abscess are the leading causes of death in patients after the first week of illness. A **pancreatic pseudocyst** is a cystic collection of inflammatory fluid and pancreatic secretions, which unlike true cysts do not have an epithelial lining. Most pancreatic pseudocysts resolve spontaneously within 6 weeks, especially if they are smaller than 6 cm. However, if they are causing pain, are large or expanding, or become infected, they usually require drainage. Any of these local complications of pancreatitis should be suspected if persistent pain, fever, abdominal mass, or persistent hyperamylasemia occurs.

Gallstones

Gallstones usually form as a consequence of precipitation of cholesterol microcrystals in bile. They are very common, occurring in 10%-20% of patients older than 65 years. Patients often are asymptomatic. When discovered incidentally, they can be followed without intervention, as only 10% of patients will develop any symptoms related to their stones within 10 years. When patients do develop symptoms because of a stone in the cystic duct or Hartmann pouch, the typical attack of **biliary colic** usually has a sudden onset, often precipitated by a large or fatty meal, with severe steady pain in the right upper quadrant or epigastrium, lasting between 1 and 4 hours. They may have mild elevations of the alkaline phosphatase level and slight hyperbilirubinemia, but elevations of the bilirubin level over 3 g/dL suggest a common duct stone. The first diagnostic test in a patient with suspected gallstones usually is an **ultrasonogram**. The test is noninvasive and very sensitive for detecting stones in the gallbladder as well as intrahepatic or extrahepatic biliary duct dilation.

One of the most common complications of gallstones is **acute cholecystitis**, which occurs when a stone becomes impacted in the cystic duct, and edema and inflammation develop behind the obstruction. This is apparent ultrasonographically as gallbladder wall thickening and pericholecystic fluid, and is characterized clinically as a persistent right upper quadrant abdominal pain, with fever and leukocytosis. Cultures of bile in the gallbladder often yield enteric flora such as *Escherichia coli* and *Klebsiella*. If the diagnosis is in question, nuclear scintigraphy with a **hepatobiliary iminodiacetic acid (HIDA) scan** may be performed. The positive test shows visualization of the liver by the isotope, but nonvisualization of the gallbladder may indicate an obstructed cystic duct. Treatment of acute cholecystitis usually involves making the patient nil per os (NPO), intravenous fluids and antibiotics, and early cholecystectomy within 48-72 hours.

Another complication of gallstones is cholangitis, which occurs when there is intermittent obstruction of the common bile duct, allowing reflux of bacteria up the biliary tree, followed by development of purulent infection behind the obstruction. If the patient is septic, the condition requires urgent decompression of the biliary tree, either surgically or by ERCP, to remove the stones endoscopically after performing a papillotomy, which allows the other stones to pass.

CASE CORRELATION

- For a differential diagnosis of abdominal pain, see also Case 20 (Peptic Ulcer Disease) and Case 22 (Acute Diverticulitis).

COMPREHENSION QUESTIONS

25.1 A 43-year-old man who is an alcoholic is admitted to the hospital with acute pancreatitis. He is given intravenous hydration and is placed NPO. Which of the following findings is a predictor of higher mortality?

A. His age

B. Initial serum glucose level of 60 mg/dL

C. BUN of 18 mg/dL

D. Disorientation, with Glasgow Coma Scale score of 10

E. Amylase level of 1000 IU/L

25.2 A 37-year-old woman is noted to have gallstones on ultrasonography. She is placed on a low-fat diet. After 3 months she is noted to have severe right upper quadrant pain, fever to 102°F, and nausea. Which of the following is the most likely diagnosis?

A. Acute cholangitis

B. Acute cholecystitis

C. Acute pancreatitis

D. Acute perforation of the gallbladder

25.3 A 45-year-old man was admitted for acute pancreatitis, thought to be a result of blunt abdominal trauma. After 3 months he still has epigastric pain but is able to eat solid food. His amylase level is elevated at 260 IU/L. Which of the following is the most likely diagnosis?

A. Recurrent pancreatitis

B. Diverticulitis

C. Peptic ulcer disease

D. Pancreatic pseudocyst

ANSWERS

25.1 **D.** Impaired mental status is a poor prognostic sign. Other findings associated with higher mortality include a BUN > or = to 25, presence of SIRS, age over 60 and presence of a pleural effusion. Notably, the amylase level does not correlate to the severity of the disease.

25.2 **B.** Acute cholecystitis is one of the most common complications of gallstones. This patient with fever, right upper quadrant pain, and a history of gallstones likely has acute cholecystitis. Acute cholangitis usually presents with Charcot's triad (RUQ pain, jaundice, and fever/chills) due to an ascending infection proximal to an obstructed bile duct.

25.3 **D.** A pancreatic pseudocyst has a clinical presentation of abdominal pain and mass and persistent hyperamylasemia in a patient with prior pancreatitis.

CLINICAL PEARLS

▶ The three most common causes of acute pancreatitis in the United States are gallstones, alcohol consumption, and hypertriglyceridemia.

▶ Acute pancreatitis usually is managed with pancreatic rest, intravenous hydration, and analgesia, often with narcotics.

▶ Pancreatic complications (phlegmon, necrosis, abscess, pseudocyst) should be suspected if persistent pain, fever, abdominal mass, or persistent hyperamylasemia occurs.

▶ Patients with asymptomatic gallstones do not require treatment; they can be observed and treated if symptoms develop. Cholecystectomy is performed for patients with symptoms of biliary colic or for those with complications.

▶ Acute cholecystitis is best treated with antibiotics and then cholecystectomy, generally within 48-72 hours.

REFERENCES

Ahmed A, Cheung RC, Keefe EB. Management of gallstones and their complications. *Am Fam Physician*. 2000;61:1673-1680.

Greenberger NJ, Conwell DL. Acute and chronic pancreatitis. In: Kasper DL, Fauci AS, Hauser SL, et al., eds. *Harrison's Principles of Internal Medicine*. 19th ed. New York, NY: McGraw-Hill; 2015:2090-2102.

Greenberger NJ, Paumgartner G. Diseases of the gallbladder and bile ducts. In: Kasper DL, Fauci AS, Hauser SL, et al., eds. *Harrison's Principles of Internal Medicine*. 19th ed. New York, NY: McGraw-Hill; 2015:2075-2086.

Tenner S. Initial management of acute pancreatitis: critical issues during the first 72 hours. *Am J Gastroenterol*. 2004;99:2489-2494.

A 28-year-old man comes to your clinic complaining of a 5-day history of nausea, vomiting, diffuse abdominal pain, fever to 101°F, and muscle aches. He has lost his appetite, but he is able to tolerate liquids and has no diarrhea. He has no significant medical history or family history, and he has not traveled outside the United States. He admits to having 12 different lifetime sexual partners, denies illicit drug use, and drinks alcohol occasionally, but not since this illness began. He takes no medications routinely, but he has been taking acetaminophen, approximately 30 tablets per day for 2 days for fever and body aches since this illness began. On examination, his temperature is 100.8°F, heart rate is 98 bpm, and blood pressure is 120/74 mm Hg. He appears jaundiced, his chest is clear to auscultation, and his heart rhythm is regular without murmurs. His liver percusses 12 cm, and is smooth and slightly tender to palpation. He has no abdominal distention or peripheral edema. Laboratory values are significant for a normal complete blood count, creatinine 1.1 mg/dL, alanine aminotransferase (ALT) 3440 IU/L, aspartate aminotransferase (AST) 2705 IU/L, total bilirubin 24.5 mg/dL, direct bilirubin 18.2 mg/dL, alkaline phosphatase 349 IU/L, serum albumin 3.0 g/dL, and prothrombin time 14 seconds.

▶ What is the most likely diagnosis?
▶ What is the most important immediate diagnostic test?

ANSWERS TO CASE 26:

Acute Viral Hepatitis, Possible Acetaminophen Hepatotoxicity

Summary: A 28-year-old man complains of nausea, vomiting, diffuse abdominal pain, fever, and myalgias. He has had 12 different lifetime sexual partners and currently is taking acetaminophen. He appears icteric and has a low-grade fever and tender hepatomegaly. Results of his laboratory studies are consistent with severe hepatocellular injury.

- **Most likely diagnosis:** Acute hepatitis, either viral infection or toxic injury, possibly exacerbated by acetaminophen (APAP) use.

- **Most important immediate diagnostic test:** Acetaminophen level, because acetaminophen toxicity may greatly exacerbate liver injury but is treatable.

ANALYSIS

Objectives

1. Understand the use of viral serologic studies for diagnosing hepatitis A, B, and C infections.

2. Know the prognosis for acute viral hepatitis and recognize fulminant hepatic failure.

3. Know measures to prevent hepatitis A and B infections.

4. Understand the use of the acetaminophen nomogram and the treatment of acetaminophen hepatotoxicity.

Considerations

This patient has an acute onset of hepatic injury and systemic symptoms that predate his acetaminophen use. The markedly elevated hepatic transaminase and bilirubin levels are consistent with viral hepatitis or possibly toxic injury. This patient denied intravenous drug use, which would be a risk factor for hepatitis B and C infections. His sexual history is a possible clue. The degree and pattern of transaminase ALT and AST elevation can provide some clues to help differentiate possible etiologies. Transaminase levels more than 1000 IU/L are seen in conditions that produce extensive hepatic necrosis, such as toxic injury, viral hepatitis, and ischemia ("shock liver"). Patients with alcoholic hepatitis almost always have levels less than 500 IU/L and often have an AST/ALT ratio of 2:1. In this case, it is important to consider the possibility of acetaminophen toxicity, both because the condition can produce fatal liver failure and because an effective antidote is available. By obtaining a serum acetaminophen level and knowing the time of his last ingestion, these data can be plotted on a nomogram (Figure 26–1) to help predict acetaminophen-related liver damage and the possible need for N-acetylcysteine, which is the antidote.

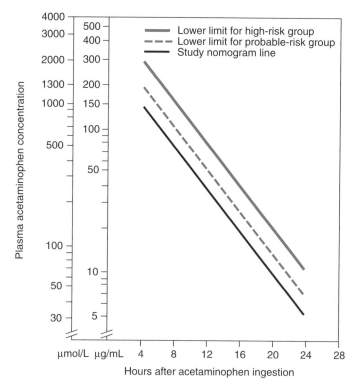

Figure 26–1. Acetaminophen nomogram. (Reproduced, with permission, from JL Dienstag, KJ Isselbacher. Poisoning and drug overdose. In: Braunwald E, Fauci AS, Kasper DL, et al, eds. *Harrison's Principles of Internal Medicine,* 15th ed. New York: McGraw-Hill, 2001:2602.)

APPROACH TO:

Suspected Hepatitis

DEFINITIONS

ACUTE HEPATITIS: An inflammation of the liver that may be caused by infection, ischemia, or toxic exposure. At least six viruses that cause hepatitis have been identified, referred to as hepatitis A, B, C, D, E, and G. Characteristically, hepatitis A, C, E, and G are caused by RNA viruses and hepatitis B and D are caused by DNA viruses.

CHRONIC HEPATITIS: A syndrome that is defined clinically by evidence of liver disease with inflammation and necrosis for at least 6 consecutive months, most commonly with hepatitis B, C, and D infections.

CIRRHOSIS: Diffuse damage to hepatocytes that show evidence of chronic inflammation with fibrosis and loss of hepatocyte function.

FULMINANT HEPATIC FAILURE: A rare but devastating syndrome that progresses within 8 weeks of symptom onset to rapidly include arrest of normal hepatic function and manifests clinically with jaundice, coagulopathy, and hepatic encephalopathy.

CLINICAL APPROACH

Viral Hepatitis

Most cases of acute hepatitis are caused by infection with one of the five viruses: hepatitis A, B, C, D, or E. They can produce virtually indistinguishable clinical syndromes, although it is unusual to observe acute hepatitis C. Affected individuals often complain of a prodrome of nonspecific constitutional symptoms, including fever, nausea, fatigue, arthralgias, myalgias, headache, and sometimes pharyngitis and coryza. This is followed by the onset of visible jaundice caused by hyperbilirubinemia, with tenderness and enlargement of the liver, and dark urine caused by bilirubinuria. The clinical course and prognosis vary based on the type of virus causing the hepatitis.

Hepatitis A and E both are very contagious and transmitted by fecal-oral route, usually by contaminated food or water where sanitation is poor, and in daycare settings by children. **Hepatitis A** is found worldwide and is the **most common cause of acute viral hepatitis in the United States. Hepatitis E** is much less common and is found in Asia, Africa, Central America, and the Caribbean. Both hepatitis A and E infections usually lead to self-limited illnesses and generally resolve within weeks. Almost all patients with hepatitis A recover completely and have no long-term complications. A few may have fulminant disease resulting in liver failure. Most patients with hepatitis E also have uncomplicated courses, but some patients, particularly pregnant women, have been reported to develop severe hepatic necrosis and fatal liver failure.

Hepatitis B is the second most common type of viral hepatitis in the United States, and it is **usually sexually transmitted.** It also may be acquired parenterally, such as by intravenous drug use, and during birth from chronically infected mothers. The outcome depends on the age at which the infection was acquired. Up to 90% of infected newborns develop chronic hepatitis B infection, which places the affected infant at significant risk of hepatocellular carcinoma later in adulthood. For individuals infected later in life, approximately 95% of patients will recover completely without sequelae. Between 5% and 10% of patients will develop chronic hepatitis, which may progress to cirrhosis. A chronic carrier state may be seen in which the virus continues to replicate, but it does not cause irreversible hepatic damage in the host.

Hepatitis C is transmitted **parenterally by blood transfusions or intravenous drug use,** and rarely by sexual contact. The mode of transmission is unknown in approximately 40% of cases. It is uncommonly diagnosed as a cause of acute hepatitis, often producing subclinical infection, but is frequently diagnosed later as a cause of chronic hepatitis and possibly liver cirrhosis.

Hepatitis D is a defective RNA virus that requires the presence of the hepatitis B virus to replicate. It can be acquired as a coinfection simultaneously with acute hepatitis B or as a later superinfection in a person with a chronic hepatitis B infection. Patients afflicted with chronic hepatitis B virus who then become infected with hepatitis D may suffer clinical deterioration; in 10% to 20% of these cases, individuals develop severe fatal hepatic failure.

Fortunately, in most cases of acute viral hepatitis, patients recover completely, so the treatment is generally supportive. However, **fulminant hepatic failure** as a result of massive hepatic necrosis may progress over a period of weeks. This usually may be caused by infection by the hepatitis B and D viruses, or can be drug induced. **Toxin- or drug-induced liver injury is the cause of the majority of cases of acute liver failure** and may be due to direct toxic effects of substances on the liver parenchyma (acetaminophen, *Amanita phalloides*), or due to idiosyncratic reactions of medications (halothane, isoniazid, phenytoin). Direct toxic effects are predictable and dose dependent, but idiosyncratic reactions are not.

Acute hepatic failure is characterized by rapid progression of encephalopathy from confusion or somnolence to coma. Patients also have worsening coagulopathy as measured by increasing prothrombin times, rising bilirubin levels, ascites and peripheral edema, hypoglycemia, hyperammonemia, and lactic acidosis. Fulminant hepatitis failure carries a poor prognosis (the mortality for comatose patients is 80%) and often is fatal without an emergent liver transplant.

Diagnosis Clinical presentation does not reliably distinguish a specific viral etiology, so serologic studies are used to establish a diagnosis. Anti-hepatitis A immunoglobulin M (IgM) establishes an acute hepatitis A infection. Anti-hepatitis C antibody is present in acute hepatitis C, but the test result may be negative for several weeks. The hepatitis C RNA assay, which becomes positive earlier in the disease course, often aids in the diagnosis. Acute hepatitis B infection is diagnosed by the presence of hepatitis B surface antigen (HBsAg) in the clinical context of elevated serum transaminase levels and jaundice. HBsAg later disappears when the antibody (anti-HBs) is produced (Figure 26–2). There is often an interval of a few weeks between the disappearance of HBsAg and the appearance of anti-HBsAb. This period is referred to as the "window period." During this interval, the presence of anti-hepatitis B core antigen IgM (anti-HBc IgM) is indicative of an acute hepatitis B infection. Hepatitis B precore antigen (HBeAg) represents a high level of viral replication and high infectivity. It is almost always present during acute infection, but its persistence after 6 weeks of illness is a sign of chronic infection and high infectivity. Persistence of HBsAg or HBeAg is a marker for chronic hepatitis or a chronic carrier state; elevated versus normal serum transaminase levels distinguish between these two entities, respectively. Patients who have been vaccinated against hepatitis B will have a positive HBsAb, but no other positive serology.

Prevention The efficacy of the hepatitis A vaccine (available in two doses given 6 months apart) exceeds 90%. It is indicated for individuals planning to travel to endemic areas. Postexposure prophylaxis with hepatitis A immunoglobulin, along with the first injection of the vaccine, should be given to household and intimate contacts within 2 weeks of exposure. The hepatitis B vaccine (given in three doses over 6 months) provides effective immunity in more than 90% of patients. It is recommended for health care workers, as well as for universal

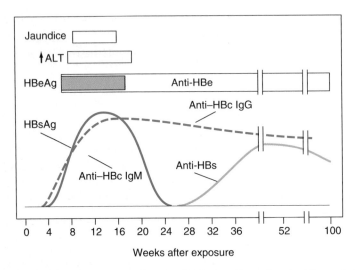

Figure 26–2. Serologic markers in acute hepatitis B infection. (Reproduced, with permission, from Deinstag JL, Isselbacher KJ. Acute viral hepatitis. In: Braunwald E, Fauci AS, Kasper DL, et al, eds. *Harrison's Principles of Internal Medicine,* 16th ed. New York: McGraw-Hill, 2005:1825.)

vaccination of infants in the United States. Hepatitis B immunoglobulin (HBIg) is given after exposure, such as a needle-stick injury from an infected patient, or to newborns of infected mothers. The first inoculation of the vaccine usually is given concurrently. There is no immunization and no proven postexposure prophylaxis for persons exposed to hepatitis C. Interferon and lamivudine are used to treat patients with chronic hepatitis B. Patients with chronic hepatitis C can be treated with peginterferon or ribavirin, and a protease inhibitor (boceprevir or telaprevir) is added if they have genotype I. Two newer treatments are Food and Drug Administration (FDA) approved for treatment of chronic viral hepatitis C: sofosbuvir (a nucleotide analog inhibitor of the hepatitis C virus) and simeprevir (a protease inhibitor specific to proteins on the hepatitis C virus) when used in combination therapy.

Acetaminophen Hepatitis

Acetaminophen-induced hepatocellular injury may result after a single, large ingestion, as in a suicide attempt, or by chronic use of over-the-counter acetaminophen-containing preparations for treatment of pain or fever. **Hepatic toxicity** most often occurs after an acute ingestion of **10 g or more**, but lower doses (4 g in 24 hours) may cause injury in patients with preexisting liver disease, particularly in those who abuse alcohol. Acetaminophen is metabolized in the liver by the cytochrome P450 enzyme system, which produces a toxic metabolite; this metabolite is detoxified by binding to glutathione. Potential hepatic injury is greater when P450 activity is augmented by drugs such as ethanol or phenobarbital, or when less glutathione is available, as in alcoholism, malnutrition, or acquired immunodeficiency syndrome (AIDS). Acetaminophen levels are measured between 4 and 24 hours after an acute ingestion and plotted on a **nomogram** to predict possible hepatotoxicity and determine if treatment is necessary (Figure 26–1). Sometimes, empiric therapy is started even before laboratory results return.

If acetaminophen levels are above the level that predisposes to hepatic injury, treatment is started with gastric decontamination with charcoal and administration of **N-acetylcysteine**, which provides cysteine to replenish glutathione stores. N-acetylcysteine should be started within the first 10 hours to prevent liver damage and is continued for 72 hours. Meanwhile, the patient should not receive any medications that are known to be hepatotoxic.

CASE CORRELATION

- See also Case 24 (Cirrhosis) and Case 27 (Painless Jaundice).

COMPREHENSION QUESTIONS

26.1 A 25-year-old medical student is stuck with a hollow needle during a procedure performed on a patient known to have hepatitis B and C viral infection, but who is HIV negative. The student's baseline laboratory studies include serology: HBsAg negative, anti-HBsAb positive, anti-HBc IgG negative. Which of the following regarding this medical student's hepatitis status is true?

A. Prior vaccination with hepatitis B vaccine

B. Acute infection with hepatitis B virus

C. Prior infection with hepatitis B virus

D. The student was vaccinated for hepatitis B but is not immune

26.2 What postexposure prophylaxis should the student described in Question 26.1 receive?

A. HBIg

B. Oral lamivudine

C. Intravenous immunoglobulin (IVIG)

D. Reassurance

26.3 In a suicide attempt, an 18-year-old woman took 4 g of acetaminophen, approximately 8 hours previously. Her acetaminophen level is 30 μg/mL. Which of the following is the best next step to be performed for this patient?

A. Immediately start N-acetylcysteine

B. Observation

C. Alkalinize the urine

D. Administer intravenous activated charcoal

ANSWERS

26.1 **A.** This student's serology is most consistent with vaccination and not prior infection. Like all health care workers, the student should have been vaccinated against the hepatitis B virus, which induces anti-HBs IgG antibody, which is thought to be protective. Not all people receiving the vaccine develop an adequate antibody titer; if none were detected, it would indicate the need for revaccination. Patients with prior hepatitis B infection will also likely have anti-HBsAb but will also have anti-HBc IgG. Acute infection would be signified by the presence of either HBsAg or anti-HBc IgM.

26.2 **D.** No postexposure prophylaxis is definitively indicated. The student has detectable protective antibody levels against the hepatitis B virus, and if the levels are judged to be adequate, the student is protected against infection. Oral lamivudine is a treatment for chronic hepatitis B infection and is part of an antiretroviral prophylaxis if the patient was HIV positive. There is no effective prophylaxis for hepatitis C exposure.

26.3 **B.** The serum acetaminophen level of 30 μg/mL, with last ingestion 8 hours previously, is plotted on the nomogram and falls below the "danger zone" of possible hepatic injury. Thus, this patient should be observed. Sometimes, patients will take more than one medication so that serum and/or urine drug testing may be worthwhile. Gastrointestinal activated charcoal, not intravenous charcoal, is used for other ingestions.

CLINICAL PEARLS

▶ The most common cause of acute hepatic failure is toxin or drug injury, which may be due to direct toxic effects or idiosyncratic reaction.

▶ The likelihood of toxic acetaminophen injury and the need for treatment can be predicted from a nomogram based on serum level and the time since last ingestion.

▶ The large majority of adults with acute hepatitis B viral infection recover completely, but 5% to 10% develop chronic hepatitis.

▶ Vaccination for hepatitis B should produce measurable HBsAb. Presence of anti-HBc IgG indicates evidence of prior infection. Anti-HBc IgM can be positive during the "window period" of acute infection.

▶ Prevention of hepatitis B viral infection hinges on long-term immunity with a highly effective recombinant vaccine or postexposure prophylaxis with HBIg. There is no postexposure prophylaxis or vaccine for hepatitis C.

REFERENCES

Bass NM. Toxic and drug-induced liver disease. In: Cecil RL, Bennett JC, Goldman L, eds. *Cecil's Textbook of Medicine*. 21st ed. Philadelphia, PA: WB Saunders; 2000:781-782.

Chopp S, Vanderwall R, Hult A, Klepser M. Simeprevir and sofosbuvir for treatment of hepatitis C infection. *Am J Health Syst Pharm*. 2015;17:1445-1455.

Deinstag JL. Acute viral hepatitis. In: Longo DL, Fauci AS, Kasper, DL, et al., eds. *Harrison's Principles of Internal Medicine*. 18th ed. New York, NY: McGraw-Hill; 2012:2357-2557.

Dienstag JL. Toxic and drug-induced hepatitis. In: Longo DL, Fauci AS, Kasper, DL, et al., eds. *Harrison's Principles of Internal Medicine*. 18th ed. New York, NY: McGraw-Hill; 2012:2558-2566.

Lawitz E, Mangia A, Wyles D, et al. Sofosbuvir for previously untreated chronic hepatitis C infection. *N Engl J Med*. 2013;368:1878-1887.

Luis S, Marsano MD. Hepatitis. *Prim Care Clin Office Pract*. 2003;30:81-107.

A 57-year-old man comes to the clinic complaining of malaise for several weeks. He says that he has not been feeling well for some time, with fatigue, depressed mood, loss of appetite, and a 20-lb unintentional weight loss. In addition, he has been bothered by generalized itching of his skin and has tried moisturizing lotions and creams without improvement. He denies fevers, abdominal pain, nausea, vomiting, or diarrhea. He does think his stools have been lighter in color recently. He has no other medical history and takes no medications except for a multivitamin. He drinks alcohol occasionally and smokes cigars.

On examination, he is afebrile, with heart rate 68 bpm and blood pressure 128/74 mm Hg. He has a flat affect and a somewhat disheveled appearance. He has noticeable icterus of his sclera and skin. His chest is clear, and his heart rhythm is regular without murmurs. His abdomen is soft and nontender with active bowel sounds, a liver span of 10 cm, and no splenomegaly or masses. His skin has a few excoriations on his arms and back, but no rashes or telangiectasias.

Blood is obtained for laboratory analysis; the results are available the next day. His serum albumin is 3.1 g/dL, alkaline phosphatase 588 IU/L, total bilirubin 8.5 mg/dL, direct bilirubin 6 mg/dL, alanine aminotransferase (ALT) 175 IU/L, and aspartate aminotransferase (AST) 140 IU/L. His hemoglobin level is 13.5 g/dL. Prothrombin time (PT) is 15 seconds, and partial thromboplastin time (PTT) is 32 seconds.

▶ What is the most likely diagnosis?
▶ What is the next step?

ANSWERS TO CASE 27:

Painless Jaundice, Pancreatic Cancer

Summary: A 57-year-old man presents with pruritus, weight loss, and light-colored stools. He is found to be jaundiced with markedly elevated alkaline phosphatase level and conjugated hyperbilirubinemia. All of these findings point toward cholestasis. The light-colored, or acholic, stools suggest the cholestasis is most likely caused by biliary obstruction. The absence of abdominal pain makes gallstone disease less likely.

- **Most likely diagnosis:** Biliary obstruction, most likely caused by malignancy.

- **Next step:** Imaging procedure of his biliary system, either ultrasonography or computed tomographic (CT) scan.

ANALYSIS

Objectives

1. Know the causes and evaluation of a patient with unconjugated hyperbilirubinemia.

2. For a patient with conjugated hyperbilirubinemia, be able to distinguish between hepatocellular disease and biliary obstruction.

3. Understand the evaluation of a patient with cholestasis.

4. Know the treatment and complications of biliary obstruction.

Considerations

In patients with jaundice, one must try to distinguish between hepatocellular and biliary disease. In the patient with suspected biliary obstruction, without the pain typically associated with gallstones, one should be suspicious of malignancy or strictures. In the case presented, the clinical picture is worrisome for a malignant cause of biliary obstruction, such as pancreatic cancer.

APPROACH TO:

Painless Jaundice

DEFINITIONS

CHOLESTASIS: Deficient bile flow that can result from intrahepatic disease or extrahepatic obstruction.

CONJUGATED BILIRUBIN (DIRECT-REACTING BILIRUBIN): Bilirubin that has entered the liver and has been enzymatically bound to glucuronic acid forming bilirubin monoglucuronide or diglucuronide.

JAUNDICE OR ICTERUS: Yellowing of the skin or whites of the eyes, indicating hyperbilirubinemia.

UNCONJUGATED BILIRUBIN (INDIRECT-REACTING BILIRUBIN): Bilirubin that has not been enzymatically bound to glucuronic acid by the liver and is in the serum reversibly and noncovalently bound to albumin.

CLINICAL APPROACH

Jaundice, or icterus, is the visible manifestation of **hyperbilirubinemia** and usually can be noticed by physical examination when the serum bilirubin level exceeds 2.0 to 2.5 mg/dL. Traditional instruction regarding the jaundiced patient divides the mechanism of hyperbilirubinemia into prehepatic (excessive production of bilirubin), intrahepatic, or extrahepatic (as in biliary obstruction). For most patients with jaundice, it probably is more clinically useful to think about hepatic or biliary diseases that cause conjugated (direct) hyperbilirubinemia, because they represent the most clinically important causes of jaundice.

The term **unconjugated (indirect) hyperbilirubinemia** is used when the conjugated (or direct-reacting fraction) does not exceed 15% of the total bilirubin. It is almost always caused by hemolysis or Gilbert syndrome. In these conditions, the serum bilirubin level almost always is less than 5 mg/dL, and there are usually no other clinical signs of liver disease. In addition, there should be no bilirubinuria (only conjugated bilirubin can be filtered and renally excreted). **Hemolysis** usually is clinically apparent, as in sickle cell disease or autoimmune hemolytic anemia. **Gilbert syndrome** is a benign condition caused by a deficiency of hepatic enzymatic conjugation of bilirubin, which results in intermittent unconjugated hyperbilirubinemia. Total bilirubin is usually less than 4 g/dL, and is often precipitated by events such as stress, fasting, and febrile illnesses. It is not associated with liver dysfunction and requires no therapy.

Conjugated (direct) hyperbilirubinemia almost always reflects either hepatocellular disease or biliary obstruction. These two conditions can be differentiated by the pattern of elevation of the liver enzymes. Elevation of serum AST and ALT levels is characteristic of hepatocellular disease as a result of the inflammation/destruction of the hepatocytes and the release of these enzymes into the blood. The serum alkaline phosphatase level is elevated in cholestatic disease as a consequence of inflammation, destruction, or obstruction of the intrahepatic or extrahepatic bile ducts with relative sparing of the hepatocytes. The serum AST and ALT levels may be mildly elevated in cholestasis but usually not to the levels seen in primary acute hepatocellular disease. Other tests, such as serum albumin or PT, generally reflect the capacity of hepatocytes to synthesize proteins such as clotting factors. When they are abnormal, they most often reflect hepatocellular disease. Table 27–1 summarizes the liver test patterns seen in various categories of hepatobiliary disorders.

The patient discussed in this case has a pattern consistent with cholestasis, and the **first diagnostic test in a patient with cholestasis usually is an ultrasound.** It is noninvasive and is very sensitive for detecting stones in the gallbladder as well as intrahepatic or extrahepatic biliary ductal dilation. The **most common cause of biliary obstruction in the United States is gallstones**, which may become lodged in the

Table 27–1 • LABORATORY FINDINGS IN HEPATOBILIARY DISORDERS

Type of Disorder	Bilirubin	Aminotransferases	Alkaline Phosphatase	Albumin	Prothrombin Time
Hemolysis/Gilbert syndrome	Normal to 5 mg/dL; 85% due to indirect fractions. No bilirubinuria.	Normal	Normal	Normal	Normal
Acute hepatocellular necrosis (viral and drug hepatitis, hepatotoxins, acute heart failure)	Both fractions may be elevated. Peak usually follows aminotransferases. Bilirubinuria.	Elevated, often >500 IU/L; ALT > AST	Normal to <3 times normal elevation	Normal	Usually normal. If >5 times above control and not corrected by vitamin K, suggests poor prognosis
Chronic hepatocellular disease (ie, cirrhosis, cancer)	Both fractions may be elevated. Bilirubinuria.	Elevated, but usually <300 IU/L	Normal to<3 times normal elevation	Often decreased	Often prolonged; fails to correct with parenteral vitamin K
Intra- and extrahepatic cholestasis (obstructive jaundice)	Both fractions may be elevated. Bilirubinuria.	Normal to moderate elevation, rarely >500 IU/L	Elevated, often >4 times normal elevation	Normal, unless chronic	Normal; if prolonged, will correct with parenteral vitamin K
Infiltrative diseases (tumor, granulomata): partial bile duct obstruction	Usually normal.	Normal to slight elevation	Elevated, often >4 times normal elevation fractionate, or confirm liver origin with 5′-nucleotidase, or gamma-glutamyl transpeptidase	Normal	Normal

(Reproduced, with permission, from Braunwald E, Fauci AS, Kasper KL, et al, eds. Harrison's Principles of Internal Medicine, 17th ed. New York: McGraw-Hill, 2008:1926.)

common bile duct. However, obstructing stones causing jaundice usually are associated with epigastric or right upper quadrant colicky pain. Extrahepatic dilatation without evidence of stones warrants further study with CT or endoscopic retrograde cholangiopancreatography (ERCP) to detect occult stones or strictures, and to exclude malignant causes of common bile duct and pancreatic duct obstruction including cholangiocarcinoma, pancreatic cancer, and ampullary cancer (ampulla of Vater).

Other possible causes include strictures, which can result from prior biliary surgery, prior inflammatory conditions such as pancreatitis (rarely), inflammatory diseases of the biliary tree, and infection in the setting of acquired immunodeficiency syndrome (AIDS). Two important primary biliary conditions are **primary sclerosing cholangitis** and **primary biliary cirrhosis**. Table 27–2 compares features of these two entities.

The complications of biliary obstruction include development of acute cholangitis as a result of ascending infection, or secondary hepatic cirrhosis, if the obstruction is chronic or recurrent. The patient in this case scenario has painless jaundice, liver enzymes consistent with a cholestatic process, and light-colored stools, suggesting obstruction of bile flow into the intestine. Because he has no history of abdominal or biliary surgery that might have caused a stricture, malignancy is the most likely cause of his biliary obstruction. The most common malignancy to present in this way is **pancreatic cancer**. The patient should undergo an imaging procedure of his abdomen, including a right upper quadrant ultrasound to evaluate the biliary tree, as well as a **CT scan** or magnetic resonance imaging (MRI) to visualize the pancreas. Endoscopic ultrasound with fine-needle aspiration of the pancreas is highly accurate in establishing a tissue diagnosis.

Pancreatic cancer is the fifth leading cause of cancer death in the United States. Peak incidence is in the seventh decade of life, with two-thirds of cases occurring in persons older than 65 years. The median survival is 9 months, with an overall 5-year survival rate of 3%. Clinically apparent metastatic disease is found in 80% of patients at the time of diagnosis. For patients without obvious metastases, the best hope for cure is surgical resection by pancreaticoduodenectomy (Whipple procedure), which in experienced hands has a perioperative mortality rate less than 5%. Even when the cancer is considered to be resectable, there is a high rate

Table 27–2 • COMPARISON OF PRIMARY SCLEROSING CHOLANGITIS AND PRIMARY BILIARY CIRRHOSIS		
	Younger Males	**Older Females**
Disease	Primary sclerosing cholangitis	Primary biliary cirrhosis
Location of disease	Larger intra- and extrahepatic ducts	Smaller intrahepatic bile ducts
Associated conditions	Ulcerative colitis	Autoimmune diseases such as rheumatoid arthritis
Serologic markers	None	Antimitochondrial antibody (AMA)
Complications	Stricture; infection (cholangitis); cholangiocarcinoma	Cirrhosis

of recurrence; so many treatment programs include neoadjuvant chemotherapy. Palliative measures may include common bile duct stenting to relieve the biliary obstruction.

> ## CASE CORRELATION
> - See also Case 24 (Cirrhosis) and Case 26 (Acute Viral Hepatitis).

COMPREHENSION QUESTIONS

For Questions 27.1 to 27.4, choose the one diagnosis (A-F) that best matches with the most likely clinical situation.

A. Hemolysis

B. Alcoholic hepatitis

C. Gilbert disease

D. Pancreatic cancer

E. Gallstones

F. Primary sclerosing cholangitis

27.1 A 38-year-old man with a 12 pack of beer per day alcohol history presents with jaundice, ascites, and dark urine. His laboratory results are AST 350 U/mL, ALT 150 U/mL, alkaline phosphatase 120 U/mL, total bilirubin 25 mg/dL, direct bilirubin 12 mg/dL, and albumin 2.1 g/dL.

27.2 A 40-year-old moderately obese woman presents with abdominal pain after eating and mild scleral icterus. Her laboratory results are AST 200 U/L, ALT 150 U/L, alkaline phosphatase 355 U/L, total bilirubin 3.5 mg/dL, direct bilirubin 1.8 mg/dL, and albumin 3.5 g/dL.

27.3 A 25-year-old man presents with 3 days of scleral icterus but has been otherwise feeling well. His laboratory results are AST 45 U/L, ALT 48 U/L, alkaline phosphatase 100 U/L, total bilirubin 3.2 mg/dL, direct bilirubin 0.2 mg/dL, and albumin 3.5 g/dL. Complete blood count and lactate dehydrogenase (LDH) are normal.

27.4 A 32-year-old man with a 5-year history of episodic bloody diarrhea and abdominal cramping pain presents with scleral icterus and fever. His laboratory results are AST 100 U/L, ALT 125 U/L, alkaline phosphatase 550 U/L, total bilirubin 5.5 mg/dL, direct bilirubin 3.0 mg/dL, and albumin 2.9 g/dL.

ANSWERS

27.1 **B.** The patient's laboratory results show a conjugated hyperbilirubinemia with evidence of hepatocellular disease (hypoalbuminemia, ascites). The AST and ALT levels show the 2:1 ratio consistent with alcohol-related liver disease.

27.2 **E.** The patient's laboratory results show a conjugated hyperbilirubinemia consistent with an obstructive pattern. She has the risk factors for gallstones (middle age, female, obese) and has symptoms of postprandial abdominal pain.

27.3 **C.** The patient's laboratory results show an unconjugated hyperbilirubinemia without other abnormality. He is otherwise healthy without symptoms of systemic disease or hemolytic anemia. No treatment is necessary.

27.4 **F.** The patient's laboratory results show a conjugated hyperbilirubinemia with an obstructive pattern. The history is consistent with inflammatory bowel disease, which is associated with primary sclerosing cholangitis. The initial evaluation should include ultrasonography to rule out gallstones; if negative, ERCP could confirm the diagnosis by demonstrating multiple strictures of the extrahepatic bile ducts. Treatment options include stenting of the larger bile duct strictures and immunosuppression to slow the progression of the disease.

CLINICAL PEARLS

▶ Unconjugated (indirect) hyperbilirubinemia usually is caused by hemolysis or Gilbert syndrome.

▶ Conjugated (direct) hyperbilirubinemia is commonly caused by hepato-cellular disease, with elevated AST and ALT levels, or biliary obstruction, with elevated alkaline phosphatase level.

▶ An imaging procedure such as ultrasonography is the initial study of choice in a patient with cholestasis to evaluate for intrahepatic or extra-hepatic biliary obstruction.

▶ The most common causes of biliary obstruction are gallstones, which are painful if obstructing, and strictures or neoplasms, which may be painless.

▶ Pancreatic cancer is initially diagnosed and staged by CT; the best hope for cure is resection by a pancreaticoduodenectomy (Whipple procedure).

REFERENCES

Brugge WR, Dam JV. Medical progress: pancreatic and biliary endoscopy. *N Engl J Med*. 1999;341: 1808-1916.

Kosuri K, Muscarella P, Bekaii-Saab TS. Updates and controversies in the treatment of pancreatic cancer. *Clin Adv Hematol Oncol*. 2006;4:47-54.

Pratt DS. Evaluation of liver function. In: Kasper DL, Fauci AS, Hauser SL, et al., eds. *Harrison's Principles of Internal Medicine*. 19th ed. New York, NY: McGraw-Hill Education; 2015:1995-1999.

Wolkoff AW. The hyperbilirubinemias. In: Kasper DL, Fauci AS, Hauser SL, et al., eds. *Harrison's Principles of Internal Medicine*. 19th ed. New York, NY: McGraw-Hill Education; 2015:1999-2004.

A 27-year-old man presents to the outpatient clinic complaining of 2 days of facial and hand swelling. He first noticed swelling around his eyes 2 days ago, along with difficulty putting on his wedding ring because of swollen fingers. Additionally, he noticed that his urine appears reddish-brown and that he has had less urine output over the last several days. He has no significant medical history. His only medication is ibuprofen that he took 2 weeks ago for fever and a sore throat, which have since resolved. On examination, he is afebrile, with heart rate 85 bpm and blood pressure 164/98 mm Hg. He has periorbital edema; his funduscopic examination is normal without arteriovenous nicking or papilledema. His chest is clear to auscultation, his heart rhythm is regular with a nondisplaced point of maximal impulse (PMI), and he has no abdominal masses or bruits. He does have edema of his feet, hands, and face. A dipstick urinalysis in the clinic shows specific gravity of 1.025 with 3+ blood and 2+ protein, but it is otherwise negative.

► What is the most likely diagnosis?
► What is your next diagnostic step?

ANSWERS TO CASE 28:
Acute Glomerulonephritis, Poststreptococcal Infection

Summary: A 27-year-old man complains of several days of facial and hand swelling, decreased urine output, and reddish-brown urine. He took ibuprofen for fever and a sore throat 2 weeks ago. He is afebrile, hypertensive, and has periorbital edema but a normal funduscopic examination. His cardiac, pulmonary, and abdominal examinations are normal, but he does have edema of his feet, hands, and face. A dipstick urinalysis in the clinic shows hematuria and proteinuria.

- **Most likely diagnosis:** Acute glomerulonephritis (GN).

- **Next diagnostic step:** Examine a fresh spun urine specimen to look for red blood cell (RBC) casts or dysmorphic red blood cells.

ANALYSIS
Objectives

1. Be able to differentiate glomerular from nonglomerular bleeding.

2. Understand the clinical features of GN.

3. Know how to evaluate and treat a patient with GN.

4. Be familiar with the evaluation of a patient with nonglomerular hematuria.

Considerations

A young man without a significant medical history now presents with new onset of hypertension, edema, and hematuria following an upper respiratory tract infection. He has no history of renal disease, does not have manifestations of chronic hypertension, and has not received any nephrotoxins. He does not have other symptoms of inflammatory diseases such as systemic lupus erythematosus (SLE). The presentation of acute renal failure, hypertension, edema, and hematuria in a young man with no significant medical history is highly suggestive of glomerular injury (GN). He likely has acute GN, either postinfectious (streptococcal) or immunoglobulin (Ig)A nephropathy. The reddish-brown appearance of the urine could represent hematuria, which was later suggested by dipstick urinalysis (3+ blood); hence, microscopic examination of the urine for RBCs is very important. Together, the history and the examination suggest that the patient likely has acute GN, either primary GN of unknown etiology (no concomitant systemic disease is mentioned) or secondary GN as a result of recent upper respiratory infection (postinfectious GN). The next logical step in diagnosing GN should be to examine the precipitate of a freshly spun urine sample for active sediment (cellular components, red cell casts, dysmorphic red cells). If present, these are signs of inflammation and establish the diagnosis of acute GN. Although likely to be present, these markers do not distinguish among the distinct immune-mediated causes of GN; they merely allow us to make the diagnosis of acute GN (primary or secondary). Further evaluation

Table 28–1 • SEROLOGIC MARKERS OF GLOMERULONEPHRITIS
Complement levels (C3, C4): low in complement-mediated GN (SLE, MPGN, infective endocarditis, poststreptococcal/postinfectious GN, cryoglobulin-induced GN)
Antineutrophil cytoplasmic antibody levels (p-ANCA and c-ANCA): c-ANCA positive in Wegener, p-ANCA positive in microscopic polyangiitis and Churg-Strauss
ANA: positive in SLE (anti-dsDNA, anti-Smith)
Antiglomerular basement membrane (anti-GBM) antibody levels: positive in anti-GBM GN and Goodpasture
ASO titers: elevated in poststreptococcal GN
Blood cultures: positive in infective endocarditis
Cryoglobulin titers: positive in cryoglobulin-induced GN
Hepatitis serologies: hepatitis C and hepatitis B associated with cryo-induced GN

with serologic markers, such as complement levels and antistreptolysin-O (ASO) titers (Table 28–1), may help to further classify the GN.

APPROACH TO:
Suspected Glomerulonephritis

DEFINITIONS

HEMATURIA: Presence of blood in the urine.

GROSS HEMATURIA: Blood in the urine visible to the eye.

MICROSCOPIC HEMATURIA: Red blood cells in the urine that require microscopy for diagnosis.

CLINICAL APPROACH

The term *hematuria* describes the presence of blood in the urine. Although direct visualization of a urine sample (gross hematuria) or dipstick examination (positive blood) can be helpful, the **diagnosis of hematuria is made by microscopic confirmation of the presence of red blood cells** (microscopic hematuria). The first step in evaluating a patient who complains of red-dark urine is to differentiate between true hematuria (presence of RBCs in urine) and pigmented urine (red-dark urine). The breakdown products of muscle cells and red blood cells (myoglobin and hemoglobin, respectively) are heme-containing compounds capable of turning the color of urine dark red or brown in the absence of true hematuria (red blood cells). A dipstick urinalysis positive for blood without the presence of RBCs (negative microscopic cellular sediment) is suggestive of hemoglobinuria or myoglobinuria.

After confirmation, the etiology of the hematuria should be determined. **Hematuria** can be classified into two broad categories: **intrarenal and extrarenal** (Table 28–2). The history and physical examination are very helpful in the

Table 28–2 • COMMON CAUSES OF HEMATURIA
Intrarenal hematuria • Kidney trauma • Renal stones and crystals • Glomerulonephritis • Infection (pyelonephritis) • Neoplasia (renal cell carcinoma) • Vascular injury (vasculitis, renal thrombosis)
Extrarenal hematuria • Trauma (eg, Foley placement) • Infections (urethritis, prostatitis, cystitis) • Nephrolithiasis (ureteral stones) • Neoplasia (prostate, bladder)

evaluation (age, fever, pain, family history). Laboratory analysis and imaging studies often are necessary, and considering the potential clinical implications, the etiology of hematuria should be pursued in all cases. First, examination of the cellular urine sediment can help to differentiate glomerular from nonglomerular hematuria. The presence of **dysmorphic/fragmented RBCs or red cell casts** is indicative of **glomerular origin** (GN). Second, the urine Gram stain and culture can aid in the diagnosis of infectious hematuria. Third, the urine sample should be sent for cytologic evaluation when the diagnosis of malignancy is suspected. Finally, renal imaging via ultrasound or CT scan can help in the visualization of the renal parenchyma and vascular structures. Cystoscopy can be used to assess the bladder.

Glomerular Disease

Glomerular disease is encountered mainly in the form of two distinct syndromes: nephritic or nephrotic (or sometimes an overlap of the two syndromes). **Nephritis** (nephritic syndrome) is defined as an **inflammatory** renal syndrome that presents as hematuria, edema, hypertension, and a low degree of proteinuria (<1-2 g/d). **Nephrosis** (or the nephrotic syndrome) is a **noninflammatory** (no active sediment in the urine) glomerulopathy that causes heavy proteinuria. Nephrotic syndrome is distinguished by four features: (1) edema, (2) hypoalbuminemia, (3) hyperlipidemia, and (4) proteinuria (>3 g/d). Glomerular injury may result from a variety of insults and presents either as the sole clinical finding in a patient (primary renal disease) or as part of a complex syndrome of a systemic disorder (secondary glomerular disease). For the purpose of this discussion, *glomerulonephritis* includes only the inflammatory glomerulopathies.

Nephritic Syndrome

The presentation of acute renal failure with associated hypertension, hematuria, and edema is consistent with acute GN. Acute kidney injury, as manifested by a decrease in urine output and azotemia, results from impaired urine production and ineffective filtration of nitrogenous waste by the glomerulus. Common signs suggesting an inflammatory glomerular cause of renal failure (ie, acute GN) include hematuria (caused by ruptured capillaries in the glomerulus), proteinuria (caused by altered permeability of the capillary walls), edema (caused by salt and water retention), and hypertension (caused by fluid retention and disturbed renal homeostasis of blood pressure). The presence of this constellation of signs in a patient makes the diagnosis of glomerulonephritis very likely. However, it is important to note that often patients present with an overlap syndrome, sharing signs of both nephritis and nephrosis. Moreover, the presence of hematuria in itself is not pathognomonic for GN because there are multiple causes of hematuria of non-glomerular origin. Therefore, confirmation of the presumptive diagnosis of acute glomerulonephritis requires microscopic examination of a urine sample from the suspected patient. The presence of **red cell casts** (inflammatory cast) or **dysmorphic RBCs** (caused by filtration through damaged glomeruli) in a sample of spun urine establishes the diagnosis of GN.

Once the diagnosis of acute GN is made, it can be broadly classified as either *primary* (present clinically as a renal disorder) or *secondary* (renal injury caused by a systemic disease). The specific diagnosis can usually be established by clinical history and serologic evaluation, and often requires a kidney biopsy (Table 28–3).

Diagnostic Approach to Glomerulonephritis

The approach to the patient with glomerular disease should be systematic and undertaken in a stepwise fashion. The history should be approached meticulously, looking for evidence of preexisting renal disease, exposure to nephrotoxins, and especially any underlying systemic illness. Serologic markers of systemic diseases should be obtained, if indicated (Figure 28–1) in order to further classify the GN. Once the appropriate serologic tests have been reviewed, a kidney biopsy may be required. A biopsy sample can be examined under the light microscope in order to determine the primary histopathologic injury to the nephron (MPGN, crescentic GN, etc). Further examination of an immunofluorescent stained sample for immune recognition (IgG, IgA, IgM, C3, C4, or pauci-immune staining) of the affected glomerular membrane (capillary, epithelial, etc) and under electron

---

Table 28–3 • CLASSIFICATION OF GLOMERULONEPHRITIS

Primary renal disorders (based on histopathology)
Membranoproliferative glomerulonephritis (MPGN, types I and II)
Mesangioproliferative glomerulonephritis (MSGN)
Crescentic glomerulonephritis
• Immune deposit (anti-GBM)
• Pauci-immune (ANCA)
Fibrillary glomerulonephritis
Proliferative glomerulonephritis (IgA nephropathy)

Secondary renal disorders (based on clinical presentation)
Lupus nephritis
Postinfectious glomerulonephritis (poststreptococcal GN)
Hepatitis C/hepatitis B-related glomerulonephritis (cryo-GN)
Vasculitis-related glomerulonephritis (Wegener, Churg-Strauss, polyarteritis nodosa, microscopic polyangiitis, Henoch-Schönlein purpura)
Infective endocarditis-related glomerulonephritis

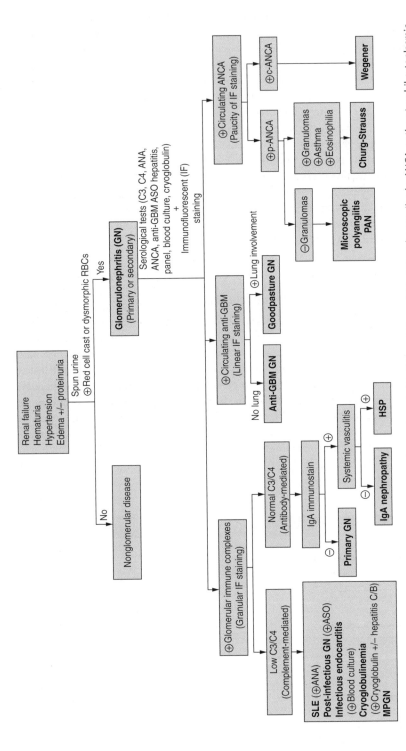

Figure 28–1. Algorithm of approach to the patient with acute glomerulonephritis. Abbreviations: ANA, antinuclear antibody; ANCA, antineutrophil cytoplasmic antibody; ASO, antistreptolysin-O; c-ANCA, cytoplasmic antineutrophil cytoplasmic antibody; GBM, glomerular basement membrane; HSP, Henoch–Schönlein purpura; MPGN, membranoproliferative glomerulonephritis; PAN, periarteritis nodosa; p-ANCA, perinuclear antineutrophil cytoplasmic antibody; SLE, systemic lupus erythematosus.

microscopy for characteristic patterns of immune deposition (granular, linear GN) may provide a definitive diagnosis of the immune-mediated injury to the glomeruli. Figure 28–1 shows an algorithmic approach to the patient with acute GN.

A common clinical scenario is to distinguish between **postinfectious (usually streptococcal) GN** versus **IgA nephropathy.** Both illnesses can present with GN occurring after an upper respiratory illness. The history can sometimes provide a clue. In poststreptococcal GN (PSGN), the glomerulonephritis typically does not set in until several weeks after the initial infection. In contrast, IgA nephropathy may present with pharyngitis and glomerulonephritis at the same time. In addition, PSGN classically presents with hypocomplementemia, and if the patient undergoes a renal biopsy there is evidence of an immune complex-mediated process. In contrast, IgA nephropathy has normal complement levels and negative ASO titer (IgA levels may be elevated in about a third of patients, but this is nonspecific) and the renal biopsy will show mesangial IgA.

Treatment of Glomerulonephritis

Treatment depends on the diagnosis of the glomerulonephritis, whether it is a primary renal disease or secondary to a systemic illness. When appropriate, the underlying disease should be treated (infective endocarditis, hepatitis, SLE, or vasculitis). The use of steroids and cyclophosphamide has been advocated in the treatment of antineutrophil cytoplasmic antibody (ANCA)-induced GN, while other antibody-mediated GNs might require plasmapheresis in order to eliminate the inciting antibody–immune complex. Treatment for poststreptococcal GN is usually supportive, with control of hypertension and edema, with a very good prognosis. There is no clearly defined treatment for IgA nephropathy, although angiotensin-converting enzyme (ACE) inhibitors, fish oils, and steroids have all been used.

> ## CASE CORRELATION
>
> • See also Case 29 (Nephrotic Syndrome) and Case 30 (Acute Renal Failure).

COMPREHENSION QUESTIONS

28.1 An 18-year-old marathon runner has been training during the summer. He is brought to the emergency room disoriented after collapsing on the track. His temperature is 102°F. A Foley catheter is placed and reveals reddish urine with 3+ blood on dipstick and no cells seen microscopically. Which of the following is the most likely explanation for his urine?

    A.   Underlying renal disease

    B.   Prerenal azotemia

    C.   Myoglobinuria

    D.   Glomerulonephritis

28.2 Which of the following laboratory findings is most consistent with post-streptococcal glomerulonephritis?

A. Elevated serum complement levels

B. Positive antinuclear antibody titers

C. Elevated ASO titers

D. Positive blood cultures

E. Positive cryoglobulin titers

28.3 A 22-year-old man complains of acute hemoptysis over the past week. He denies smoking or pulmonary disease. His blood pressure is 130/70 mm Hg, and his physical examination is normal. His urinalysis also shows microscopic hematuria and red blood cell casts. Which of the following is the most likely etiology?

A. Metastatic renal cell carcinoma to the lungs

B. Acute tuberculosis of the kidneys and lungs

C. Systemic lupus erythematosus

D. Goodpasture disease (antiglomerular basement membrane)

ANSWERS

28.1 **C.** This individual is suffering from heat exhaustion, which can lead to rhabdomyolysis and release of myoglobin. Myoglobinuria leads to a reddish appearance and positive urine dipstick reaction for blood, but microscopic analysis of the urine likely will demonstrate no red cells.

28.2 **C.** The antistreptolysin-O titers typically are elevated and serum complement levels are decreased in poststreptococcal GN. Answer B would be more likely to be seen in a patient with Lupus Nephritis along with decreased complement levels (C3 and C4). Answer D is more likely in a patient with glomerulonephritis secondary to endocarditis where valvular disease would also be present. Answer E is appropriate for glomerulonephritis secondary to cryoglobulinemia where the patient is also likely to test positive for Hepatitis C.

28.3 **D.** Goodpasture (antiglomerular basement membrane) disease typically affects young males, who present with hemoptysis and hematuria. Antibody against type IV collagen, expressed in the pulmonary alveolar and glomerular basement membrane, leads to the pulmonary and renal manifestations. Wegener granulomatosis typically affects older adults, and includes more systemic symptoms such as arthralgias, myalgias, and sinonasal symptoms, and these patients are positive for ANCA.

CLINICAL PEARLS

▶ Finding red blood cell casts or dysmorphic red blood cells on urinalysis differentiates glomerular bleeding (eg, glomerulonephritis) from non-glomerular bleeding (eg, kidney stones).

▶ Glomerulonephritis is characterized by hematuria, edema, and hypertension caused by volume retention.

▶ Gross hematuria following an upper respiratory illness suggests either immunoglobulin A nephropathy or poststreptococcal glomerulonephritis.

▶ Patients with nonglomerular hematuria and no evidence of infection should undergo investigation with imaging (ultrasound or intravenous pyelogram) or cystoscopy to evaluate for stones or malignancy.

REFERENCES

Hricik DE, Chung-Park M, Sedor JR, et al. Glomerulonephritis. *N Engl J Med*. 1998;339:888-899.

Johnson RJ, Freehally J, eds. *Comprehensive Clinical Nephrology*. St. Louis, MO: CV Mosby; 2000.

Lewis JB, Neilson EG. Glomerular diseases. In: Longo DL, Fauci AS, Kasper DL, et al., eds. *Harrison's Principles of Internal Medicine*. 18th ed. New York, NY: McGraw-Hill Education; 2012:2334-2354.

A 58-year-old Hispanic woman presents to your office complaining of persistent swelling of her feet and ankles, so much so that she cannot put on her shoes. She first noted mild ankle swelling approximately 2 to 3 months ago. She borrowed a few diuretic pills from a friend; the pills seemed to help, but now she has run out. She also reports that she has gained 20 to 25 lb over the last few months, despite regular exercise and trying to adhere to a healthy diet. Her medical history is significant for type 2 diabetes, for which she takes a sulfonylurea agent. She neither sees a doctor regularly nor monitors her blood glucose at home. She denies dysuria, urinary frequency, or urgency, but she does report that her urine has appeared foamy. She had no fevers, joint pain, skin rashes, or gastrointestinal (GI) symptoms.

Her physical examination is significant for mild periorbital edema, multiple hard exudates, and dot hemorrhages on funduscopic examination, and pitting edema of her hands, feet, and legs. Her chest is clear, her heart rhythm is regular without murmurs, and her abdominal examination is benign. She has diminished sensation to light touch in her feet and legs to mid-calf. A urine dipstick performed in the office shows 2+ glucose, 3+ protein, and negative leukocyte esterase, nitrates, and blood.

▶ What is the most likely diagnosis?
▶ What is the best intervention to slow disease progression?

ANSWERS TO CASE 29:

Nephrotic Syndrome, Diabetic Nephropathy

Summary: A 58-year-old woman with long-standing diabetes now presents with edema and significant proteinuria on a urine dipstick. She has diabetic retinopathy, some peripheral neuropathy, and no other findings suggestive of any other systemic disease.

- **Most likely diagnosis:** Nephrotic syndrome as a consequence of diabetic nephropathy

- **Best intervention:** Angiotensin inhibition with either an angiotensin-converting enzyme (ACE) inhibitor or angiotensin receptor blocker (ARB)

ANALYSIS

Objectives

1. Recognize the clinical features and complications of nephrotic syndrome.

2. Know the most common causes of nephrotic syndrome.

3. Understand the natural history of diabetic renal disease and how to diagnose and manage it.

4. Learn the principles of treatment of nephrotic syndrome.

Considerations

Patients develop significant proteinuria as a result of glomerular damage, which can result from many systemic diseases. It is important to screen for diseases such as human immunodeficiency virus (HIV), autoimmune diseases, and malignancy by history, physical examination, and sometimes laboratory investigation to determine the underlying cause and appropriate treatment of the renal manifestations.

APPROACH TO:

Nephrotic Syndrome

DEFINITION

NEPHROTIC SYNDROME: Urine protein excretion more than 3.5 g over 24 hours, serum hypoalbuminemia (<3 g/dL), hyperlipidemia, and edema.

CLINICAL APPROACH

Normally, the kidneys do not excrete appreciable amounts of protein (<150 mg/d) because serum proteins are excluded from the urine by the glomerular filter both by their large size and their net negative charge. Thus, the appearance of significant proteinuria heralds glomerular disease, with disruption of its normal barrier function. Proteinuria in excess of 3 to 3.5 g of protein per day is considered to be in the nephrotic range. The key feature of nephrotic syndrome is the heavy proteinuria, which leads to loss of albumin and other serum proteins. The hypoalbuminemia and hypoproteinemia result in decreased intravascular oncotic pressure, leading to tissue edema that usually starts in dependent areas such as the feet but may progress to involve the face, hands, and ultimately the whole body (anasarca). Both increased synthesis and decreased clearance of lipoproteins may lead to hyperlipidemia.

Patients typically present to the doctor complaining of the edema and have the laboratory features described earlier. Urinalysis usually shows few or no cellular elements and may show waxy casts and oval fat bodies (which look similar to Maltese crosses under polarized light) if hyperlipidemia is present.

In adults, one-third of patients with nephrotic syndrome have a systemic disease that involves the kidneys, such as diabetes or lupus; the rest have a primary renal disease, with one of four pathologic lesions: minimal change disease, membranous nephropathy, focal segmental glomerulosclerosis (FSGS), or membranoproliferative glomerulonephritis (MPGN). Thus, a new diagnosis of nephrotic syndrome warrants further investigation into an underlying systemic disease. Common tests include serum glucose and glycosylated hemoglobin levels to evaluate for diabetes, antinuclear antibody (ANA) to screen for systemic lupus erythematosus (SLE), serum and urine protein electrophoresis to look for multiple myeloma or amyloidosis, and viral serologies, because HIV and hepatitis B or C can cause nephrosis. Less common causes include various cancers, medications such as nonsteroidal anti-inflammatory drugs (NSAIDs), heavy metals such as mercury, and hereditary renal conditions. Of these causes, diabetes mellitus is by far the most common, as in the patient presented in this scenario.

Adults with nephrotic syndrome usually undergo renal biopsy, especially if the underlying diagnosis is unclear, or if there is a possibility of a treatable or reversible condition. Patients with advanced diabetes who have heavy proteinuria and microvascular disease, such as retinopathy, but no active cellular components on a urinary sediment are generally presumed to have diabetic nephropathy. These patients typically do not undergo renal biopsy because the nephrotic proteinuria represents irreversible glomerular damage.

Treatment of nephrotic syndrome consists of treatment of the underlying disease, if present, as well as management of the edema and attempts to limit the progression of the renal disease. For edema, all patients require strict **salt restriction**, but most patients will also need **diuretics**. Because both thiazide and loop diuretics are highly protein bound, there is reduced delivery to the kidney, and often very large doses are required to manage the edema. **Dietary protein restriction** usually is recommended for patients with moderate proteinuria and chronic kidney disease, and is thought to protect against the progression of glomerular scarring.

Besides the edema, patients with nephrotic syndrome have other consequences of renal protein wasting. They have **decreased levels of antithrombin III and proteins C and S,** and often are **hypercoagulable**, with formation of venous thromboembolism, including renal vein thrombosis. Patients with evidence of thrombus formation require anticoagulation, often for life. Other complications include hypogammaglobulinemia with **increased infection risk** (especially pneumococcal infection), iron deficiency anemia caused by hypotransferrinemia, and vitamin D deficiency because of loss of vitamin D–binding protein.

In the progression of diabetic nephropathy, initially the glomerular filtration rate (GFR) is elevated and then declines over time. Prior to the decline in GFR, the earliest stages of diabetic nephropathy can be detected as **microalbuminuria.** This is defined as a urine albumin excretion between 30 and 300 mg/d. It is possible to measure this in a random urine sample rather than a timed collection, because a ratio of albumin (in milligrams) to creatinine (in grams) of 30 to 300 usually correlates with the total excretion described. When albuminuria exceeds 300 mg/d, it is detectable on ordinary urine dipsticks (macroalbuminuria), and the patient is said to have **overt nephropathy.**

After the development of microalbuminuria, most patients will remain asymptomatic, but the glomerulopathy will continue to progress over the subsequent 5 to 10 years until overt nephropathy develops. At this point, many patients have some edema, and nearly all patients have developed hypertension. The presence of hypertension will markedly accelerate the decline of renal function. If left untreated, patients then progress to **end-stage renal disease** (**ESRD**), requiring dialysis or transplant, within a 5- to 15-year period.

The development of nephropathy and proteinuria is very significant because they are associated with a much higher risk for cardiovascular disease, which is the leading cause of death in patients with diabetes. By the time patients with diabetes develop ESRD and require dialysis, the average life expectancy is less than 2 years. Thus, the development of microalbuminuria in diabetic patients is extremely important because of the progressive disease it heralds.

Tight glycemic control with a **goal hemoglobin A$_{1c}$ less than 7%** has been shown to slow or prevent the progression of renal disease in patients with microalbuminuria Once macroalbuminuria has developed, however, it is not clear whether improved glycemic control affects the course of renal disease. In addition, as renal function declines, insulin requirements typically fall, and some oral medications such as sulfonylureas and metformin can be dangerous in advanced renal insufficiency.

Strict blood pressure control with a goal less than 140/90 mm Hg in all patients with diabetes is essential to slow progression. Many guidelines recommend lower goal blood pressures of less than 130/80 mm Hg in patients with diabetic nephropathy and proteinuria >500 mg/d.

Angiotensin inhibition, with either an ACE inhibitor or ARB, has been shown to reduce the progression of renal disease independent of blood pressure control by reducing intraglomerular filtration and proteinuria. If additional blood pressure control is needed, nondihydropyridine calcium channel blockers, beta-blockers, or diuretics may be added.

In addition, because cardiovascular disease is the major killer of patients with diabetes, aggressive risk factor reduction should be attempted, including smoking cessation and reduction of hypercholesterolemia. Patients with diabetes are regarded as the highest risk category, and should be treated with diet and **statins** with a goal of low-density lipoprotein (**LDL**) **cholesterol less than 100 mg/dL.** If diabetic patients are known to have atherosclerotic coronary disease, they should achieve an LDL goal of less than 70 mg/dL.

CASE CORRELATION

- See also Case 28 (Acute Glomerulonephritis) and Case 30 (Acute Renal Failure).

COMPREHENSION QUESTIONS

29.1 A 49-year-old woman with type 2 diabetes presents to your office for new-onset swelling in her legs and face. She has no other medical problems and says that at her last ophthalmologic appointment she was told that the diabetes had started to affect her eyes. She takes glyburide daily for her diabetes. Physical examination is normal except for hard exudates and dot hemorrhages on funduscopic examination, and diminished sensation up to the mid-shin bilaterally. Her blood pressure is normal. Urine analysis shows 2+ protein and 2+ glucose (otherwise negative). Which of the following is the best treatment for this patient?

   A. Have the patient return in 6 weeks and check a repeat urine analysis at that time.

   B. Start metoprolol.

   C. Change the glyburide to glipizide and have the patient return for follow-up in 6 weeks.

   D. Start lisinopril.

   E. Refer the patient to a cardiologist.

29.2 A 19-year-old man was seen at the university student health clinic a week ago complaining of pharyngitis, and now returns because he has noted discoloration of his urine. He is noted to have elevated blood pressure (178/110 mm Hg), and urinalysis reveals red blood cell (RBC) casts, dysmorphic RBCs, and 1+ proteinuria. Which of the following is the most likely diagnosis?

   A. SLE

   B. Amyloidosis

   C. Poststreptococcal glomerulonephritis

   D. HIV nephropathy

   E. Diabetic nephropathy

29.3 Which of the following is the best screening test for early diabetic nephropathy?

   A. Urine microalbuminuria

   B. Dipstick urinalysis

   C. Renal biopsy

   D. Fasting blood glucose

   E. Twenty-four-hour urine collection for creatinine clearance

29.4 A 58-year-old man with type 2 diabetes is normotensive, has no known heart disease, and has a baseline creatinine of 1.8 mg/dL. His fasting lipid profile shows triglycerides 205 mg/dL, total cholesterol 220 mg/dL, high-density lipoprotein (HDL) 35 mg/dL, and LDL 148 mg/dL. What is the most appropriate treatment?

A. Niacin

B. Low-protein diet

C. Gemfibrozil

D. Simvastatin

ANSWERS

29.1 **D.** In this patient with diabetes and nephropathy described in the clinical vignette, the benefit of an ACE inhibitor for decreasing proteinuria makes this the best choice for initial treatment. Changing from one sulfonylurea to another is of no benefit because all are equally efficacious. There is no indication for referral to a cardiologist based on the information provided in the vignette.

29.2 **C.** The patient has hypertension, and urinary sediment consistent with a nephritic rather than nephrotic syndrome (RBC casts, mild degree of proteinuria). Given his recent episode of pharyngitis, the most likely cause would be postinfectious, probably due to streptococcal infection. SLE can produce a variety of renal diseases, including both nephritic and nephrotic manifestations, but it would be unlikely in a male patient, especially without other clinical manifestations of lupus such as arthritis. Amyloidosis, diabetes, and HIV all cause renal disease, but usually produce the nephrotic syndrome (heavy proteinuria >3 g/d, edema, hypoalbuminemia).

29.3 **A.** Although a 24-hour urine collection for creatinine may be useful in assessing declining GFR, it is not the best screening test for the diagnosis of early diabetic nephropathy. In the outpatient setting, a dipstick urinalysis is readily available but will detect only patients with overt nephropathy (proteinuria >300 mg/d). Thus, a random urinary albumin/creatinine ratio of 30/300 is the best test to screen for early diabetic nephropathy. A fasting blood glucose may aid in the diagnosis of diabetes but not nephropathy. Finally, although most patients with nephrotic syndrome require a renal biopsy for diagnosis, a patient with worsening renal function who has had long-standing diabetes is assumed to have renal disease secondary to diabetic nephropathy, and the majority of these patients do not undergo a renal biopsy.

29.4 **D.** Patients with diabetes are considered at high risk for the development of coronary artery disease, and should be treated with lipid-lowering agents such as statins to achieve an LDL less than 100 mg/dL.

CLINICAL PEARLS

▶ Nephrotic syndrome is characterized by more than 3.5 g proteinuria over 24 hours, hypoalbuminemia, and edema. Often, hypercoagulability and hyperlipidemia are present.

▶ Nephrotic syndrome can be a result of a primary renal disease but is often a manifestation of a systemic disease such as diabetes, HIV infection, an autoimmune disease, or a malignancy.

▶ Patients with diabetes should be screened for microalbuminuria (albumin excretion 30-300 mg/d); if present, treatment should be initiated with an ACE inhibitor or ARB even if the patient is normotensive.

▶ Patients with diabetic nephropathy are at very high risk for cardiovascular disease, so aggressive risk factor reduction, such as use of statins, is important, with a goal LDL less than 100 mg/dL.

REFERENCES

Bargman JM, Skorecki K. Chronic kidney disease. In: Kasper DL, Fauci AS, Hauser SL, et al., eds. *Harrison's Principles of Internal Medicine*. 19th ed. New York, NY: McGraw-Hill Education; 2015: 1811-1821.

Gross JL, de Azevedo MJ, Silveiro SP, Canani LH, Caramori ML, Zelmanovitz T. Diabetic nephropathy: diagnosis, prevention, and treatment. *Diabetes Care*. 2005;28:164-176.

Lewis JB, Neilson EG. Glomerular diseases. In: Kasper DL, Fauci AS, Hauser SL, et al., eds. *Harrison's Principles of Internal Medicine*. 19th ed. New York, NY: McGraw-Hill Education; 2015: 1831-1850.

A 54-year-old man with a history of type 2 diabetes and coronary artery disease is admitted to the coronary care unit with worsening angina and hypertension. His pain is controlled with intravenous nitroglycerin, and he is treated with aspirin, beta-blockers to lower his heart rate, and angiotensin-converting enzyme (ACE) inhibitors to lower his blood pressure. Cardiac enzymes are normal. He undergoes coronary angiography, which reveals no significant stenosis. By the next day, his urine output has diminished to 200 mL over 24 hours. Examination at that time reveals that he is afebrile, his heart rate is regular at 56 bpm, and his blood pressure is 109/65 mm Hg. His fundus reveals dot hemorrhages and hard exudates, his neck veins are flat, his chest is clear, and his heart rhythm is normal with an S_4 gallop and no murmur or friction rub. His abdomen is soft without masses or bruits. He has no peripheral edema or rashes, with normal pulses in all extremities. Current laboratory studies include Na 140 mEq/L, K 5.3 mEq/L, Cl 104 mEq/L, CO_2 19 mEq/L, and blood urea nitrogen (BUN) 69 mg/dL. His creatinine (Cr) level has risen to 2.9 mg/dL from 1.6 mg/dL on admission.

▶ What is the patient's new clinical problem?
▶ What is your next diagnostic step?

ANSWERS TO CASE 30:

Acute Kidney Injury

Summary: A 54-year-old diabetic man is receiving medical therapy consisting of oral aspirin, beta-blockers, ACE inhibitor, and intravenous nitroglycerin for treatment of his angina and hypertension. He undergoes coronary angiography, which reveals no significant stenosis. He is normotensive. His funduscopic examination shows dot hemorrhages and hard exudates, evidence of diabetic retinopathy. In this setting, the baseline elevated creatinine level on admission likely represents diabetic nephropathy as well. His creatinine level has risen to 2.9 mg/dL from 1.6 mg/dL on admission. By the next day, he has become oliguric.

- **New clinical problem:** Acute kidney injury (AKI).

- **Next step:** Urinalysis and urine chemistries to determine whether the process is prerenal or renal, or less likely postrenal.

ANALYSIS

Objectives

1. Be familiar with the common causes, evaluation, and prevention of AKI in hospitalized patients.

2. Know how to use urinalysis and serum chemistry values in the diagnostic approach of AKI so as to be able to categorize the etiology as prerenal, renal, or postrenal.

3. Be familiar with the management of hyperkalemia and indications for acute dialysis.

Considerations

A 54-year-old man with diabetes, retinopathy, and some chronic kidney disease develops AKI in the hospital, as indicated by the elevated serum creatinine level to 2.9 mg/dL and BUN of 69 mg/dL. He has undergone several medical therapies and procedures, all of which might be potentially contributory: acute lowering of his blood pressure, an ACE inhibitor, radiocontrast media, and arterial catheterization with possible atheroemboli. The mortality rate associated with critically ill patients who develop AKI is high; thus, identifying and treating the underlying etiology of this patient's kidney failure and taking measures to protect the kidneys from further damage are essential.

APPROACH TO:
Acute Renal Failure

DEFINITIONS

ACUTE KIDNEY INJURY: Abrupt decline in kidney function, measured as glomerular filtration rate (GFR). True GFR is difficult to measure, so we rely on increases in serum creatinine levels to indicate a fall in GFR. Because creatinine is both filtered and secreted by the kidneys, changes in serum creatinine concentrations always lag behind and underestimate the decline in the GFR. In other words, **by the time the serum creatinine level rises, the GFR has already fallen significantly.**

ANURIA: Less than 50 mL of urine output in 24 hours. Acute obstruction, cortical necrosis, and vascular catastrophes such as aortic dissection should be considered in the differential diagnosis.

OLIGURIA: Less than 400 mL of urine output in 24 hours. Physiologically, it is the lowest amount of urine a person on a normal diet can make if he or she is severely dehydrated and does not retain uremic waste products. **Oliguria is a poor prognostic sign in acute renal failure (ARF).** Patients with **oliguric renal failure have higher mortality rates** and less renal recovery than do patients who are nonoliguric.

UREMIA: Nonspecific symptoms of fatigue, weakness, nausea and early morning vomiting, itchiness, confusion, pericarditis, and coma attributed to the retention of waste products in renal failure but do not always correlate with the BUN level. A highly malnourished patient with renal failure may have a modestly elevated BUN and be uremic. Another patient may have a highly elevated BUN and be asymptomatic. Elevated BUN without symptoms is called **azotemia.**

CLINICAL APPROACH

The differential diagnosis of AKI proceeds from consideration of three basic pathophysiologic mechanisms: **prerenal failure, postrenal failure, and intrinsic renal failure.** Individuals with **prerenal failure** experience diminished GFR as a result of a marked **decreased renal blood perfusion** so that less glomerular filtrate is formed. Sometimes, the clinical presentation is straightforward, such as volume depletion from gastrointestinal fluid loss or hemorrhage; at other times, the presentation of patients with prerenal failure can be more confusing. For example, a patient with severe nephrotic syndrome may appear to be volume overloaded because of the massive peripheral edema present, while the effective arterial blood volume may be very low as a consequence of the severe hypoalbuminemia. Yet the mechanism of this individual's AKI is prerenal. Similarly, a patient with severe congestive heart failure may have prerenal failure because of a low cardiac ejection fraction, yet be fluid overloaded with peripheral and pulmonary edema. **The key is to assess "what the kidneys see" versus the remainder of the body.** Typically, the BUN:Cr ratio is more than 20 in prerenal failure. Medications such as aspirin, nonsteroidal anti-inflammatory drugs (NSAIDs), and ACE inhibitors can alter intrarenal blood flow

Table 30-1 • CAUSES OF PRERENAL ACUTE KIDNEY INJURY
True volume depletion
• Gastrointestinal losses
• Renal losses (diuretics)
Reduced effective arterial blood volume
• Nephrotic syndrome
• Cirrhosis with portal hypertension
• Severe burns
• Sepsis
• Systemic inflammatory response syndrome (SIRS)
Medications
• ACE inhibitors
• NSAIDs
Decreased cardiac output
• Congestive heart failure
• Pericardial tamponade

and result in prerenal failure. Table 30–1 provides an abbreviated listing of the etiologies of prerenal failure.

Postrenal failure, also referred to as obstructive nephropathy, implies **blockage of urinary flow**. The site of obstruction can be anywhere along the urinary system, including the intratubular region (crystals), ureters (stones, extrinsic compression by tumor), bladder, or urethra. By far, the most common causes of obstructive nephropathy are ureteral obstruction due to malignancy, or prostatic obstruction due to benign or malignant hypertrophy. The patient's symptoms depend on whether or not both kidneys are involved, the degree of obstruction, and the time course of the blockage. This is usually diagnosed by seeing **hydronephrosis on renal ultrasound.**

Intrinsic renal failure is caused by disorders that injure the renal glomeruli or tubules directly. These include glomerulonephritis, tubulointerstitial nephritis, and acute tubular necrosis (ATN) from either ischemia or nephrotoxic drugs. Table 30–2 lists major causes of intrinsic AKI.

Evaluation of a patient with AKI starts with a detailed history and physical examination. Does the patient have signs or symptoms of a systemic disease, such as heart failure or cirrhosis, that could cause prerenal failure? Does the patient have symptoms of a disease, such as lupus, that could cause a glomerulonephritis? Did the patient receive something in the hospital that could cause ATN, such as intravenous contrast or an aminoglycoside? While in the operating room did the patient become hypotensive from sepsis or from hemorrhage that caused ischemic ATN? Is the patient receiving an antibiotic and now has allergic interstitial nephritis? In addition to the history and physical examination, **urinalysis and measurement of urinary electrolytes** are helpful in making the diagnosis.

Urinalysis

The urine findings based on testing with reagent paper and microscopic examination help with the diagnosis of ARF (Table 30–3). In **prerenal failure**, urinalysis

Table 30–2 • CAUSES OF INTRINSIC ACUTE KIDNEY INJURY

Acute tubular necrosis
Nephrotoxic agents
• Aminoglycosides
• Radiocontrast
• Chemotherapy
Ischemic
• Hypotension
• Vascular catastrophe

Glomerulonephritis
Postinfectious
Vasculitis
Immune complex diseases (lupus, MPGN [mesangioproliferative glomerulonephritis], cryoglobulinemia)
Cholesterol emboli syndrome
Hemolytic uremic syndrome/thrombotic thrombocytopenic purpura

Tubulointerstitial nephritis
Medications (cephalosporins, methicillin, rifampin)
Infection (pyelonephritis, HIV)

usually reveals a **high specific gravity** and **normal microscopic findings.** Individuals with **postrenal failure** typically are **unable to concentrate the urine,** so the urine osmolality is equal to the serum osmolality (**isosthenuria**) and the **specific gravity is 1.010.** The **microscopic findings vary** depending on the cause of the obstruction: hematuria (crystals or stones), leukocytes (prostatic hypertrophy), or normal (extrinsic ureteral compression from a tumor). Urinalysis of various intrinsic renal disorders may be helpful. **Ischemic and nephrotoxic ATN** usually is associated with urine that is **isosthenuric,** often with **proteinuria,** and containing **"muddy brown" granular casts** on microscopy. In **glomerulonephritis,** the urine generally reveals

Table 30–3 • EVALUATION OF ACUTE RENAL FAILURE

Etiology of Renal Failure	Urinalysis	FE_{NA}	U_{NA}
Prerenal failure	Concentrated (high specific gravity) with normal sediment	<1%	<20 mEq/L
ATN	Isosthenuric with muddy brown granular casts	>1%	>20 mEq/L
Glomerulonephritis	Moderate to severe proteinuria with red blood cells and red blood cell casts	<1%	Variable
Interstitial nephritis	Mild to moderate proteinuria with red and white blood cells and white blood cell casts	>1%	>20 mEq/L
Postrenal failure	Variable depending on cause	<1% (early) >1% (later)	<20 mEq/L (early) >20 mEq/L (later)

Abbreviation: U_{Na}, urinary concentration of sodium.

moderate to severe **proteinuria,** sometimes in the nephrotic range, and **microscopic hematuria and red blood cell (RBC) casts.** Tubulointerstitial nephritis classically produces urine that is **isosthenuric** (the tubules are unable to concentrate the urine), with **mild proteinuria,** and on microscopy, reveals **leukocytes, white cell casts, and urinary eosinophils.**

Urinary Electrolytes

Measurement of urinary electrolytes and calculation of the fractional excretion of sodium (FE_{Na}) were devised to differentiate oliguric prerenal failure from oliguric ATN; they are of little use in other circumstances. FE_{Na} represents the amount of sodium filtered by the kidneys that is not reabsorbed. The **kidneys of a healthy person on a normal diet** usually reabsorb more than 99% of the sodium that is filtered, with a corresponding FE_{Na} less than **1%.** Normally, the excreted sodium represents the dietary intake of sodium, maintaining sodium homeostasis. In prerenal failure, decreased renal perfusion leads to a diminished GFR; if the renal tubular function is intact, FE_{Na} remains less than 1%. Furthermore, because the patient has either true volume depletion or "effective" volume depletion, serum aldosterone will stimulate the kidneys to retain sodium, and the urinary sodium will be low (<20 mEq/L). On the other hand, in oliguric ATN, the renal failure is caused by tubular injury. Hence, there is **tubular dysfunction** with an associated **inability to reabsorb sodium,** leading to an FE_{Na} more than **2%** and a **urinary sodium** exceeding **20 mEq/L.**

Measurements of FE_{Na} and urinary sodium are less helpful in other circumstances. For example, in nonoliguric ATN, the injury usually is less severe, so the kidneys still may maintain sodium reabsorption and be able to produce an FE_{Na} less than 1%. Diuretic medications, which interfere with sodium reabsorption, are often used in congestive heart failure or nephrotic syndrome. Although these patients may have prerenal failure, the use of diuretics will increase the urinary sodium and FE_{Na}. In acute glomerulonephritis, the kidneys often avidly resorb sodium, leading to very low urinary sodium levels and FE_{Na}. Early in the course of postobstructive renal failure caused by ureteral obstruction, the afferent arteriole typically undergoes intense vasoconstriction, with consequent, low urinary sodium levels (Table 30–3).

The **indications for dialysis** in AKI include **fluid overload, such as pulmonary edema, metabolic acidosis, hyperkalemia, uremic pericarditis, severe hyperphosphatemia, and uremic symptoms.** Because of the risk of fatal cardiac arrhythmias, severe hyperkalemia is considered an emergency, best treated acutely medically and not with dialysis. An urgent electrocardiogram (ECG) should be performed on any patient with suspected hyperkalemia; if the classic peaked or "tented" T waves are present, intravenous calcium should be administered immediately. Although it will not lower the serum potassium level, the calcium will oppose the membrane effects of the high potassium concentration on the heart, allowing time for other methods to lower the potassium level. One of the most effective methods for treating hyperkalemia is administration of intravenous insulin (usually 10 units), along with 50 to 100 mL of 50% glucose solution to prevent hypoglycemia. Insulin drives potassium into cells, lowering levels within 30 minutes. Potassium also can be driven intracellularly with a beta-agonist, such as albuterol, by nebulizer. In the presence of a severe metabolic acidosis, administration of intravenous sodium bicarbonate also promotes intracellular diffusion of potassium, albeit less effectively. All three therapies have only a transient effect on serum potassium levels, because the total body potassium balance is unchanged, and the potassium eventually leaks back out of the cells. Definitive treatment of hyperkalemia, removal of potassium from the body, is accomplished by one of three methods: (1) administration of a loop diuretic such as furosemide to increase urinary flow and excretion of potassium, or, if the patient does not make sufficient urine, (2) administration of sodium poly-styrene sulfonate (Kayexalate), a cationic exchange resin that lowers potassium by exchanging sodium for potassium in the colon, or, finally, (3) emergency dialysis.

> ## CASE CORRELATION
> - See also Case 28 (Acute Glomerulonephritis) and Case 29 (Nephrotic Syndrome).

COMPREHENSION QUESTIONS

30.1 A 63-year-old woman with a history of cervical cancer treated with hysterec-tomy and pelvic irradiation now presents with acute oliguric renal failure. On physical examination, she has normal jugular venous pressure, is normoten-sive without orthostasis, and has a benign abdominal examination. Her uri-nalysis shows a specific gravity of 1.010, with no cells or casts on microscopy. Urinary FE_{Na} is 2% and the Na level is 35 mEq/L. Which of the following is the best next step?

A. Bolus of intravenous fluids

B. Renal ultrasound

C. Computed tomographic (CT) scan of the abdomen with intravenous contrast

D. Administration of furosemide to increase her urine output

30.2 A 49-year-old man with a long-standing history of chronic renal failure as a consequence of diabetic nephropathy is brought to the emergency room for nausea, lethargy, and confusion. His physical examination is significant for an elevated jugular venous pressure, clear lung fields, and harsh systolic and diastolic sounds heard over the precordium. Serum chemistries reveal K 5.1 mEq/L, CO_2 17 mEq/L, BUN 145 mg/dL, and creatinine 9.8 mg/dL. Which of the following is the most appropriate therapy?

A. Administer IV insulin and glucose.

B. Administer IV sodium bicarbonate.

C. Administer IV furosemide.

D. Urgent hemodialysis.

30.3 A 62-year-old diabetic man underwent an abdominal aortic aneurysm repair 2 days ago. He is being treated with gentamicin for a urinary tract infection. His urine output has fallen to 300 mL over 24 hours, and his serum creatinine has risen from 1.1 mg/dL on admission to 1.9 mg/dL. Which of the following laboratory values would be most consistent with a prerenal etiology of his renal insufficiency?

A. FE_{Na} of 3%

B. Urinary sodium level of 10 mEq/L

C. Central venous pressure reading of 10 mm Hg

D. Gentamicin trough level of 4 µg/mL

ANSWERS

30.1 **B.** Renal ultrasound is the next appropriate step to assess for hydronephrosis and to evaluate for bilateral ureteral obstructions, which are common sites of metastases of cervical cancer. Her physical examination and urine studies (showing an FE >1%) are inconsistent with hypovolemia, so intravenous infusion is unlikely to improve her renal function. Use of loop diuretics may increase her urine output somewhat but does not help to diagnose the cause of her renal failure or to improve her outcome. Further imaging may be necessary after the ultrasound, but use of intravenous contrast at this point may actually worsen her renal failure.

30.2 **D.** The patient has uremia, hyperkalemia, and (likely) uremic pericarditis, which may progress to life-threatening cardiac tamponade unless the underlying renal failure is treated with dialysis. As for the other treatments, insulin plus glucose would treat hyperkalemia, and bicarbonate would help with both metabolic acidosis and hyperkalemia, but in this patient, his potassium and bicarbonate levels are only mildly abnormal and are not immediately life threatening. Furosemide will not help because he does not have pulmonary edema and has renal insufficiency.

30.3 **B.** Prerenal insufficiency connotes insufficient blood volume, typically with FE_{Na} less than 1% and urinary sodium less than 20 mEq/L. Supporting information would be a low central venous pressure reading (normal central venous pressure is 4-8 mm Hg). The gentamicin level of 4 µg/mL is elevated (normal <2 µg/mL) and may predispose to kidney damage.

CLINICAL PEARLS

▶ The two main causes of AKI in hospitalized patients are prerenal azotemia and acute tubular necrosis.

▶ In the anuric patient, one must quickly determine if the kidneys are obstructed or if the vascular supply is interrupted.

▶ Treatment of prerenal renal failure is volume replacement; treatment of postrenal failure is relief of the obstruction.

▶ The main causes of postrenal failure are obstruction caused by prostatic hypertrophy in men and bilateral ureteral obstruction caused by abdominal or pelvic malignancy in either gender.

▶ Uremic pericarditis is an indication for urgent hemodialysis. Other indications include hyperkalemia, metabolic acidosis, severe hyperphosphatemia, and volume overload when refractory to medical management.

▶ Treatment of hyperkalemia: **C BIG K** (calcium, bicarbonate/beta-agonist, insulin, glucose, Kayexalate).

▶ Hyperkalemia is treated initially with calcium to stabilize cardiac membranes; insulin and beta-agonists to redistribute potassium intracellularly (sodium bicarbonate if there is a severe metabolic acidosis); and then loop diuretics, a potassium exchange resin, or hemodialysis to remove excess potassium from the body.

▶ Indications for dialysis: **AEIOU** (acidosis, electrolyte disturbances, ingestions, overload, uremia).

REFERENCES

Lameire N, Van Biesen W, Vanholder R. Acute renal failure. *Lancet.* 2005;365:417-430.

Liu KD, Chertow GM. Acute renal failure. In: Longo DL, Fauci AS, Kasper DL, et al., eds. *Harrison's Principles of Internal Medicine.* 18th ed. New York, NY: McGraw-Hill Education; 2012:1867-1877.

Rose BD, Post TW. Hyperkalemia. In: *Clinical Physiology of Acid-Base and Electrolyte Disorders.* 5th ed. New York, NY: McGraw-Hill Education; 2001:913-919.

A 56-year-old woman presents to her doctor's office complaining of gradually progressive, nonpainful enlargement of the terminal joint on her left hand over a 9-month period. She has some stiffness with typing but not first thing in the morning. She also reports pain in her right knee, which occasionally "locks up." The right knee also hurts after long walks. On examination, her blood pressure is 130/85 mm Hg, heart rate is 80 bpm, and weight is 285 lb. Examination reveals only a nontender enlargement of her left distal interphalangeal (DIP) joint, and the right knee is noted to have crepitus and slightly decreased range of motion. There is no redness or swelling.

▶ What is your next step?
▶ What is the most likely diagnosis?
▶ What is the best initial treatment?

ANSWERS TO CASE 31:
Osteoarthritis

Summary: The patient is a 56-year-old obese woman with complaints of activity-related joint disease in the left DIP and right knee. There is no evidence of synovitis on examination.

- **Next step:** Obtain erythrocyte sedimentation rate (ESR) and plain x-rays of the hand and knee.
- **Most likely diagnosis:** Osteoarthritis (OA).
- **Best initial treatment:** NSAID or acetaminophen.

ANALYSIS
Objectives

1. Know the major clinical characteristics of OA.
2. Be familiar with management approaches to OA.
3. Understand the major classes of medications used for OA.
4. Know how to differentiate OA from inflammatory arthritis.

Considerations

This patient's history and examination are characteristic of OA. Laboratory work, typically negative for inflammatory arthritis, and x-rays will confirm the diagnosis. The most important features are the gradual onset, the lack of active synovitis, and the fact that her symptoms worsen with activity. If there were evidence of inflammation or joint effusion, then the best next step would be to aspirate the fluid from the joint and send it for various studies, including Gram stain and culture to assess for infection, crystal analysis to assess for gout or pseudogout, and cell count to assess for inflammation.

APPROACH TO:
Osteoarthritis

DEFINITIONS

BOUCHARD NODES: Bony enlargement of proximal interphalangeal (PIP) joints, often asymptomatic.

CREPITUS: A creaking or hook and loop (Velcro)-like sound made by a joint in motion, typically not painful.

HEBERDEN NODES: Bony enlargement of DIP joints, often asymptomatic.

SYNOVITIS: Inflammation of the joint space characterized by redness, swelling, and tenderness to touch.

CLINICAL APPROACH

OA is the most common joint disease in adults. It is uncommon before age 40, but highly prevalent over age 60. The disease affects women more often than men. OA begins insidiously, progresses slowly, and eventually may lead to disability, recurrent falls, inability to live independently, and significant morbidity.

Patients with OA often experience joint stiffness, which occurs with activity or after inactivity ("gel phenomena") and lasts for less than 15 to 30 minutes. This is in contrast to the morning stiffness of patients with an inflammatory arthritis, such as rheumatoid arthritis (RA), which often lasts for 1 to 2 hours and often requires warming, such as soaking in a hot tub, to improve. Early in the disease, there are no obvious findings. There may be some crepitus (creaking sound) in the joint, and, unlike inflammatory arthritis, there is often no or minimal tissue swelling (except in the most advanced disease). Bony prominences, especially in the DIP/PIP joints, can occur later. Figure 34–1 shows a typical joint involvement in OA versus RA. Pain seen in OA typically can be reproduced with passive motion of the joint. Table 31–1 lists the patterns of typical joint involvement.

Laboratory examination typically is unremarkable; inflammatory markers such as ESR, C-reactive protein, and white blood cells (WBCs) all are normal. Likewise, autoimmune studies such as antinuclear antibody (ANA), rheumatoid factor, and complement levels also are normal. If the joint is aspirated, then examination of the synovial fluid also reflects a lack of inflammation: WBCs less than $2000/mm^3$, protein less than 45 mg/dL without crystals, and glucose equal to serum. X-ray evaluation in **OA may show osteophytes that are the most specific finding in the disease but might not be found early.** Other characteristics seen on x-rays include joint space narrowing, subchondral sclerosis, and subchondral cysts.

It is critical to differentiate OA from other conditions that may present similarly. Periarticular pain that is not reproduced with passive motion suggests bursitis or tendonitis. Prolonged pain lasting for more than 1 hour points toward an inflammatory arthritis. Intense inflammation suggests one of the microcrystalline

Table 31–1 • JOINT INVOLVEMENT IN OSTEOARTHRITIS	
Joints Affected in OA	Joints Spared
Hands (often asymmetric) • DIP (Heberden nodes) • PIP (Bouchard nodes) • Carpal metacarpophalangeal (CMP) of thumb	MCP joints Wrist Elbow Shoulder
Knee, hip	
Cervical and lumbar spine	
Feet (usually first toe metatarsophalangeal joint)	

Abbreviations: DIP, distal interphalangeal; MCP, metacarpophalangeal; PIP, proximal interphalangeal.

diseases (gout/pseudogout) or infectious arthritis. Systemic constitutional symptoms, such as weight loss, fatigue, fever, anorexia, and malaise, indicate an underlying inflammatory condition, such as polymyalgia rheumatica, rheumatoid arthritis, systemic lupus erythematosus (SLE), or a malignancy, and generally demand aggressive evaluation.

Management

Education is critical. Encourage the patient to stay active, because not using the joint can cause further immobility. Multiple short periods of rest throughout the day are better than one large period. In patients with OA who are overweight, **weight loss** of even modest degree may produce improvement in lower extremity joint pain and function. Other methods of unloading an osteoarthritic joint include canes and walkers, which can reduce joint forces at the hip by as much as 50%.

Equipment such as canes and/or walkers are helpful for patients with advanced disease because these patients are less stable and, as a result, have frequent falls. Physical therapy in the form of heat applied to the affected joints in early disease often is helpful. Perhaps the most important intervention is having the patient **maintain full/near-full range of motion with regular exercise.** Physical therapy and exercise improve functional outcome and pain in OA by improving flexibility and by strengthening muscles that support the affected joints. Moist superficial heat can raise the threshold for pain, produce analgesia by acting on free nerve endings, and decrease muscle spasm.

Pharmacotherapy early in the course of the disease consists primarily of **acetaminophen**, the first line of therapy. Acetaminophen can be used on an as needed basis, or on a schedule for patients with persistent symptoms. Regular dosing of up to **3 g/d** (eg, 1000 mg every 6 hours while awake) is considered safe. Patients using this dosing should be cautioned about concurrent heavy alcohol use, which may produce higher risk of hepatotoxicity. Those taking chronic daily acetaminophen, or with any underlying liver disease, should have periodic laboratory monitoring for hepatotoxicity. **At the time of this writing, a large meta-analysis published in the Lancet in 2016 suggested that acetaminophen was ineffective in treating the pain of OA, and that NSAIDs should be considered first line.**

For patients with an inadequate response to acetaminophen, or with more severe pain can be advised to try a nonselective nonsteroidal anti-inflammatory drug (NSAID) or a cyclooxygenase 2 (COX-2) selective NSAID (commonly termed a "coxib"), which offer higher efficacy for pain relief. NSAIDs have a higher risk of gastrointestinal irritation and bleeding, and both NSAIDs and COX-2 inhibitors are associated with increased risk of adverse cardiovascular effects. Because of these risks, if NSAIDs or COX-2 inhibitors are used, they should be used in the lowest dose necessary and for the shortest period in order to achieve symptom control.

Topical medications such as diclofenac, lidocaine, or capsaicin may be considered in patients who cannot tolerate oral NSAIDs or for those at higher risk for adverse effects (eg, patients over 75 years or those with significant cardiovascular disease).

The use of glucosamine and chondroitin for OA has been controversial, and results of randomized trials have varied. Most findings suggest that glucosamine and chondroitin have little benefit in patients with osteoarthritis. There appear to be few risks associated with their use, however, so patients who wish to try those remedies can be advised that they appear to be relatively safe.

Oral steroids are generally not used to treat OA. Intra-articular steroids may be rarely useful for long-term treatment and can be helpful for the rare inflammation of a loose cartilage fragment, which may cause the joint to "lock up."

Surgery is reserved for only the most severe cases, which include patients who have major instability, a loose body in the joint, intractable pain of advanced disease, or severe functional limitation. Arthroscopic debridement is widely used for those with symptomatic OA of the knee, especially with a meniscal tear, but clinical benefit is not supported by randomized clinical trials. Total joint arthroplasty (eg, knee replacement) is recommended for patients with severe symptomatic OA, who fail to respond to optimal nonpharmacologic and medical therapy, and for whom OA causes significant impairment in quality of life.

CASE CORRELATION

- See also Case 32 (Low Back Pain), Case 33 (Acute Monoarticular Arthritis), and Case 34 (Rheumatoid Arthritis).

COMPREHENSION QUESTIONS

31.1 Which of the following is most likely to be associated with advanced OA?

A. Disability with recurrent falls and inability to live alone

B. Joints with redness and effusion

C. Best treated with oral steroids

D. Improvement throughout the day after approximately 1 to 2 hours of "unfreezing the joint"

Match the following disease processes (A-F) to the clinical setting described in Questions 31.2 to 31.5.

A. Gonococcal arthritis

B. Gout

C. Pseudogout

D. Osteoarthritis

E. Rheumatoid arthritis

F. Systemic lupus erythematosus

31.2 Symmetric bilateral ulnar deviation of both hands in a 42-year-old woman

31.3 Painful, swollen metatarsophalangeal great toe (unilateral) with redness and warmth after eating a steak and shrimp dinner in a 45-year-old man

31.4 Acute onset of unilateral elbow swelling, warmth, and tenderness and cervical discharge in a 25-year-old woman

31.5 Unilateral nontender bony enlargement of the first DIP and activity-related right hip pain in a 68-year-old woman

31.6 A 72-year-old man complains of painful joints in his hips and knees, which you have diagnosed as osteoarthritis. Which of the following is the best first medication to prescribe for this patient?

A. Naproxen sodium

B. Celecoxib

C. Oral prednisone

D. Intra-articular prednisone

E. Acetaminophen

ANSWERS

31.1 **A.** Osteoarthritis is a major cause of decreased functional status in elderly patients and requires ongoing treatment and evaluation by the physician to try to improve symptoms and to promote mobility. Oral steroids are not helpful in this condition. Joints that exhibit redness and effusion are less likely to be due OA.

31.2 **E.** Rheumatoid arthritis gives the ulnar deviation of the fingers. Other deformities associated with RA include the swan neck (MCP flexion with PIP hyperextension and DIP flexion) and boutonniere (PIP flexion, DIP hyperextension) deformities.

31.3 **B.** Gouty arthritis often affects the first metatarsophalangeal joint and can be precipitated by various foods or alcohol.

31.4 **A.** Cervical discharge and inflammatory joint are consistent with gonococcal arthritis, which can also present as a migratory arthritis.

31.5 **D.** The location and asymmetry of joint involvement, lack of inflammatory signs, and worsening with exertion all are characteristic of OA.

31.6 **E.** Acetaminophen is the first agent of choice in the treatment of early osteoarthritis.

CLINICAL PEARLS

▶ Osteoarthritis is the most common articular disease of adults, most often affecting the distal interphalangeal joints, proximal interphalangeal joints, knees, hip joints, and cervical and lumbar spine.

▶ Pain in osteoarthritis is worsened with activity and is not associated with morning stiffness.

▶ No pharmacologic agents that modify or stop disease progression are available. Treatment is aimed at symptom relief.

▶ Initial pharmacologic therapy should be acetaminophen. Joint replacement for severe osteoarthritis is reserved for patients with intractable pain despite medical therapy and for those with severe functional limitations.

REFERENCES

Felson DT. Osteoarthritis. In: Kasper DL, Fauci AS, Hauser SL, et al., eds. *Harrison's Principles of Internal Medicine*. 19th ed. New York, NY: McGraw-Hill Education; 2015:2226-2232.

Felson DT. Osteoarthritis of the knee. *N Engl J Med*. 2006;354:841-848.

Zhang W, Jones A, Doherty M. Does paracetamol (acetaminophen) reduce the pain of osteoarthritis? A meta-analysis of randomized controlled trials. *Ann Rheum Dis*. 2004;63:901-907.

An obese 45-year-old housekeeper presents with low back pain and requests an x-ray. She has had this pain off and on for several years; however, for the past 2 days it is worse than it has ever been. It started after she vigorously vacuumed a rug, is primarily on the right lower side, radiates down her posterior right thigh to her knee, but is not associated with any numbness or tingling. It is relieved by laying flat on her back with her legs slightly elevated and lessened somewhat when she takes ibuprofen 400 mg. Except for moderate obesity and difficulty maneuvering onto the examination table because of pain, her examination is fairly normal. The only abnormalities you note are a positive straight leg raise test, with raising the right leg eliciting more pain than the left. Her strength, sensation, and deep tendon reflexes in all extremities are normal.

▶ What is your diagnosis?
▶ What is your next step?

ANSWERS TO CASE 32:

Low Back Pain

Summary: An obese 45-year-old woman with acute worsening of chronic low back pain complains of shooting pain down her right leg. Her physical examination is normal.

- **Most likely diagnosis:** Musculoskeletal low back pain, possible sciatica without neurologic deficits.

- **Next step:** Encourage continuation of usual activity, avoiding twisting motions or heavy lifting. Use nonsteroidal anti-inflammatory drugs (NSAIDs) on a scheduled basis; you can also recommend muscle relaxants, although these drugs may cause sleepiness. Massage or physical therapy might be helpful. Follow up in 4 weeks. Long-term advice includes weight loss and back-strengthening exercises.

ANALYSIS

Objectives

1. Learn the history and physical examination findings that help to distinguish benign musculoskeletal low back pain from more serious causes of low back pain.

2. Understand the variety of treatment options and their effectiveness in low back pain.

3. Learn the judicious use of laboratory and imaging tests in evaluating low back pain.

Considerations

This 45 year old patient with chronic back pain has an acute exacerbation with pain radiating down her leg, which may indicate possible sciatic nerve compression. She has no other neurologic abnormalities, such as sensory deficits, motor weakness, or "red flag" symptoms of more serious etiologies of back pain, which if present would demand a more urgent evaluation. Thus, this individual has a good prognosis for recovery with conservative therapy, perhaps time being the most important factor. If she does not improve after 6 weeks, then imaging studies can be considered.

APPROACH TO:

Low Back Pain

DEFINITIONS

CAUDA EQUINA SYNDROME: Lower back pain, saddle anesthesia, and bowel or bladder dysfunction with possible lower extremity weakness and loss of reflexes caused by compression of multiple sacral nerve roots. Cauda equina syndrome is a surgical emergency.

SCIATICA: Pain in the distribution of the lumbar or sacral nerve roots, with or without motor or sensory deficits.

SPONDYLOLISTHESIS: Anterior displacement of a vertebra on the one beneath it, which can cause symptoms and signs of spinal stenosis.

SPONDYLOSIS: Osteoarthritic spine disease, typically affecting cervical and lumbosacral spine, seen radiographically as disc space narrowing and arthritic changes of the facet joints.

CLINICAL APPROACH

Low back pain is experienced by two-thirds of all adults at some point in their lives. Approximately 2% of adults miss work each year because of low back pain. This complaint is most common in adults in their working years, usually affecting patients between 30 and 60 years. Although it is common in workers required to perform lifting and twisting, it is also a common complaint in those who sit or stand for prolonged periods. Low back pain is a recurrent disease that tends to be mild in younger patients, often resolving within 2 weeks, but can be more severe and prolonged as the patient ages. It is one of the most common reasons for young adults to seek medical care, second only to upper respiratory infections, and millions of health care dollars are expended on this problem each year. In evaluating patients with low back pain, the clinician needs to exclude potentially serious conditions, such as **malignancy, infection,** and dangerous neurologic processes, such as **spinal cord compression or cauda equina syndrome.** Individuals without these conditions are initially managed with conservative therapy. Nearly all patients recover spontaneously within 4 to 6 weeks; only 3% to 5% remain disabled for more than 3 months. If patients do not improve within 4 weeks with conservative management, they should undergo further evaluation to rule out systemic or rheumatic disease and to clarify the anatomic cause, especially patients with localized pain, nocturnal pain, or sciatica.

The potential causes of back pain are numerous (Table 32–1). Pain can emanate from the bones, ligaments, muscles, or nerves. Rarely, it can be a result of referred pain from a visceral organ or other structure. Back pain with **radiation down the back of the leg** suggests **sciatic nerve root compression,** generally caused by a herniated intervertebral disk at the **L4-L5** or **L5-S1** level. Patients typically report aching pain in the buttock and paresthesias radiating into the posterior thigh and calf or lateral foreleg. When pain radiates below the knee, it is more likely to indicate a true radiculopathy than radiation only to the posterior thigh. A history of persistent leg numbness or weakness further increases the likelihood of neurologic involvement.

Most cases of back pain are idiopathic, and this group, in general, is referred to as nonspecific low back pain, which is usually of musculoskeletal origin. **In patients with back pain <4 weeks duration and no associated symptoms, imaging studies and other diagnostic tests are generally not helpful in managing these cases.** Studies show that the history and physical examination can help separate the majority of patients with simple and self-limited musculoskeletal back pain from the minority with

Table 32-1 • ETIOLOGIES OF LOW BACK PAIN	
Causes of Low Back Pain	Incidence
Musculoskeletal low back or leg pain	97%
• Lumbar sprain or strain	70%
• Degenerative disk disease	10%
• Herniated disk	4%
• Spinal stenosis	3%
• Trauma	1%
• Congenital disease, eg, kyphoscoliosis	<1%
Referred or visceral pain	2%
• Pelvic disease	
• Renal disease	
• Aortic aneurysm	
• Gastrointestinal disease	
Nonmechanical low back pain	1%
• Neoplasia	
• Infection	
• Inflammatory arthritis	
• Paget disease	

(Data from Deyo RA. Low back pain. N Engl J Med 2001;344:365.)

more serious underlying causes. Searching for "red flag" symptoms can help the physician use diagnostic tests in a more judicious manner (Table 32–2). **Malignancy should be considered in patients with systemic symptoms and who have pain at night or pain that is not relieved by lying** in a supine position. **Primary cancers** that commonly metastasize to the spine include **lung, breast, prostate, lymphoma, and gastrointestinal (GI) tumors and melanoma. Multiple myeloma** is a plasma cell neoplasm that can present with **bone pain, renal failure, and anemia.** When the patient has worrisome symptoms or signs, in most cases, the most effective initial evaluation is plain anteroposterior and lateral radiographs of the involved area of the spine, a sedimentation rate, and a complete blood count. More advanced imaging, such as magnetic resonance imaging (MRI), should be reserved for those patients for whom surgery is being considered, because it is not usually required to make most diagnoses. Another caveat to remember is that imaging studies often have abnormal findings, even in patients without low back pain, making it difficult to correlate symptoms with imaging findings.

Table 32-2 • "RED FLAG" SIGNS AND SYMPTOMS OF LOW BACK PAIN
New onset of pain in a patient older than 50 y or younger than 20 y
Fever
Unintentional weight loss
Severe nighttime pain or pain that is worse in the supine position
Bowel or bladder incontinence
History of cancer
Immunosuppression (chemotherapy or HIV)
Saddle anesthesia
Major motor weakness

It is rare that the patient can recall a precipitating event. Patients often have a history of recurrent episodes of low back pain. Psychological causes have not been consistently related to low back pain; however, there does seem to be an association with job satisfaction. During the physical examination, palpable point tenderness over the spinous processes may indicate a destructive lesion of the spine itself; in contrast, those with musculoskeletal back pain most often have tenderness in the muscular paraspinal area. Strength, sensation, and reflexes should be assessed, especially in those with complaints of radicular or radiating pain. **Straight leg raise testing,** in which the examiner holds the patient's ankle and passively elevates the patient's leg to 45°, is helpful if it elicits pain in the lower back suggesting nerve root compression. However, it is **not a very sensitive or specific test.** The Patrick maneuver, in which the patient externally rotates the hip, flexes the knee, and crosses the knee of the other leg with the ankle (like a number 4) while the examiner simultaneously presses down on the flexed knee and the opposite side of the pelvis, can help distinguish pain emanating from the sacroiliac joint.

In treating idiopathic low back pain, various modalities have been shown to be equally effective in the long run. Randomized, controlled trials have shown that encouraging the patient to continue his or her **usual activity is superior to recommendations for bed rest.** Patients without disability and without evidence of nerve root compression probably can maintain judicious activity rather than undergoing bed rest. Bed rest probably is appropriate only for individuals with severe pain or neurologic deficits. Nonsteroidal anti-inflammatory medications (on a scheduled rather than on an as-needed basis), nonaspirin analgesics, and muscle relaxants may help in the acute phase. Because most cases of disk herniation with radiculopathy resolve spontaneously within 4 to 6 weeks without surgery, these conservative measures are initial regimen recommended for these patients as well. Narcotic analgesics are also an option in cases of severe pain; however, because idiopathic low back pain is often a chronic problem, their prolonged use beyond the initial phase is discouraged. Chiropractic therapy, physical therapy, massage therapy, and acupuncture have been studied (in trials of varying quality), with results comparable to traditional approaches. **Referral** to a surgeon may be considered for those patients with radicular pain with or without neuropathy that **does not resolve with 4 to 6 weeks of conservative management.**

Patients with concerning clinical features, such as a history of malignancy, fever, or examination findings suggestive of spinal cord compression or cauda equina syndrome, should be referred for urgent imaging, either MRI or computed tomography (CT) of the spine, to evaluate for conditions such as vertebral metastases, vertebral osteomyelitis, or spinal epidural abscess that require urgent treatment.

CASE CORRELATION

- See also Case 31 (Osteoarthritis), Case 33 (Monoarticular Arthritis), and Case 34 (Rheumatoid Arthritis).

COMPREHENSION QUESTIONS

32.1 A 35-year-old obese hotel housekeeper presents with 1 week of lower back pain. Her history and examination are without "red flag" symptoms and completely normal, except for her weight. Which of the following is the best next step?

A. Regular doses of a NSAID, and activity as tolerated

B. Six weeks of bed rest

C. MRI of the lumbar spine

D. Plain film x-ray of lumbosacral spine

32.2 A 28-year-old woman from Nigeria presents with a 6-month history of persistent lower lumbar back pain, associated with a low-grade fever and night sweats. She denies any extremity weakness or human immunodeficiency virus (HIV) risk factors. Her examination is normal except for point tenderness over the spinous processes of L4-L5. Which of the following is the most likely diagnosis?

A. *Staphylococcus aureus* osteomyelitis

B. Tuberculous osteomyelitis

C. Given her age, idiopathic low back pain

D. Metastatic breast cancer

E. Multiple myeloma

32.3 A 70-year-old woman presents with a 4-week history of low back pain, generalized weakness, and a 15-lb weight loss over the last 2 months. Her medical history is unremarkable, and her examination is normal except that she is generally weak. Initial laboratory tests reveal an elevated sedimentation rate, mild anemia, creatinine level 1.8 mg/dL, and calcium level 11.2 mg/dL. Which of the following is the most likely diagnosis?

A. Osteoporosis with compression fractures

B. Renal failure with osteodystrophy

C. Multiple myeloma

D. Lumbar strain

E. Osteomyelitis

32.4 A 45-year-old man complains of decreased sensation in his buttocks and inability to achieve an erection. On examination he has decreased anal sphincter tone and decreased ankle reflexes bilaterally. Which of the following is the next best step in management?

A. Bed rest and follow-up in 4 to 6 weeks

B. Plain film x-ray of lumbosacral spine

C. Sedimentation rate and complete blood count

D. Immediate referral for advanced imaging and surgical evaluation

ANSWERS

32.1 **A.** Bed rest has not been shown to improve outcome in idiopathic low back pain compared to encouraging usual activities that do not exacerbate the pain. Imaging is not necessary with uncomplicated back pain.

32.2 **B.** The patient's country of origin, the chronic and slowly progressive nature of the pain in association with fever, and night sweats are highly suggestive of tuberculous osteomyelitis of the spine, or Pott disease. Bacterial osteomyelitis presents more acutely, often with high, spiking fevers. Metastatic breast cancer and multiple myeloma are extremely rare in this age group. The fevers, night sweats, and persistent and progressive nature of her back pain make a musculoskeletal cause unlikely.

32.3 **C.** This patient has many "red flag" symptoms in her presentation: her age, new-onset pain, and history of weight loss. The elevated calcium level and mild renal failure are suggestive of multiple myeloma. Plain radiographs of the axial and appendicular skeleton may illustrate the lytic bone lesions often seen in this disease.

32.4 **D.** This individual has cauda equina syndrome and requires immediate surgical decompression to avoid long-term nerve denervation and incontinence/lower extremity weakness.

CLINICAL PEARLS

► Acute low back pain, even with sciatic nerve involvement, resolves within 4 to 6 weeks in 90% of patients.

► Analgesics, such as nonsteroidal anti-inflammatory drugs or acetaminophen, muscle relaxants, and attempts at maintaining some level of activity are helpful in managing acute low back pain; bed rest does not help.

► Pain that interferes with sleep, significant unintentional weight loss, or fever suggests an infectious or neoplastic cause of back pain.

► Imaging studies, such as magnetic resonance imaging, are useful only if surgery is being considered (persistent pain and neurologic symptoms after 4-6 weeks of conservative care in patients with herniated disks) or if a neoplastic or infectious cause of back pain is being considered.

► Signs for cauda equina syndrome are a clinical emergency and require immediate referral to surgery for decompression.

REFERENCES

Deyo RA, Weinstein JN. Low back pain. *N Engl J Med*. 2001;344:363-370.

Engstrom JW, Deyo RA. Back and neck pain. In: Kasper DL, Fauci AS, Hauser SL, et al., eds. *Harrison's Principles of Internal Medicine*. 19th ed. New York, NY: McGraw-Hill; 2015:111-123

Jarvik JG, Deyo RA. Diagnostic evaluation of low back pain with emphasis on imaging. *Ann Intern Med*. 2002;137:586-597.

Staal JB, Hlobil H, Twisk JW, et al. Graded activity for low back pain in occupational health care: a randomized, controlled trial. *Ann Intern Med*. 2004;140:77-84.

A 48-year-old man comes to your office complaining of severe right knee pain for 8 hours. He states that the pain, which started abruptly at 2 AM and woke him from sleep, was quite severe—so painful that even the weight of the bed sheets on his knee was unbearable. By the morning, the knee had become warm, swollen, and tender. He prefers to keep his knee bent, since straightening the knee causes the pain to worsen. He has never had pain, surgery, or injury to his knees. A year ago, he did have some pain and swelling at the base of his great toe on the left foot, which was not as severe as this episode, and resolved in 2 or 3 days after taking ibuprofen. His only medical history is hypertension, which is controlled with hydrochlorothiazide. He is a nonsmoker, and reports moderate social alcohol use.

On examination, his temperature is 99.4°F, heart rate is 104 bpm, and blood pressure is 136/78 mm Hg. His head and neck examinations are unremarkable, his chest is clear, and his heart is tachycardic but regular, with no gallops or murmurs. His right knee is swollen, with a moderate effusion, and appears erythematous, warm, and very tender to palpation. He is unable to fully extend the knee because of pain. He has no other joint swelling, pain, or deformity, and no skin rashes.

- ▶ What is the most likely diagnosis?
- ▶ What is your next step?
- ▶ What is the best initial treatment?

ANSWERS TO CASE 33:

Acute Monoarticular Arthritis—Gout

Summary: A 48-year-old hypertensive man complains of acute onset of severe right knee pain of 8-hour duration. He denies previous pain, surgery, or injury to his knees. One year ago, he had pain and swelling at the base of his great toe for several days that resolved with ibuprofen. His right knee is swollen, with a moderate effusion, and appears erythematous, warm, and very tender to palpation. He is unable to fully extend the knee because of pain. He has no other joint swelling, pain, or deformity, and no skin rashes.

- **Most likely diagnosis:** Acute monoarticular arthritis, likely crystalline or infectious, most likely gout because of history.

- **Next step:** Aspiration of the knee joint to send fluid for cell count, culture, and crystal analysis.

- **Best initial treatment:** If the joint fluid analysis is consistent with infection, he needs drainage of the infected fluid by aspiration and administration of antibiotics. If analysis is suggestive of crystal-induced arthritis, he can be treated with colchicine, nonsteroidal anti-inflammatory drugs (NSAIDs), or corticosteroids.

ANALYSIS

Objectives

1. Be familiar with the use of synovial fluid analysis to determine the etiology of arthritis.

2. Know the stages of gout and the appropriate treatment for each stage.

3. Know about the similarities and differences between gout and pseudogout.

Considerations

A middle-aged man presents with an acute attack of monoarticular arthritis, as evidenced by knee effusion, limited range of motion, and signs of inflammation (low-grade fever, erythema, warmth, tenderness). The two most likely causes are infection (eg, *Staphylococcus aureus*) and crystalline arthritis (eg, gout or pseudogout). If the patient is at risk, gonococcal arthritis is also a possibility. The previous less severe episode involving his first metatarsophalangeal (MTP) joint sounds like **podagra**, the most common presentation of gout. The rapid onset of severe symptoms during the current attack is consistent with acute gouty arthritis. In this patient, the attack could have been precipitated by the use of alcohol, which increases uric acid production, and his use of thiazide diuretics, which decrease renal excretion of uric acid.

Although the first attack was typical of gout, which makes this episode very likely to also be acute gouty arthritis, the current presentation could also be consistent with bacterial infection. Untreated septic arthritis could lead to rapid destruction of the joint, so joint aspiration and empiric antibiotic therapy are appropriate until his cultures and crystal analysis are available.

APPROACH TO:
Monoarticular Arthritis

DEFINITIONS

MONOARTHRITIS: Inflammation of a single joint.

GOUT: A disturbance of uric acid metabolism occurring mainly in men, characterized by hyperuricemia and the deposition of monosodium urate crystals in the joints, as well as in connective tissues.

PSEUDOGOUT: Arthritis caused by deposition of calcium pyrophosphate dihydrate crystals.

CLINICAL APPROACH

Almost any joint disorder may begin as monoarthritis; however, the primary concern is always **infectious arthritis**, because it may lead to **joint destruction and resultant severe morbidity**. For that reason, **acute monoarthritis should be considered a medical emergency** and investigated and treated aggressively.

Accurate diagnosis starts with a good history and physical examination supplemented by additional diagnostic testing, such as **synovial fluid analysis, radiography**, and occasionally **synovial biopsy**. Patients with crystal-induced arthritis may give a history of recurrent, self-limited episodes. Precipitation of an attack by surgery or some other stress can occur with both crystalline disorders, but **gout is far more common than is pseudogout**. The clinical course can provide some clues to the etiology: septic arthritis usually worsens unless treated; osteoarthritis worsens with physical activity.

The location of joint involvement may be helpful. **Gout** most commonly involves the **first MTP joint (podagra), ankle, mid-foot, or knee**. Pseudogout most commonly affects the large joints, such as the knee; it may also affect the wrist or the first MTP joint (hence the name pseudogout). In **gonococcal** arthritis, there are often **migratory arthralgias and tenosynovitis**, often involving the wrist and hands, associated with **pustular skin lesions**, before progressing to a purulent monoarthritis or oligoarthritis. Nongonococcal causes of septic arthritis often involve large weight-bearing joints, such as the knee and hip.

The basic approach in physical examination is to differentiate arthritis from inflammatory conditions adjacent to the joint, such as cellulitis or bursitis. **True arthritis** is characterized by **swelling and redness around the joint, and painful limitation of motion in all planes**, during **active and passive motion. Joint movement that is not limited by passive motion** suggests **a soft tissue disorder such as bursitis** rather than arthritis.

Table 33-1 • JOINT ASPIRATE CHARACTERISTICS				
Gross Examination	Normal	Noninflammatory	Inflammatory	Septic
Volume (knee)	<1 mL	Often >1 mL	Often >1 mL	Often >1 mL
Viscosity	High	High	Low	Variable
Color	Colorless to straw	Straw to yellow	Yellow	Variable
Clarity	Transparent	Transparent	Translucent	Opaque
Leukocytes/mm³	<200	50-1000	2000-75 000	Often >100 000
Polymorphonuclear cells	<25%	<25%	Often >50%	>85%
Culture results	Negative	Negative	Negative	Often positive
Glucose	Nearly equal to blood	Nearly equal to blood	<50 mg/dL lower than blood	<50 mg/dL lower than blood

(*Data from Koch AE. Approach to the patient with pain in one or a few joints. In*: Kelly's Textbook of Internal Medicine. *New York: Lippincott Williams and Wilkins, 2000:1322.*)

Diagnostic arthrocentesis is usually necessary when evaluating an acute monoarthritis, and is essential when infection is suspected. Synovial fluid analysis helps to differentiate between inflammatory and noninflammatory causes of arthritis. Fluid analysis typically includes gross examination, cell count and differential, Gram stain and culture, and crystal analysis. Table 33–1 gives the typical results that can help one distinguish between noninflammatory conditions such as osteoarthritis, inflammatory arthritis such as crystalline disease, and septic arthritis, which is most often a bacterial infection.

Normal joints contain a small amount of fluid that is essentially acellular. Noninflammatory effusions should have a white blood cell count less than 1000 to 2000/mm³ with less than 25% to 50% polymorphonuclear (PMN) cells. **If the fluid is inflammatory, the joint should be considered infected until proven otherwise,** especially if the patient is febrile.

Crystal analysis requires the use of a polarizing light microscope. Monosodium urate crystals, the cause of **gout,** are **needle shaped,** typically **intracellular** within a PMN cell, and are **negatively birefringent, appearing yellow** under the polarizing microscope. Calcium pyrophosphate dihydrate (CPPD) crystals, the cause of **pseudogout,** are **short and rhomboid,** and are **weakly positively birefringent,** appearing blue under polarized light. **Even if crystals are seen, infection must be excluded when the synovial fluid is inflammatory!** Crystals and infection may coexist in the same joint, and chronic arthritis or previous joint damage, such as occurs in gout, may predispose that joint to hematogenous infection.

In septic arthritis, Gram stain and culture of the synovial fluid is positive in 60% to 80% of cases. False-negative results may be related to prior antibiotic use or fastidious microorganisms. For example, in **gonococcal arthritis, joint fluid cultures typically are negative, whereas cultures of blood or the pustular skin lesions may be**

positive. Sometimes, the diagnosis rests on demonstration of gonococcal infection in another site, such as urethritis, with the typical arthritis-dermatitis syndrome. **Synovial biopsy** may be required when the cause of monoarthritis remains unclear, and is usually **necessary to diagnose arthritis caused by tuberculosis or hemochromatosis.**

Plain radiographs usually are unremarkable in cases of inflammatory arthritis; the typical finding is soft tissue swelling. **Chondrocalcinosis** or linear calcium deposition in joint cartilage suggests pseudogout.

Generally, patients require initiation of treatment before all test results are available. When septic arthritis is suspected, the clinician should culture the joint fluid and start antibiotic therapy; the antibiotic choice should be initially based on the Gram stain and, when available, the culture results. If the Gram stain is negative, the clinical picture should dictate antimicrobial selection. For example, if the patient has the typical presentation of **gonococcal arthritis, intravenous ceftriaxone** is the usual initial therapy, usually with rapid improvement in symptoms. Nongonococcal septic arthritis usually is caused by gram-positive organisms, most often *S aureus*, so treatment would involve an **antistaphylococcal antibiotic such as** vancomycin, daptomycin, or linezolid. If cultures demonstrate organisms that are sensitive to beta-lactams, antibiotic therapy can be guided by the culture and susceptibility results. **It is essential to drain the purulent joint fluid, usually by repeated percutaneous aspiration.** Open surgical drainage or arthroscopy is required when joint fluid is loculated, or when shoulders, hips, or sacroiliac joints are involved.

Gout classically progresses through four stages:

Stage 1 is **asymptomatic hyperuricemia.** Patients have elevated uric acid levels without arthritis or kidney stones. The majority of patients with hyperuricemia never develop any symptoms, but the higher the uric acid level and the longer the duration of hyperuricemia, the greater the likelihood of the patient developing gouty arthritis.

Stage 2 is **acute gouty arthritis,** which most often involves the acute onset of severe **monoarticular pain,** often occurring at night, in the first MTP joint, ankle, or knee, with rapid development of joint swelling and erythema and sometimes associated with systemic symptoms such as fever and chills. This usually follows decades of asymptomatic hyperuricemia. Attacks may last hours or up to 2 weeks.

Stage 3 is **intercritical gout** or the period between acute attacks. Patients are generally completely asymptomatic. However, 60% to 70% of patients will have another acute attack within 1 to 2 years. The presence of these completely asymptomatic periods between monoarthritic attacks is so uncommon, except in crystalline arthritis, that it is often used as a diagnostic criterion for gout.

Stage 4 is **chronic tophaceous gout,** which usually occurs after 10 or more years of acute intermittent gout. In this stage, the intercritical periods are no longer asymptomatic; the involved joints now have chronic swelling and discomfort, which worsens over time. Patients also develop subcutaneous tophaceous deposits of monosodium urate.

In general, **asymptomatic hyperuricemia requires no specific treatment.** Lowering the urate level does not necessarily prevent the development of gout, and most of these patients will never develop any symptoms. Acute gouty arthritis is treated with therapies to reduce the inflammatory reaction to the presence of the crystals, all of which are most effective if started early in the attack. **Potent NSAIDs, such as indomethacin, are the mainstay of therapy** during an acute attack. Alternatively, oral colchicine can be taken TID until the joint symptoms abate, but dosing is limited by gastrointestinal side effects such as nausea and diarrhea. Individuals affected by acute joint pain with **renal insufficiency,** for which a **NSAID or colchicine** is relatively **contraindicated,** usually benefit **from intra-articular glucocorticoid injection or oral steroid therapy.** Steroids should be used only if infection has been excluded. Treatment to lower uric acid levels is inappropriate during an acute episode because any sudden increase or decrease in urate levels may precipitate further attacks.

During intercritical gout, the focus shifts to **preventing further attacks by lowering uric acid levels to less than 6 mg/dL.** Dietary restriction is mainly aimed at avoiding organ-rich foods, such as liver, and alcohol. Patients taking thiazide diuretics should be switched to another antihypertensive if possible. Urate lowering can be accomplished by therapy to increase uric acid excretion by the kidney, such as with probenecid. Uricosuric agents such as probenecid are ineffective in patients with renal failure, however, and are contraindicated in patients with a history of uric acid kidney stones. In these patients, **allopurinol** can be used to diminish uric acid production, but given at lower doses in patients with renal disease. Febuxostat is a new xanthine oxidase inhibitor that does not require dose adjustment in renal insufficiency.

Patients with tophaceous gout are managed as previously described during acute attacks and subsequently treated with allopurinol to help tophaceous deposits resolve. Surgery may be indicated if the mass effect of tophi causes nerve compression, joint deformity, or chronic skin ulceration with resultant infection.

Patients with pseudogout are treated similarly for acute attacks (NSAIDs, colchicine, systemic, or intra-articular steroids). Prophylaxis with colchicine may be helpful in patients with chronic recurrent attacks, but there is no effective therapy for preventing CPPD crystal formation or deposition.

CASE CORRELATION

- See also Case 31 (Osteoarthritis), Case 32 (Low Back Pain), and Case 34 (Rheumatoid Arthritis).

COMPREHENSION QUESTIONS

33.1 A previously healthy 18-year-old college freshman presents to the student health clinic complaining of pain on the dorsum of her left wrist and in her right ankle, fever, and a pustular rash on the extensor surfaces of both her forearms. She has mild swelling and erythema of her ankle, and pain on passive flexion of her wrist. Less than 1 mL of joint fluid is aspirated from her ankle, which shows 8000 PMN cells per high-power field (hpf) but no organisms on Gram stain. Which of the following is the best initial treatment?

A. Indomethacin orally

B. Intravenous ampicillin

C. Colchicine orally

D. Intra-articular prednisone

E. Intravenous ceftriaxone

33.2 Which of the following diagnostic tests is most likely to give the diagnosis for the case in Question 33.1?

A. Crystal analysis of the joint fluid

B. Culture of joint fluid

C. Blood culture

D. Cervical culture

33.3 A 30-year-old man is noted to have an acutely swollen and red knee. Joint aspirate reveals numerous leukocytes and polymorphonuclear leukocytes, but no organisms on Gram stain. Analysis shows few negatively birefringent crystals. Which of the following is the best initial treatment?

A. Oral corticosteroids

B. Intra-articular corticosteroids

C. Intravenous antibiotic therapy

D. Oral colchicine

ANSWERS

33. **E.** The patient described best fits the picture of disseminated gonococcal infection. She has the rash, which typically is located on extensor surfaces of distal extremities. Pain on passive flexion of her wrist indicates likely tenosynovitis of that area. The fluid is inflammatory, but gonococci are typically not seen on Gram stain. Ceftriaxone is the usual treatment of choice for gonococcal infection. Nafcillin would be useful for staphylococcal arthritis and would be the more likely choice if she were older, had some chronic joint disease such as rheumatoid arthritis, or were immunocompromised. **Gonococcal arthritis is the most common cause of infectious arthritis in patients younger than 40 years.** Indomethacin or colchicine would be useful if she had a crystalline arthritis, but that is unlikely in this clinical picture. Intra-articular prednisone is contraindicated until infectious arthritis is ruled out.

33.2 **D.** Synovial fluid cultures usually are sterile in gonococcal arthritis (in fact, the arthritis is more likely caused by immune complex deposition than by actual joint infection), and blood cultures are positive less than 50% of the time. Diagnosis is more often made by finding gonococcal infection in a more typical site, such as urethra, cervix, or pharynx.

33.3 **C.** Corticosteroids should not be used until infection is ruled out. The inflammatory arthritis as shown by Gram stain of the joint aspirate is suspicious for infection, even with no organisms seen on Gram stain. Also, the presence of a few crystals does not eliminate an infection.

CLINICAL PEARLS

▶ In the absence of trauma, acute monoarthritis is most likely to be caused by septic or crystalline arthritis.

▶ In a febrile patient with a joint effusion, diagnostic arthrocentesis is mandatory. Inflammatory fluid (white blood cell count more than 2000/mm³) should be considered infected until proven otherwise.

▶ Gonococcal arthritis usually presents as a migratory tenosynovitis, often involving the wrists and hands, with few vesiculopustular skin lesions.

▶ Nongonococcal septic arthritis is most often caused by *S aureus* and most often affects large weight-bearing joints.

▶ Monosodium urate crystals in gout are needle shaped and negatively birefringent (yellow) under the polarizing microscope. Calcium pyrophosphate dihydrate crystals in pseudogout are rhomboid and positively birefringent (blue).

▶ Treatment of gout depends on the stage: NSAIDs, specifically indomethacin colchicine, or steroids for an acute gouty arthritis, and urate lowering with probenecid or allopurinol during the intercritical period.

REFERENCES

Campion EW, Glynn RJ, DeLabray LO. Asymptomatic hyperuricemia: risk and consequences in the Normative Aging Study. *Am J Med.* 1987;82:421-426.

Madoff LC. Infectious arthritis. In: Kasper DL, Fauci AS, Hauser SL, et al., eds. *Harrison's Principles of Internal Medicine.* 19th ed. New York, NY: McGraw-Hill; 2015:833-838.

Schumacher HR, Chen LX. Gout and other crystal-associated arthropathies. In: Kasper DL, Fauci AS, Hauser SL, et al., eds. *Harrison's Principles of Internal Medicine.* 19th ed. New York, NY: McGraw-Hill; 2015: 2233-2237.

Terkeltaub RA. Gout. *N Engl J Med.* 2003;349:1647-1655.

A 32-year-old nurse presents to your office with a complaint of intermittent episodes of pain, stiffness, and swelling in both hands and wrists for approximately 1 year. The episodes last for several weeks and then resolve. More recently, she noticed similar symptoms in her knees and ankles. Joint pain and stiffness are making it harder for her to get out of bed in the morning and are interfering with her ability to perform her duties at work. The joint stiffness usually lasts for several hours before improving. She also reports malaise and easy fatigability for the past few months, but she denies having fever, chills, skin rashes, and weight loss. Physical examination reveals a well-developed woman, with blood pressure 120/70 mm Hg, heart rate 82 bpm, and respiratory rate 14 bpm. Her skin does not reveal any rashes. Head, neck, cardiovascular, chest, and abdominal examinations are normal. There is no hepatosplenomegaly. The joint examination reveals the presence of bilateral swelling, redness, and tenderness of most proximal interphalangeal (PIP) joints, metacarpophalangeal (MCP) joints, the wrists, and the knees. Laboratory studies show a mild anemia with hemoglobin 11.2 g/dL, hematocrit 32.5%, mean corpuscular volume (MCV) 85.7 fL, white blood cell (WBC) count 7.9/mm³ with a normal differential, and platelet count 300,000/mm³. The urinalysis is clear with no protein and no red blood cells (RBCs). The erythrocyte sedimentation rate (ESR) is 75 mm/h, and the kidney and liver function tests are normal.

▶ What is your most likely diagnosis?
▶ What is your next diagnostic step?

ANSWERS TO CASE 34:
Rheumatoid Arthritis

Summary: This is a 32-year-old woman with a 1-year history of symmetric polyarticular arthritis and morning stiffness. Joint examination reveals the presence of bilateral swelling, redness, and tenderness of her PIP joints, MCP joints, wrists, and knees. She has a mild normocytic anemia with an otherwise normal complete blood count (CBC). Urinalysis, renal, and liver function tests are normal. The ESR is elevated, suggesting an inflammatory cause of her arthritis.

- **Most likely diagnosis:** Rheumatoid arthritis (RA).

- **Next diagnostic step:** Rheumatoid factor and antinuclear antibody titer.

ANALYSIS
Objectives

1. Discern between the clinical presentation of RA and other symmetric polyarthritis syndromes.

2. Learn about the clinical course and treatment of RA.

Considerations

This patient's history, including the symmetric peripheral polyarthritis and duration of symptoms, is suggestive of RA. Rheumatoid arthritis is a systemic autoimmune disorder of unknown etiology. Its major distinctive feature is a chronic, symmetric, and erosive synovitis of peripheral joints, which, if untreated, leads to deformity and destruction of joints due to erosion of cartilage and bone. The diagnosis of RA is a clinical one, based on the presence of a combination of clinical findings, laboratory abnormalities, and, in later stages, radiographic erosions.

APPROACH TO:
Polyarticular Arthritis

CLINICAL APPROACH

The first and most important step in evaluating a patient with polyarticular joint pain is determining whether or not **synovitis/arthritis** is present, producing soft tissue swelling, joint effusion, tenderness, warmth of the joint, and limitation of both active and passive range of motion. If the only finding is pain without inflammatory changes, then the diagnostic considerations include noninflammatory diseases such as osteoarthritis (OA), fibromyalgia, hypothyroidism, neuropathic pain, and depression. The presence of soft tissue swelling and tenderness with limited active range of motion but normal passive range of motion suggests the problem is extra-articular soft tissue inflammation, such as bursitis or tendonitis.

If there is active synovitis/arthritis, it is clinically useful to distinguish between monoarticular/oligoarticular arthritis (see Case 33) and polyarticular arthritis. In polyarticular disease, the next diagnostic clue is the duration of symptoms. If symptoms are relatively acute (<**6 weeks**), the major considerations are arthritis due to **viral infection** (such as hepatitis B or C, rubella, or parvovirus B19) or the earliest manifestation of a true rheumatic disease. Viral serologies and compatible clinical history of exposure often can make the diagnosis at this point and obviate need for further rheumatologic evaluation. Treatment of a viral arthritis usually is limited to symptom relief with nonsteroidal anti-inflammatory drugs (NSAIDs) because the conditions are generally self-limited.

Symmetric peripheral polyarthritis is the most characteristic feature of RA. Other autoimmune rheumatic diseases, such as systemic lupus erythematosus (SLE) and psoriatic arthritis, are often asymmetric. **Lupus**, which may present with a symmetric polyarthritis, usually is characterized by the presence of other symptoms, such as malar rash, serositis (pleuritis and pericarditis), renal disease with proteinuria or hematuria, central nervous system (CNS) manifestations, as well as hematologic disorders, such as hemolytic anemia, leukopenia, lymphopenia, or thrombocytopenia. **Rheumatic fever**, which can cause symmetric polyarthritis, is an acute febrile illness lasting only 6 to 8 weeks. In **psoriatic arthritis** the pattern of joint involvement varies widely. The vast majority of patients have peripheral joint involvement of more than five joints. Others have a pauciarticular asymmetric arthritis or exclusive distal interphalangeal (DIP) involvement. Inflammation is not limited to the joints but also occurs at the periosteum, along tendons, and at the insertion points into the bone, resulting in the development of **"sausage digits," which are typical of psoriatic arthritis (and Reiter syndrome).** Although the arthritis can precede the development of a skin rash, the definite diagnosis of psoriatic arthritis cannot be made without the evidence of skin or nail changes typical of psoriasis (nail pitting, scaly plaques). **Reactive arthritis** is an asymmetric inflammatory arthritis that follows infection of the gastrointestinal (GI) or genitourinary (GU) tract with bacteria such as *Salmonella, Shigella, Campylobacter, Yersinia,* or *Chlamydia*. **Reiter syndrome** is a form of reactive arthritis with the **triad of arthritis, uveitis, and urethritis.**

The peripheral polyarthritis of **RA** most typically involves the wrists and the MCP or **PIP joints** of both hands; the DIP joints usually are spared. It is useful to contrast the typical pattern of joint involvement of RA from that of degenerative OA. Degenerative joint disease may affect multiple joints, but it occurs in older age groups, is usually not associated with inflammation or constitutional symptoms, and tends not to be episodic. Also, in **OA** the hand joints most commonly involved are the **DIP joints**, where the formation of **Heberden nodes** can be noted (Figure 34–1). In RA, **ulnar deviation of the MCP joints** is often associated with **radial deviation of the wrists; swan-neck deformities** as well as the **boutonnière deformity** can develop (**Figure 34–2**). Swan-neck deformity results from contracture of the interosseous and flexor muscles and tendons, which causes a flexion contracture of the MCP joint, hyperextension of the PIP joint, and flexion of the DIP joint. In the boutonnière deformity, there is a flexion of the PIP and hyperextension of the DIP joints. These findings are typical of advanced RA.

Figure 34–1. Rheumatoid arthritis versus osteoarthritis.

Morning stiffness or stiffness after any prolonged inactivity is a common feature of many arthritic disorders. However, stiffness that lasts more than 1 hour is seen only in inflammatory conditions such as RA and reflects the severity of joint inflammation.

Rheumatoid nodules are subcutaneous nodules typically found over extensor surfaces of the proximal ulna or other pressure points. They only occur in 20%

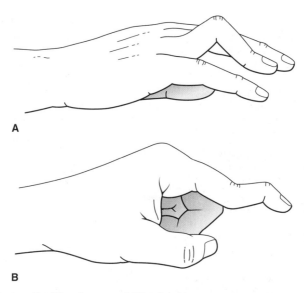

Figure 34–2. Boutonnière (A) and swan-neck (B) deformities.

to 30% of patients with RA but are believed to have a high diagnostic specificity for RA.

Rheumatoid factors (RFs) are **immunoglobulins** that react to the F_C **portion of immunoglobulin (Ig)G molecules.** The usual serologic tests used in clinical laboratories detect IgM RFs, which are found in 80% to 85% of patients with RA. Rheumatoid factor is not specific for RA, as it is found in 5% of healthy patients, but it can support the diagnosis when clinical features are suggestive. High RF titers have a prognostic utility for more severe systemic and progressive disease.

Antibodies to cyclic citrullinated peptides (**anti-CCP**) are now recognized as very useful biomarkers with diagnostic and prognostic significance. Anti-CCP antibodies have the same sensitivity as RF, but are highly specific, about 95%. The presence of anti-CCP also portends worse outcomes in RA. Current classification criteria for the diagnosis of RA are listed in Table 34–1.

Radiologic findings in RA, such as erosion of periarticular bone and cartilage destruction with loss of joint space, may help the diagnosis. Usually, though, the typical x-ray findings do not develop until later in the disease process after a diagnosis has been made based on clinical findings. Joint deformities in RA occur from several different mechanisms, all related to synovitis and pannus formation with resulting cartilage destruction and erosion of periarticular bone. The structural damage to the joint is irreversible and worsens with disease progression.

There are several **extra-articular manifestations in RA,** including vasculitic lesions with the development of ischemic ulcers, which implies systemic involvement; ocular manifestations with symptoms of **keratoconjunctivitis sicca** (Sjögren syndrome); respiratory manifestations caused by **interstitial lung disease;** cardiac manifestations; and several neurologic manifestations, such as myelopathy, related to cervical spine instability. Although not common, the continuous bone erosion may

Table 34-1 • CLASSIFICATION CRITERIA FOR RHEUMATOID ARTHRITIS A SCORE OF ≥ 6 FULFILLS REQUIREMENTS FOR DEFINITE RA		Score
Joint involvement	1 Large joint	0
	2-10 Large joints	1
	1-3 Small joints	2
	4-10 Small joints	3
	> 10 joints (at least 1 small joint)	5
Serology	Negative RF, negative anti-CCP Ab	0
	Low positive RF or low positive anti-CCP Ab	2
	High-positive RF or high-positive anti-CCP Ab	3
Acute phase reactants	Normal CRP and normal ESR	0
	Abnormal CRP or abnormal ESR	1
Duration of symptoms	< 6 weeks	0
	≥ 6 weeks	1

Notes:
Large joint: shoulder, elbow, hip, knee, ankle
Small joints: MCP, PIP, thumb IP, MTP, wrists
Low-positive serology: ≤ 3X ULN
High-positive serology: > 3X ULN
RF: rheumatoid factor
Anti-CCP Ab: anti-citrullinated peptide antibody

result in an atlantoaxial subluxation with cervical dislocation and spinal cord compression. Entrapment neuropathy may develop, such as carpal tunnel syndrome. Hematologic manifestations include anemia, typically anemia of chronic disease. The combination of **RA, splenomegaly, leukopenia, lymphadenopathy**, and **thrombocytopenia** is called **Felty syndrome**. Felty syndrome is most common with severe nodule-forming RA.

At this stage in the disease process, our patient is presenting with joint complaints, fatigue, and malaise. No other extra-articular manifestations have developed yet. At the very onset of RA, the characteristic symmetric inflammation of the joints and the typical serologic findings may not be evident. Therefore, initially distinguishing RA from other conditions, such as lupus, may be difficult. Usually, the development of extra-articular phenomenon allows the physician to make a more specific diagnosis.

Treatment

Several drugs are currently used for treatment of RA. **NSAIDs** or cyclooxygenase 2 (COX-2) inhibitors such as celecoxib may control local inflammatory symptoms. **Corticosteroids** have an immediate and dramatic effect on joint symptoms, but were historically thought not to alter the natural progression of the disease. Recent evidence suggests that low-dose corticosteroids may retard the progression of bone erosions.

Disease-modifying antirheumatic drugs (DMARDs) may have a favorable impact on the natural course of the disease, reducing joint inflammation and disease activity, and slow or prevent the structural progression of RA. The nonbiologic DMARDs include methotrexate, hydroxychloroquine, sulfasalazine, minocycline, and leflunomide. There is controversy regarding which DMARD is the most effective, but **methotrexate** is often used as the first drug of choice because of its rapid onset of action and higher tolerability and patient compliance. Toxicity of the various DMARDs is often the most important determinant of which drug is used, and if the patient fails to respond or develops unacceptable side effects, the patient may be tried on a different agent.

In the last decade, the **biologic** DMARDs have revolutionized the treatment of RA. **Tumor necrosis factor (TNF) antagonists** (etanercept, infliximab, adalimumab, golimumab, and certolizumab) have been found to reduce disease activity within weeks, unlike other DMARDs, which may take several months to act, and may also control signs and symptoms in patients who have failed conventional DMARD therapy. Side effects of TNF blockers may include increased risk of infection, such as reactivation tuberculosis (TB), so all patients should first be screened for latent TB. Other biologics currently in use include **anakinra**, a recombinant interleukin 1 (IL-1) receptor antagonist, **abatacept**, a soluble fusion protein of IgG and human cytotoxic T-lymphocyte-associated antigen 4 (CTLA-4), and **rituximab**, a chimeric monoclonal antibody against CD20, a cell-surface molecule of B-lymphocytes.

COMPREHENSION QUESTIONS

34.1 A 72-year-old man develops severe pain and swelling in both knees, shortly after undergoing an abdominal hernia repair surgery. Physical examination shows warmth and swelling of both knees with large effusions. Arthrocentesis of the right knee reveals the presence of intracellular and extracellular *weakly positive birefringent crystals* in the synovial fluid. Gram stain is negative. Which of the following is the most likely diagnosis?

A. Gout

B. Septic arthritis

C. Calcium oxalate deposition disease

D. Reactive arthritis

E. Pseudogout

34.2 A 65-year-old man with a history of chronic hypertension, diabetes mellitus, and degenerative joint disease presents with acute onset of severe pain of the metatarsophalangeal (MTP) joint and swelling of the left first toe. Physical examination shows exquisite tenderness of the joint, with swelling, warmth, and erythema. The patient has no history of trauma or other significant medical problems. Synovial fluid analysis and aspiration are most likely to show which of the following?

A. Hemorrhagic fluid

B. Needle-shaped, negatively birefringent crystals

C. Gram-negative organisms

D. Noninflammatory fluid

E. Rhomboidal, positively birefringent crystals

34.3 A 17-year-old sexually active adolescent boy presents with a 5-day history of fever, chills, and persistent left ankle pain and swelling. On physical examination, maculopapular and pustular skin lesions are noted on the trunk and extremities. He denies any symptoms of genitourinary tract infection. Synovial fluid analysis is most likely to show which of the following?

A. WBCs 75,000/mm^3 with 95% polymorphonuclear leukocytes

B. RBCs 100,000/mm^3, WBCs 1000/mm^3

C. WBCs 48,000/mm^3 with 80% lymphocytes

D. WBCs 500/mm^3 with 25% polymorphonuclear leukocytes

34.4 A 22-year-old man presents with complaints of low back pain for 3 to 4 months and stiffness of the lumbar area, which worsen with inactivity. He reports difficulty in getting out of bed in the morning and may have to roll out sideways, trying not to flex or rotate the spine to minimize pain. A lumbosacral (LS) spine x-ray film would most likely show which of the following?

A. Degenerative joint disease with spur formation

B. Sacroiliitis with increased sclerosis around the sacroiliac joints

C. Vertebral body destruction with wedge fractures

D. Osteoporosis with compression fractures of L3-L5

E. Diffuse osteonecrosis of the LS spine

34.5 A 36-year-old woman was seen by her physician due to pain in her hands, wrists, and knees. She is diagnosed with rheumatoid arthritis. Which of the following treatments will reduce joint inflammation and slow progression of the disease?

A. NSAIDs

B. Joint aspiration

C. Methotrexate

D. Systemic corticosteroids

ANSWERS

34.1 **E.** Pseudogout is diagnosed by positive birefringent crystals. Arthrocentesis revealing needle-shaped, negatively birefringent crystals would be more consistent with gout. Septic arthritis is more likely to present as a monoarticular arthritis and synovial fluid will be filled with WBCs often with a left shift rather than crystals.

34.2 **B.** The involvement of the great toe is most likely gout, and the synovial fluid is likely to show **needle-shaped, negatively birefringent crystals.**

34.3 **A.** This history is suggestive of gonococcal arthritis, and the rash is suggestive of disseminated gonococcal disease. The synovial fluid would most likely show an acute inflammatory exudate, WBCs 72,000/mm³ with 75% polymorphonuclear cells.

34.4 **B.** A young man is not likely to have osteoporosis, osteoarthritis, or compression fractures. His morning stiffness, which worsens with rest, suggests an inflammatory arthritis, such as ankylosing spondylitis, which would include sacroiliitis with increased sclerosis around the sacroiliac joints.

34.5 **C.** Although NSAIDs and corticosteroids may help to relieve symptoms, they typically do not slow or prevent structural progression of disease. Disease-Modifying Anti-Rheumatic Drugs (DMARDs) include methotrexate, hydroxychloroquine, sulfasalazine, leflunomide, and biologic agents. Of these agents, methotrexate is usually the drug of choice, and is the anchor drug of most combination therapies.

CLINICAL PEARLS

▶ Rheumatoid arthritis is a chronic systemic inflammatory disorder characterized by the insidious onset of symmetric polyarthritis and extra-articular symptoms.

▶ Rheumatoid factor is found in the serum of 85% of patients with rheumatoid arthritis, but is less specific than anti-CCP antibodies (specificity 95%).

▶ In nearly all patients with rheumatoid arthritis, the wrist, metacarpophalangeal joints, and proximal interphalangeal joints are affected, whereas the distal interphalangeal joints are spared.

▶ Distal interphalangeal joints and large weight-bearing joints are most commonly involved in osteoarthritis.

▶ The typical x-ray finding in rheumatoid arthritis—periarticular bone erosion (loss of joint space)—may not develop until later in the disease process, when the diagnosis has already been made based on clinical findings.

▶ DMARDs for rheumatoid arthritis includes methotrexate, TNF antagonists, and other biologic agents.

REFERENCES

Aletaha D, Neogi T, Silman AJ, et al. 2010 Rheumatoid arthritis classification criteria: an ACR/EULAR collaborative initiative. *Arthritis Rheum.* 2010;62:2569-2581.

Shah A, St Clair EW. Rheumatoid arthritis. In: Kasper DL, Fauci AS, Hauser SL, et al., eds. *Harrison's Principles of Internal Medicine.* 19th ed. New York, NY: McGraw-Hill; 2015:2137-2149.

A 75-year-old white woman presents to the emergency room with right wrist pain after a fall at home. She tripped and fell while preparing dinner, and she says that she tried to stop her fall with her outstretched right hand. She heard a "snap" and felt immediate pain. Her medical history is remarkable only for three normal pregnancies, menopause at age 50, and hypertension that is well controlled with diuretics. She has a 50-pack-year history of smoking. Her weight is 100 lb, and her height is 5 ft 6 in. Her examination is remarkable for normal vital signs; a swollen, deformed right distal forearm and wrist, with limited mobility because of pain; and good radial pulses and capillary refill in the right fingernail beds. An x-ray confirms a fracture of the right radial head, and the radiologist notes osteopenia.

▶ What risk factor for fracture is this woman likely to have?
▶ What are the causes of this condition?
▶ What can her physician offer her to prevent future fractures?

ANSWERS TO CASE 35:

Osteoporosis

Summary: A 75-year-old white woman tried to stop her fall using her out-stretched right hand, heard a "snap," and felt immediate pain. Her medical history is remarkable only for menopause at age 50 and hypertension that is well controlled with diuretics. She does have a 50-pack-year history of smoking. She has a swollen, deformed, right distal forearm and wrist, with limited mobility because of pain, and good radial pulses and capillary refill in the right fingernail beds. An x-ray confirms a fracture of the right radial head, and the radiologist notes osteopenia.

- **Risk factor for fracture:** Osteoporosis.

- **Causes of this condition:** Decreased bone strength as a consequence of demineralization and increased bone turnover as a result of decreased levels of sex steroids (estrogen and testosterone), medications, other hormonal conditions, or diseases of decreased calcium absorption.

- **Preventive measures:** Several medications are available to increase bone density, which may decrease the risk of future fractures. Also, her physician would want to work with her to prevent future falls by limiting unnecessary medications that may cause instability, making changes in the home environment, and evaluating her gait, visual acuity, and peripheral sensory system. The patient should be advised to quit smoking.

ANALYSIS

Objectives

1. Understand the pathophysiology of osteoporosis.

2. Learn the risk factors that predispose both men and women to osteoporosis.

3. Be familiar with the tests used to evaluate bone density.

4. Know the treatment options for osteoporosis.

Considerations

This 75-year-old woman with a fracture after a fall likely sustained the fracture because of decreased bone density. Her risk factors for osteoporosis are her race, smoking history, postmenopausal state and thin physique. Osteoporosis puts her at risk for future fractures with substantial morbidity, such as painful vertebral compression fractures or incapacitating hip fractures. She requires intervention to reduce her risk of fractures as well as her risk of falls.

APPROACH TO:
Osteoporosis

DEFINITIONS

BISPHOSPHONATES: Synthetic carbon phosphate compounds (alendronate, risedronate, ibandronate) that build bone mass by binding to pyrophosphatase in bone and by inhibiting osteoclast bone resorption.

OSTEOPENIA: T score between −1.0 and −2.5 standard deviations (SD) below the mean.

OSTEOPOROSIS: Decrease in bone mass leading to increased bone fragility and predisposing to fracture of the hip, vertebrae, and long bones, with a defined bone mineral density (BMD) more than 2.5 SD below the mean of young healthy adults.

T SCORE: BMD comparison against young healthy adults (in standard deviations from the mean).

CLINICAL APPROACH

Osteoporosis is an important health issue because the resultant bone fractures cause a great deal of morbidity in chronic pain, loss of independence, and loss of function, as well as mortality. Risk factors for the development of osteoporotic fracture include advanced age, previous fracture, glucocorticoid therapy, rheumatoid arthritis, low body weight, loss of steroid hormone production (menopause or hypogonadism), current smoking, excessive alcohol, parental history of hip fracture. The FRAX risk calculator is available online to assess the 10-year probability of fracture. Approximately 14% of white women and 3% to 5% of white men will develop osteoporosis in their lifetime. The prevalence is lower in African Americans and higher in Asians.

Osteoporosis can be either idiopathic or a manifestation of another underlying disease process. Probably the most common form of **secondary osteoporosis** is caused by **glucocorticoid excess**, usually iatrogenic steroid use for an inflammatory disease such as rheumatoid arthritis. Patients, both men and women, with rheumatoid arthritis are susceptible to accelerated bone loss with even low doses of glucocorticoids. **Gonadal deficiency** is another common cause, which is seen physiologically in menopausal women but is seen pathologically in women who are amenorrheic (eg, female athletes such as gymnasts or marathon runners) or as a result of hyperprolactinemia. Men with gonadal failure for whatever reason also are prone to develop osteoporosis.

Osteoporosis is a common feature of several endocrinopathies. Patients with **hyperparathyroidism** will develop osteoporosis because of increased calcium mobilization from bone. Long-standing **hyperthyroidism**, either naturally occurring, as in Graves disease, or as a result of excessive replacement of levothyroxine in patients with hypothyroidism, will also lead to accelerated bone loss. Malnutrition and nutritional deficiencies are causative and are often seen in patients with malabsorption; for example, most patients, both men and women, with **celiac sprue** have osteoporosis. Certain medications, such as cyclosporine, antiepileptics, heparin, and gonadotropin-releasing hormone (GnRH) inhibitors, among others, may accelerate bone loss.

Peak bone density occurs in young adulthood under the influence of sex steroid hormone production. Other influential factors include **genetics**, which may account for 80% of total bone density, adequate calcium intake, and level of physical activity, especially **weight-bearing activity**. The type of bone growth at this stage is called *modeling*. After skeletal maturation is reached, the bone growth enters a new phase, termed *remodeling*, in which repairs are made to damaged bone, existing bone is strengthened, and calcium is released to maintain serum levels under the influence of estrogens, androgens, parathyroid hormone, vitamin D, and various cytokines and other hormones. The activity of the osteoclasts approximates the activity of the osteoblasts in that overall bone density remains stable. However, after age 35, bone breakdown begins to exceed bone replacement, and this increases **markedly after menopause** as a consequence of **increased osteoclast activity**.

Diagnostic Approach

The benefits and costs of universal screening for osteoporosis are unclear. Rather, a targeted approach is advocated. Those with a family history or other risk factors should be offered screening, as well as patients undergoing a chronic drug (steroid) therapy that may lead to osteoporosis. **Currently, all women older than 65 years, or those who have sustained a fracture before age 65, are recommended to undergo BMD testing.** Dual-energy x-ray absorptiometry (DEXA scan) is the technique used to define diagnostic thresholds; however, whether the hip, spine, or forearm is the best site for screening is not clearly established. DEXA scan results can be expressed as a Z score, which compares BMD to that in persons of the same age, and a T score, which compares to the young adult normal range. **T scores are more useful for predicting fracture risk.** Every 1 SD decrease in BMD below the mean doubles the fracture risk. As mentioned, osteoporosis is defined as a T score of −2.5 SD.

Other laboratory evaluations should routinely be considered in patients with osteoporosis. The **serum levels of calcium, phosphorus, and alkaline phosphatase are typically normal** in patients with osteoporosis, although the alkaline phosphatase level sometimes is mildly elevated in the presence of a healing fracture. Laboratory abnormalities should prompt consideration of alternative diagnoses for the bone disease: hypercalcemia in hyperparathyroidism, or hypocalcemia in osteomalacia.

If a patient suffers a pathologic fracture, that is, one with minimal trauma, other diagnoses must be excluded. **Osteomalacia** is defective mineralization of bone matrix with accumulation of unmineralized osteoid and is most often caused by vitamin D deficiency or phosphate deficiency. Patients with osteomalacia frequently have diffuse bone pain and tenderness, proximal muscle weakness, and laboratory abnormalities such as elevated alkaline phosphatase level and low to normal calcium level. In the absence of fractures, patients with osteoporosis should have no bone pain or laboratory abnormalities. Both of these disease processes can coexist. A less common bone disease is **Paget disease**, which is characterized by disorganized bone remodeling with a high alkaline phosphatase level causing weakened and enlarged bones with skeletal deformities. Other important causes of pathologic fracture that must be considered include **malignancy**, such as multiple myeloma or metastatic disease, and vertebral osteomyelitis.

Treatment

Treatment of osteoporosis takes a multifaceted approach. Adequate **calcium intake**, 1000 mg/d for premenopausal women and adult men, and 1200 mg with 400 to 800 IU of **vitamin D** per day for postmenopausal women, leads to decreased fractures. Steroid estrogen receptor moduluators such as raloxifene can increase bone density and reduce fracture risk, as can the use of bisphosphonates, both in combination with calcium and vitamin D. **Bisphosphonates** can lead to **severe esophagitis** and must be used with caution in individuals with gastric reflux disease. Oral bisphosphonates should be taken on an empty stomach, with a large quantity of water, and the patient should remain in the upright position for at least 30 minutes. Intravenous bisphosphonates are now available that can be infused quarterly or annually. There is some concern about long-term effects of bisphosphonates, including risk of osteonecrosis of the jaw and paradoxical bone fragility causing atypical subtrochanteric femur fractures. Many experts recommend a drug holiday after 5 years of treatment for patients with stable BMD. **Estrogens** have proven benefit in preventing bone loss and reducing fracture risk, but the Women's Health Initiative study demonstrated an increased risk of venous thromboembolism and cardiovascular events with conjugated equine estrogen. Consequently, postmenopausal estrogen is not commonly prescribed for this purpose. Selective estrogen receptor modifiers (raloxifene, tamoxifen) are used for treatment of osteoporosis as well.

    Weight-bearing physical activity decreases bone loss and improves coordination and muscle strength, which may prevent falls. Ensuring that patients can see adequately, that they use a cane or walker if needed, that throw rugs are removed, that patients have railings to hold on to in the shower or bath, or that they wear hip protectors can further decrease the risk of life-altering bone fractures.

> ## CASE CORRELATION
>
> - See also Case 31 (Osteoarthritis), Case 32 (Low Back Pain), Case 33 (Acute Monoarticular Arthritis), and Case 34 (Rheumatoid Arthritis).

COMPREHENSION QUESTIONS

35.1 Which of the following patients is most likely to be a candidate for bone mineral density screening?

    A. A 65-year-old, thin, white woman who smokes and is 15 years postmenopausal

    B. A 40-year-old white woman who exercises daily and still menstruates

    C. A healthy 75-year-old white man who is sedentary

    D. A 60-year-old overweight African-American woman

    E. A 35-year-old asthmatic woman who took prednisone 40 mg/d for a 2-week course 1 week ago

35.2   During which of the following periods in a woman's life is the most bone mass accumulated?

A.   Ages 15-25

B.   Ages 25-35

C.   Ages 35-45

D.   Ages 45-55

35.3   A 60-year-old woman presents with the results of her DEXA scan. She has a T score of −1.5 SD at the hip and −2.5 at the spine. Which of the following is the most accurate interpretation of these results?

A.   She has osteoporosis at the spine and osteopenia at the hip.

B.   She has osteoporosis in both areas.

C.   This is a normal examination.

D.   She has osteoporosis of the hip and osteopenia at the spine.

E.   You need to know the Z score.

35.4   You see a 70-year-old woman in your office for a routine checkup, and you order a DEXA scan for bone mineral density screening. The T score returns as −2.5 SD in the spine and −2.6 in the hip. Which of the following statements is most accurate?

A.   This patient has osteopenia.

B.   Estrogen replacement therapy should be started with an anticipated rebuilding of bone mass to near-normal within 1 year.

C.   Swimming will help build bone mass.

D.   Bisphosphonates would reduce the risk of hip fracture by 30%-50%.

ANSWERS

35.1   **A.** Of the choices, this woman is the only individual with risk factors. Risk factors include white race, age, postmenopausal status, smoking, positive family history, poor nutritional status, and chronic treatment with a drug known to predispose to bone loss.

35.2   **A.** The time of greatest accumulation of bone mass in women is during adolescence.

35.3   **A.** The T score is the number of standard deviations of a patient's bone mineral density from the mean of young, adult, white women. It is the standard measurement of bone mineral density used by the World Health Organization. Osteopenia is defined as a T score of 1 to -2.4. A score of −2.5 SD is the definition of osteoporosis. A Z score is the number of standard deviations from the mean bone mineral density of women in the same age group as the patient.

35.4 **D.** Estrogen primarily inhibits loss of bone mass, although it can help to build a modest amount of bone mass, but also may be associated with increased thrombotic and cardiovascular risk. Weight-bearing exercise, not swimming or bicycling, is important in preventing osteoporosis. Bisphosphonates decrease the incidence of hip fractures by 30% to 50%.

CLINICAL PEARLS

▶ Bone mineral density screening should be offered to all women of 65 years and older, and to younger patients with risk factors for osteo-porosis.

▶ Every 1 SD decrease in bone mineral density below the mean of young adults doubles the fracture risk. Osteoporosis is defined as a T score of −2.5 SD.

▶ Patients with osteoporosis should have normal serum calcium, phospho-rus, and alkaline phosphatase levels. Laboratory abnormalities should prompt a search for an alternative diagnosis.

▶ Fractures can have a devastating effect on a patient's quality of life, and a multifaceted approach through nutritional counseling, home improve-ments, gait stabilization through exercise and with canes or walkers, and medical interventions to improve eyesight or with medications to improve bone density should be offered to patients at risk.

▶ In patients with a pathologic fracture, osteoporosis is a diagnosis of exclusion; osteomalacia, Paget disease, and metastatic malignancies also must be considered.

REFERENCES

Lindsay R, Cosman F. Osteoporosis. In: Kasper DL, Fauci AS, Hauser SL, et al., eds. *Harrison's Principles of Internal Medicine.* 19th ed. New York, NY: McGraw-Hill; 2015:2488-2504.

Mauck KF, Clarke BL. Diagnosis, screening, prevention, and treatment of osteoporosis. *Mayo Clin Proc.* 2006;81:662-672.

Rosen CJ. Clinical practice: postmenopausal osteoporosis. *N Engl J Med.* 2005;353:595-603.

A 72-year-old man is admitted to the hospital because of the acute onset of a right facial droop, right arm weakness, and some difficulty speaking. These symptoms started 6 hours ago while he was sitting at the breakfast table. He had no headache, no diminishment of consciousness, and no abnormal involuntary movements. Two weeks ago, he had a transient painless loss of vision in his left eye, which resolved spontaneously within a few hours. His medical history is significant for long-standing hypertension and a myocardial infarction (MI) 4 years previously, which was treated with percutaneous angioplasty. His medications include a daily aspirin, metoprolol, and simvastatin. He does not smoke. When you see him in the emergency room, his symptoms have nearly resolved. He is afebrile, heart rate is 62 bpm, and blood pressure is 135/87 mm Hg. The corner of his mouth droops, with slight flattening of the right nasolabial fold, but he is able to fully elevate his eyebrows. His strength is 4/5 in his right arm and hand, and the rest of his neurologic examination is normal. He has no carotid bruits, his heart rhythm is regular with no murmur but with an S_4 gallop. The remainder of his physical examination is normal. Laboratory studies, including renal function, liver function, lipid profile, and complete blood count (CBC), all are normal. Within a few hours, all of the patient's symptoms have resolved.

▶ What is the most likely diagnosis?
▶ What is the next step?

ANSWERS TO CASE 36:
Transient Ischemic Attack

Summary: A 72-year-old man is admitted because of an acute onset of right facial droop and right arm weakness, and some difficulty speaking, which resolves within hours. He denies headache, diminishment of consciousness, or abnormal involuntary movements. Two weeks ago, he had a transient painless loss of vision in his left eye, which resolved spontaneously within a few hours. He has no carotid bruits, but he does have a known atherosclerotic disease.

- **Most likely diagnosis:** Transient ischemic attack (TIA) caused by atheroembolism from the left internal carotid artery.

- **Next step:** Perform a noncontrast computed tomography (CT) of the head.

ANALYSIS

Objectives

1. Know the most common mechanisms for ischemic stroke: carotid stenosis, cardioembolism, and small-vessel disease.

2. Understand the evaluation of a stroke patient with the goal of secondary prevention.

3. Learn which patients are best managed with medical therapy and which patients benefit from carotid endarterectomy.

Considerations

Patients who present with acute focal neurologic deficits require rapid evaluation for suspected stroke. **Noncontrast CT of the brain** is necessary to differentiate between ischemic stroke and hemorrhagic stroke, which cannot be definitively distinguished clinically. If CT shows no hemorrhage, and no large multilobar infarction (>1/3 of the cerebral hemisphere), patients with the clinical diagnosis of acute ischemic attack may receive **thrombolytics** (IV recombinant tissue plasminogen activator) as long as it can be delivered **within 3 hours** (some patients may be treated with IV thrombolytics up to 4.5 hours) of the onset of symptoms, with a reduction in mortality and disability.

This 72-year-old man presented more than 6 hours after the onset of symptoms and has had resolution of neurologic deficits, consistent with a suspected diagnosis of TIA. He has established atherosclerotic coronary disease but no known carotid artery disease. He denies headache, which is important because migraine headache may be associated with neurologic deficits; it would be rare for an elderly man to have the first presentation of migraine headache. Various neurologic diseases, such as multiple sclerosis, may be characterized by complete resolution of neurologic deficits, but the symptoms usually last longer than 24 hours. He does not have abnormal motor activity, which might suggest seizure disorder.

His evaluation will be focused on secondary prevention of another, perhaps more devastating cerebrovascular event.

After a noncontrast CT to exclude acute intracranial pathology, secondary prevention of future ischemic events will include noninvasive imaging of the carotid arteries to determine the extent of stenosis. With these symptoms, if there is more than 70% stenosis of the left internal carotid artery, the possibility of left carotid endarterectomy should be discussed.

APPROACH TO:
Transient Ischemic Attack/Stroke

DEFINITIONS

AMAUROSIS FUGAX: Transient monocular blindness that often is described as a gray shade being pulled down over the eye caused by retinal ischemia, most often due to emboli originating from the carotid artery.

STROKE: Acute onset of a focal neurologic deficit due to a cerebral infarction or hemorrhage.

TRANSIENT ISCHEMIC ATTACK: Transient neurologic deficit caused by focal brain, spinal cord, or retinal ischemia, without acute infarction.

CLINICAL APPROACH

Transient ischemic attacks, often called "mini-strokes," typically refer to the sudden onset of a focal neurologic deficit, with spontaneous resolution within 24 hours (usually within the first hour). Current definition of TIA focuses on a biological end point (tissue injury), however, rather than an arbitrary time cutoff. Recent understanding is that here is risk of tissue infarction, even when focal symptoms resolve within less than 24 hours, which may be visualized on brain magnetic resonance imaging (MRI) with diffusion-weighted or perfusion-weighted imaging.

Not all transient focal neurologic events actually represent ischemia, however. The differential diagnosis includes classic migraine, postictal paralysis, seizures, cerebral hemorrhage, or even slow-evolving intracranial processes such as subdural hematoma, abscess, or tumors, which can suddenly produce symptoms because of edema or hemorrhage or result in seizure activity. However, clinical evaluation and imaging studies of the brain should be sufficient to exclude most or all of these diagnoses.

The **focal neurologic symptoms** produced by ischemia depend on the **area of the cerebral circulation** involved and may include (1) amaurosis fugax, (2) hemiparesis, (3) hemianesthesia, (4) aphasia, or (5) dizziness/vertigo as a result of vertebrobasilar insufficiency. The significance of a TIA is not the symptoms it produces, because by definition it is self-resolved, but the risk for future events it portends. **The highest-risk patients for stroke are those with previous ischemic events such as TIA;** that is, it can be looked upon as a warning sign of recurrent stroke, which may be disabling. Table 36–1 shows the ABCD^2 scoring system, which can be used to

Table 36–1 • ABCD^2 SCORE: RISK OF STROKE FOLLOWING TIA	
Clinical Factor	Score
A: Age ≥ 60 y	1
B: BP > 140/90 mm Hg	1
C: Clinical symptoms	
Unilateral weakness	2
Speech disturbance without weakness	1
D: Duration	
≥ 60 min	2
10-59 min	1
D: Diabetes	1
Total Score	**2-Day Stroke Risk**
6-7	High (8%)
4-5	Moderate (4%)
0-3	Low (1%)

triage patients with TIA to assess their risk for recurrent events within the first 3 months (most events occur within the first 2 days).

TIAs are produced by temporary ischemia to a vascular territory, usually caused by thrombosis or embolism and less commonly by vasculitis, hematologic disorders such as sickle cell disease or vasospasm. By far, the most common causes of stroke or TIA are **carotid atherosclerosis** (large-vessel disease), **cardioembolism** usually to branches of the middle cerebral artery (medium-size vessel disease), or **lipohyalinosis** affecting small lenticulostriate arteries (small-vessel disease). Table 36–2 lists the etiologies of a TIA/stroke.

The workup for a TIA begins with a history and physical examination. Pertinent historical factors include onset, course, and duration of symptoms, atherosclerotic risk factors, and relevant medical history (ie, atrial fibrillation). Physical examination should begin with blood pressures in four extremities and should include a funduscopic examination. In this patient, the first symptom was amaurosis fugax due to cholesterol emboli, called **Hollenhorst plaques**, which often can be seen lodged in the retinal artery. Auscultation for carotid bruits, cardiac murmurs, assessment of cardiac rhythm, evidence of embolic events to other parts of the body, and a complete neurologic examination should also be assessed.

Laboratory data that should always be obtained include a complete blood count, fasting lipid profile, and serum glucose level. Other laboratory data, such as an erythrocyte sedimentation rate in elderly populations to evaluate for temporal arteritis, should be tailored to the patient. Generally, a 12-lead electrocardiogram (ECG) must be obtained to evaluate for atrial fibrillation. An echocardiogram can be useful to evaluate for valvular or mural thrombi. **A noncontrast CT scan of the brain also must be performed initially.** Noncontrast CT scans of the brain are very sensitive in detecting acute cerebral hemorrhage but are relatively insensitive to

Table 36–2 • CAUSES OF ISCHEMIC STROKE OR TIA
Embolic
Cardioembolic
• Atrial fibrillation
• Dilated cardiomyopathy, mural thrombus
• Bacterial endocarditis
• Prosthetic valve thrombosis
• Paradoxical embolus (atrial septal defect, patent foramen ovale)
Artery-to-artery embolism
• Aortic arch
• Carotid bifurcation
• Carotid or vertebral artery dissection
Thrombotic stroke
Acute thrombosis of large to medium arteries (eg, internal carotid, middle cerebral) due to atherosclerotic disease
Small-vessel stroke (lacunar stroke)
Atherothrombotic or lipohyalonotic occlusion of small penetrating arteries
Most commonly due to hypertension (80%-90%) or diabetes
Subcortical location (basal ganglia, thalamus, internal capsule)
Miscellaneous uncommon causes
Hypercoagulable disorders (protein S deficiency, homocysteinemia)
Giant cell arteritis (temporal arteritis, Takayasu arteritis)
Wegener granulomatosis, granulomatous arteritis
Sickle cell disease
Venous sinus thrombosis
Infectious vasculitis (neurovascular syphilis, Lyme disease, bacterial and fungal meningitis, tuberculous meningitis)
Moyamoya disease
Drug related

acute ischemic strokes, particularly when the area of the stroke is less than 5 mm in diameter or is located in the region of the brainstem or the stroke is less than 12 hours old. Further imaging with magnetic resonance may be considered.

Finally, imaging of the extracranial vasculature to detect severe **carotid artery stenosis is essential to guide further stroke prevention therapy.** Carotid Doppler ultrasound and magnetic resonance angiography are effective noninvasive imaging studies and are often used as first-line diagnostic tools.

Stroke prevention begins with **antiplatelet therapy,** and **aspirin** should be used in all cases unless there is a contraindication to its use. Use of **clopidogrel** or combination **aspirin and dipyridamole** may be slightly superior to aspirin for stroke prevention but at a substantially higher dollar cost. Combination therapy with aspirin and clopidogrel has not been shown to provide greater benefit in stroke prevention but does produce a higher rate of bleeding complications. For patients with TIA/stroke as a consequence of carotid atherosclerosis, medical management includes antiplatelet agents, and **aggressive risk factor reduction** with blood pressure control, treatment of hyperlipidemia, and smoking cessation. For patients with cardioembolic stroke as a result of **atrial fibrillation,** long-term **anticoagulation with warfarin** (Coumadin) reduces the risk of systemic embolization by approximately 70%. Newer oral anticoagulants (dabigatran, apixaban, rivaroxaban, and edoxaban) have recently been approved for patients with atrial fibrillation, and are comparable in efficacy to warfarin. For patients with small-vessel disease-producing lacunar infarctions, blood pressure control and antiplatelet agents are the mainstays of therapy.

Surgical endarterectomy for severe carotid artery stenosis has successfully reduced the long-term risk of stroke in both symptomatic and asymptomatic patients. The North American Symptomatic Carotid Endarterectomy Trial (NASCET) showed that in patients who had suffered a TIA or stroke and had an ipsilateral **carotid artery stenosis** greater than **70%**, endarterectomy reduced the rate of stroke from 26% to 9% over 2 years compared with standard medical management. The Asymptomatic Carotid Artery Stenosis (ACAS) trial also showed benefit from carotid endarterectomy in patients with **asymptomatic carotid artery stenoses** (those without prior TIA or stroke) **greater than 60%.** However, the risk reduction was smaller than in symptomatic patients, from 11% to 5% over 5 years compared to medical management. It should also be noted that the surgery is not without risk and can actually cause strokes. In both trials, the stipulation was made that in order to achieve the risk reduction benefit; **surgery should be performed in a center with very low surgical morbidity and mortality.** For asymptomatic patients, the benefits of the procedure do not begin to exceed the perioperative morbidity for at least 2 years, so it should be viewed as a "long-term investment" in patients with relatively low comorbidity and a long life expectancy.

Carotid angioplasty and stenting is another procedure available for patients with carotid stenosis but, like endarterectomy, also carries a risk of embolization and stroke. Angioplasty has not been proven to be superior to surgical endarterectomy, and its exact role is not yet defined. It may be considered as an alternative to surgery for symptomatic patients, those with previous TIA or stroke, whose surgical risk is believed to be too high or who are believed to have a high risk for restenosis. It is not recommended for patients with asymptomatic carotid stenosis.

CASE CORRELATION

- See also Case 38 (Headache) and Case 39 (Dizziness/Benign Positional Vertigo).

COMPREHENSION QUESTIONS

36.1 A previously healthy 75-year-old man experienced a TIA 2 weeks ago. On physical examination, he is found to have a right carotid bruit. Duplex ultrasound demonstrates a 75% stenosis of the right carotid artery. Which of the following is the best therapy?

A. Aspirin plus clopidogrel

B. Warfarin (Coumadin)

C. Carotid endarterectomy

D. Carotid artery stenting

36.2 One year ago, a 24-year-old woman had an episode of diplopia of 2 weeks' duration. The symptoms resolved completely. Currently, she complains of left arm weakness but no headache. Which of the following is the most likely diagnosis?

   A. Recurrent transient ischemic attacks

   B. Subarachnoid hemorrhage

   C. Complicated migraine

   D. Multiple sclerosis

36.3 A 67-year-old woman with extensive atherosclerotic cerebrovascular disease complains of dizziness and vertigo. Which of the following arteries is most likely to be affected?

   A. Vertebrobasilar

   B. Carotid

   C. Aorta

   D. Middle cerebral

36.4 A 62-year-old man who works at an automobile assembly line has noticed that he feels pain, fatigue, and numbness in his right arm while working for the last several months. This morning at work, he noticed vertigo, then light-headedness, then lost consciousness for a few seconds. The blood pressure in his right arm is 30 mm Hg lower than that in his left arm. What is the most likely diagnosis?

   A. Left middle cerebral artery stroke

   B. Lacunar infarction involving right internal capsule

   C. Stenosis of right subclavian artery due to atherosclerosis

   D. Multiple sclerosis

ANSWERS

36.1 **C.** This patient has symptomatic carotid disease which include symptoms such as TIAs, episodes of monocular blindness, and small, nondisabling ischemic strokes. A patient who presents with symptomatic carotid disease and stenosis between 70-99% should receive a carotid endarterectomy. It has been found that patients over the age of 70 fare better with a carotid endarterectomy rather than stenting alone. When symptomatic patients present with stenosis between 50-69%, management depends on gender. Women should receive optimal medical management where men should receive a carotid endarterectomy.

36.2 **D.** Multiple neurologic deficits separated in space and time in a young patient are suggestive of multiple sclerosis. Symptoms lasting longer than 24 hours as well as the patient's age makes transient ischemic attacks (even if recurrent) less likely to be the cause of her symptoms. A subarachnoid hemorrhage will often present with a "thunder clap headache" or "the worst headache" of the patient's life and is usually an isolated event. A complicated migraine can include symptoms such as changes in vision and arm weakness but with or before the onset of the headache.

36.3 **A.** Vertigo and dizziness can be seen in vertebrobasilar insufficiency. Transient monocular blindness or Amaurosis fugx is associated with internal carotid pathology. Face weakness, dysarthria, and hemiplegia greater in the upper extremity is associated with pathology in the middle cerebral artery.

36.4 **C.** The patient likely has subclavian steal: phenomenon of flow reversal in the vertebral artery ipsilateral to a hemodynamically significant stenosis of the subclavian artery. The neurologic symptoms can be caused by vertebrobasilar ischemia.

CLINICAL PEARLS

▶ The most common causes of cerebral infarction are carotid atherosclerotic stenosis, cardioembolism, and small-vessel disease such as lipohyalinosis.

▶ Cerebral infarction, transient ischemic attack, and amaurosis fugax all may be symptoms of carotid stenosis.

▶ In symptomatic patients with severe stenosis >70%, carotid endarterectomy is superior to medical therapy in stroke prevention provided the surgical risk is low (<6%).

▶ For other patients, stroke prevention consists mainly of antiplatelet agents (aspirin, clopidogrel) and risk factor modification, for example, lowering blood pressure, hypercholesterolemia, smoking cessation.

REFERENCES

Brott TG, Brown RD Jr, Meyer FB, et al. Carotid revascularization for prevention of stroke: carotid endarterectomy and carotid artery stenting. *Mayo Clin Proc.* 2004;79:1197-1208.

Furie KL, Kasner SE, Adams RJ, et al. Guidelines for the prevention of stroke in patients with stroke or transient ischemic attack: a guideline for healthcare professionals from the American Heart Association/American Stroke Association. *Stroke.* 2011;42(1):227.

Pulsinelli WA. Ischemic cerebrovascular disease. In: Goldman L, Bennett JC, eds. *Cecil's Textbook of Medicine.* 21st ed. Philadelphia, PA: WB Saunders; 2000:2099-2109.

Smith WS, English JD, Johnston SC. Cerebrovascular diseases. In: Kasper DL, Fauci AS, Hauser SL. et al. *Harrison's Principles of Internal Medicine.* 19th ed. New York, NY: McGraw-Hill; 2015: 2259-2586.

A 68-year-old woman is noted to have memory loss and confusion. Her daughter relates a history of progressive decline in her mother's cognitive function over the last year. The mother has lived on her own for many years, but recently she has begun to become unable to take care of herself. The daughter states that her mother has become withdrawn and has lost interest in her usual activities, such as gardening and reading. The patient was always a fastidious housekeeper; however, recently she is noted to wear the same clothes for several days, and her house is unkempt and dirty. She seems anxious and confused, and she calls her daughter several times a day, worried that the neighbors, previously good friends, are spying on her. She denies bowel or urinary incontinence, and she has had no trouble with headaches or gait instability. Overall the patient has been very healthy, and she only receives treatment with hydrochlorothiazide for hypertension. She never smoked and drank alcohol only rarely. On examination, her blood pressure is 116/56 mm Hg, heart rate is 78 bpm, temperature is 98.7°F, and respiratory rate is 18 bpm. Her weight is 160 lb and her height is 5 ft 3 in. She is noted to be well developed, but her affect throughout the examination is rather flat. She is oriented to person and place, but she is a little confused as to the date. Head, neck, and cardiovascular examinations are unremarkable. Examination of her abdomen is benign. The extremities are without edema, cyanosis, or clubbing. Neurologic examination reveals that the cranial nerves are intact, and the motor and sensory examinations are within normal limits. Cerebellar examination is unremarkable, and the gait is normal. Mini Mental State Examination (MMSE) reveals a score of 24 out of 30.

▶ What is the most likely diagnosis?
▶ What are the next diagnostic steps?
▶ What is the best treatment for this condition?

ANSWERS TO CASE 37:

Alzheimer Dementia

Summary: A 68-year-old woman has memory loss, confusion, and fatigue. She is more withdrawn and is noted to have a flat affect. She is oriented to person and place, but not to time. The remainder of the examination, including neurologic examination, is normal. Notable, however, is her low MMSE score.

- **Most likely diagnosis:** Alzheimer dementia.

- **Next diagnostic step:** Assess for depression and reversible causes of dementia.

- **Probable treatment:** Acetylcholinesterase inhibitor.

ANALYSIS

Objectives

1. Know some of the common causes and evaluation of dementia.

2. Understand the presentation and diagnosis of Alzheimer dementia.

3. Know acetylcholinesterase inhibitors may slow the progression of dementia.

Considerations

In this elderly patient with slowly progressive decline in memory and cognitive functioning, dementia due to Alzheimer disease (AD) is the most likely diagnosis. As in other cases of major organ system failure (heart and kidney failures), dementia (brain failure) necessitates investigation into treatable or reversible causes before assigning a diagnosis such as Alzheimer disease, which is progressive and incurable, and for which no highly effective therapy exists (Table 37–1).

Table 37-1 • INITIAL EVALUATION OF DEMENTIA
Routine Tests:
Complete blood count (CBC)
Electrolytes, blood urea nitrogen (BUN), creatinine, glucose
Thyroid function tests
Liver function tests
Serum vitamin B_{12} level
Computed tomography (CT) or magnetic resonance imaging (MRI) of the head
Optional Tests:
Venereal Disease Research Laboratory (VDRL) or RPR
Human immunodeficiency virus (HIV) assay
Urinalysis, urine toxin screen
Apo E genotyping for Alzheimer dementia
Lumbar puncture
Reversible Causes of Dementia:
Normal pressure hydrocephalus, alcohol dependence, medication side effects, hypothyroidism. B_{12} or thiamine deficiency

APPROACH TO:
Dementia

DEFINITIONS

DEMENTIA: (also called major neurocognitive disorder) Significant cognitive impairment in more than one of the following cognitive domains (learning and memory, language, executive function, complex attention, perceptual-motor function, social cognition). The impairment represents a decline from previous level of ability, interferes with daily functioning and independent living, and is not occurring exclusively during the course of delirium.

ALZHEIMER DISEASE: Leading cause of dementia, accounting for half of the cases involving elderly individuals, correlating to diffuse cortical atrophy and hippocampal atrophy with ventricular enlargement. The pathologic changes in the brains of patients with AD include neurofibrillary tangles with deposition of abnormal amyloid in the brain. Risk factors are advanced age, positive family history, and presence of apolipoprotein E4 allele.

VASCULAR (MULTI-INFARCT) DEMENTIA: Dementia in the setting of cerebrovascular disease, occurring after multiple cerebral infarctions, whether large or small (lacunar).

CLINICAL APPROACH

In assessing the patient with dementia, the clinician should strive to answer three questions: (1) What is the most likely diagnosis? (2) Is any treatable or reversible condition contributing to the patient's cognitive decline? (3) What interventions are available to preserve the patient's level of function and relieve the burden to caregivers?

To answer the first question, the most important investigation is the history of symptoms. If the patient has an acute or subacute onset of confusion or has a fluctuating level of consciousness, the most likely diagnosis is a **delirium** resulting from infection, intoxication, or adverse medication effects, or metabolic derangements such as hyponatremia, hypercalcemia, or hypoglycemia.

If cognitive decline occurs with prominent mood disturbance, then one consideration is **depression** or pseudodementia. Distinguishing which occurred first is often difficult because many elderly patients with cognitive decline and a declining level of independent functioning suffer from a reactive depression. History provided by involved family members regarding the onset of symptoms or history of prior depression or other psychiatric illness may help establish the diagnosis, and an empiric trial of antidepressants may be considered.

If the patient has a history of irregular stepwise decline in functioning, especially if the patient has had apparent stroke symptoms or transient ischemic events or has a known cardiovascular disease or atrial fibrillation, then vascular, or **multi-infarct, dementia** is the most likely diagnosis. This type of **vascular dementia is the second most common cause of dementia in the United States**, composing 10% to 20% of dementias. Other patients with cerebrovascular disease, especially as a result of long-standing hypertension, may develop diffuse subcortical white matter changes seen on imaging and an insidious rather than sudden stepwise decline in cognitive function. This condition is often referred to as *Binswanger disease* or *subcortical arteriosclerotic leukoencephalopathy.*

Other common causes of dementia include cognitive decline as a result of long-standing **alcoholism** or dementia associated with **parkinsonism**. Both of these underlying conditions may be discovered by the appropriate history or physical findings (eg, resting tremor with bradykinesia and masked faces of parkinsonism). Other dementia syndromes include behavioral changes with intact navigation in **frontotemporal dementia**, or rapid progression of dementia with muscular rigidity and myoclonus in **Creutzfeld-Jakob disease.**

Less common causes of dementia include medical conditions such as Wernicke encephalopathy resulting from thiamine (vitamin B_1) deficiency, vitamin B_{12} deficiency resulting from pernicious anemia, untreated **hypothyroidism**, or chronic infections such as **HIV** dementia or **neurosyphilis**. A variety of primary central nervous system (CNS) diseases can lead to dementia or other cognitive dysfunction, including Huntington disease, multiple sclerosis, neoplastic diseases such as primary or metastatic brain tumors (although they are much more likely to produce seizures or focal deficits rather than dementia), or leptomeningeal spread of various cancers.

Normal pressure hydrocephalus is a potentially reversible form of dementia in which the cerebral ventricles slowly enlarge as a result of disturbances to cerebral spinal fluid resorption. The **classic triad is dementia, gait disturbance, and urinary or bowel incontinence.** Relief of hydrocephalus through placement of a ventriculoperitoneal shunt may reverse the cognitive decline. Descriptions of the primary neurologic diseases associated with cognitive dysfunction are listed in Table 37–2.

Once likely diagnoses have been established by history and physical examination, investigation should be undertaken to look for treatable or reversible causes. The choice of laboratory or imaging tests is not straightforward because of the numerous, yet uncommon, causes of reversible dementia, so testing is generally low yield. Tests that may be considered for the evaluation of dementia are listed in Table 37–1. The American Academy of Neurology recommends routine assessment of thyroid function tests, a vitamin B_{12} level, and a neuroimaging study (either computed tomography [CT] or magnetic resonance imaging [MRI] of the brain).

For patients with AD, the average life expectancy after diagnosis is 7 to 10 years. The clinical course is characterized by progressive decline of cognitive functions (memory, orientation, attention, and concentration) and the development of psychological and behavioral symptoms (wandering, aggression, anxiety, depression, and psychosis; Table 37–3). The goals of treatment in AD are to (1) improve cognitive function, (2) reduce behavioral and psychological symptoms, and (3) improve the quality of life. **Donepezil, rivastigmine, and galantamine are *cholinesterase inhibitors* that are effective in improving cognitive function and global clinical state. Antagonists to N-methyl-D-aspartate (NMDA) receptors, such as memantine,** are effective in moderate to severe dementia. Risperidone reduces psychotic symptoms and aggression in patients with dementia.

Other issues include wakefulness, nightwalking and wandering, aggression, incontinence, and depression. A structured environment, with predictability, and

Table 37–2 • CAUSES OF DEMENTIA		
Disease	Clinical Features	Treatment
Alzheimer disease	Slow decline in cognitive and behavioral ability; pathology: neurofibrillary tangles, enlarged cerebral ventricles, atrophy	Cholinesterase inhibitors such as donepezil, rivastigmine, galantamine Add memantine for more advanced dementia
Normal-pressure hydrocephalus	Gait disturbance, dementia, incontinence; enlarged ventricles without atrophy	Ventricular shunting process
Vascular (multi-infarct) dementia	Focal deficits, stepwise loss of function; multiple areas of infarct, usually subcortical	Address atherosclerotic risk factors, identify and treat thrombus
Parkinson disease	Extrapyramidal signs (tremor, rigidity), slow onset	Dopaminergic agents
HIV infection	Systemic involvement; risk factors for acquisition; positive HIV serology	Antiretroviral therapy
Neurosyphilis	Optic atrophy, Argyll Robertson pupils, gait disturbance; positive cerebrospinal fluid serology	High-dose intravenous penicillin
Frontotemporal dementia (eg, Pick disease)	Behavioral and language deficits with spared memory; frontotemporal atrophy on MRI; intraneuronal inclusions (Pick bodies)	Supportive care, no therapy to slow progression or improve symptoms
Creutzfeldt-Jakob disease (CJD)	Rapidly progressive mental deterioration and myoclonus, death in <1 y of onset	No effective therapy; prion disease not transmissible, so no special precautions needed

judicious use of pharmacotherapy, such as a selective serotonin reuptake inhibitor (SSRI) for depression or trazodone for insomnia, are helpful. The primary caregiver is often overwhelmed and needs support. The Alzheimer Association is a national organization developed to give support to family members and can be contacted through its web site at *www.alz.org*.

Table 37–3 • CLINICAL COURSE OF ALZHEIMER DISEASE	
Clinical Stage	Manifestations
Early	Mild forgetfulness, poor concentration, fairly good function, denial, occasional disorientation
Intermediate MMSE 21-26	Drastic deficits of recent memory, can travel to familiar locations; suspicious, anxious, aware of confusion
Late MMSE 10-20	Cannot remember names of family members or close friends; may have delusions or hallucinations, agitation, aggression, wandering, disoriented to time and place; needs substantial care
Advanced MMSE <10	Totally incapacitated and disoriented, incontinent, personality and emotional changes; eventually all verbal and motor skills deteriorate, leading to need for total care

> CASE CORRELATION
>
> - See also Case 36 (Transient Ischemic Attacks) and Case 38 (Headache).

COMPREHENSION QUESTIONS

37.1 A 78-year-old woman is diagnosed with early Alzheimer disease. Which of the following agents is most likely to help with the cognitive function?

A. Haloperidol

B. Estrogen replacement therapy

C. Donepezil

D. High-dose vitamin B_{12} injections

37.2 A 74-year-old man was noted to have excellent cognitive and motor skill 12 months ago. His wife noted that 6 months ago his function deteriorated noticeably, and 2 months ago another level of deterioration was noted. Which of the following is most likely to reveal the etiology of his functional decline?

A. HIV antibody test

B. Magnetic resonance imaging of the brain

C. Cerebrospinal fluid (CSF) Venereal Disease Research Laboratory (VDRL) test

D. Serum thyroid-stimulating hormone

37.3 A 55-year-old man is noted by his family members to be forgetful and become disoriented. He has difficulty making it to the bathroom in time and complains of feeling as though "he is walking like he was drunk." Which of the following therapies is most likely to improve his condition?

A. Intravenous penicillin for 21 days

B. Rivastigmine

C. Treatment with fluoxetine for 9 to 12 months

D. Ventriculoperitoneal shunt

E. Enrollment into Alcoholics Anonymous

37.4 Which of the following are commonly seen in brain imaging of patients with Alzheimer disease?

A. Chronic subdural hematoma

B. Cortical atrophy with atrophy of medial temporal structures

C. Ventriculomegaly without cortical atrophy

D. Normal cerebral ventricles and normal brain tissue, acetylcholine deficiency

ANSWERS

37.1 **C.** Cholinesterase inhibitors help with the cognitive function in Alzheimer disease and may slow the progression. Cholinesterase inhibitors are considered first line therapy.

37.2 **B.** The stepwise decline in function is typical for multi-infarct dementia, diagnosed by viewing multiple areas of the brain infarct.

37.3 **D.** The classic triad for normal pressure hydrocephalus is dementia, incontinence, and gait disturbance; one treatment is shunting the cerebrospinal fluid.

37.4 **B.** Alzheimer disease has no pathognomonic structural imaging criteria, but may include cortical atrophy and mesial temporal atrophy, whereas normal pressure hydrocephalus has enlarged brain ventricles without significant brain atrophy. Functional imaging can detect decreased perfusion and decreased metabolism in the temporal, parietal, and prefrontal cortex in patients with AD.

CLINICAL PEARLS

▶ Alzheimer disease is the most common type of dementia, followed by multi-infarct (vascular) dementia.

▶ Approximately 5% of people older than 65 years and 20% older than 80 years have some form of dementia.

▶ Depression and reversible causes of dementia should be considered in the evaluation of a patient with memory loss and functional decline.

▶ Cholinesterase inhibitors are effective in improving cognitive function and global clinical state in patients with Alzheimer disease. The NMDA receptor antagonist is added in more advanced disease.

REFERENCES

Geldmacher DS, Whitehouse PJ. Evaluation of dementia. *N Engl J Med.* 1996;335:330-336.

Knopman DS, DeKosky ST, Cummings JL, et al. Practice parameter: diagnosis of dementia (an evidence-based review). *Neurology.* 2001;56:1143-1153.

Seeley WW, Miller BL. Alzheimer's disease and other dementias. In: Kasper DL, Fauci AS, Hauser SL. et al. *Harrison's Principles of Internal Medicine.* 19th ed. New York, NY: McGraw-Hill; 2015: 2598-2608.

A 59-year-old woman comes to your clinic because she is concerned that she might have a brain tumor. She has had a fairly severe headache for the last 3 weeks (she rates it as an 8 on a scale of 1-10). She describes the pain as constant, occasionally throbbing but mostly a dull ache, and localized to the right side of her head. She thinks the pain is worse at night, especially when she lies with that side of her head on the pillow. She has had no nausea, vomiting, photophobia, or other visual disturbances. She has had headaches before, but they were mostly occipital and frontal, which she attributed to "stress," and they were relieved with acetaminophen. Her medical history is significant for hypertension, which is controlled with hydrochlorothiazide, and "arthritis" of her neck, shoulders, and hips for which she takes ibuprofen when she feels stiff and achy. On physical examination, her temperature is 100.4°F, heart rate is 88 bpm, blood pressure is 126/75 mm Hg, and respiratory rate is 12 bpm. Her visual acuity is normal, visual fields are intact, and her funduscopic examination is significant for arteriolar narrowing but no papilledema or hemorrhage. She has moderate tenderness over the right side of her head but no obvious scalp lesions. Her chest is clear, and her heart rhythm is regular, with normal S_1 and S_2 but an S_4 gallop. Abdominal examination is benign. She has no focal deficits on neurologic examination. She has no joint swelling or deformity but is tender to palpation over her shoulders, hips, and thighs.

▶ What is the most likely diagnosis?
▶ What is the best next step to confirm the diagnosis?

ANSWERS TO CASE 38:
Headache/Temporal Arteritis

Summary: A 59-year-old woman complains of a 3-week history of severe right-side headaches that are worse at night, when she lies with that side of her head on the pillow. Her medical history is significant for hypertension and "arthritis" of her neck, shoulders, and hips, for which she takes ibuprofen. She has a temperature 100.4°F and normal neurologic and eye examinations. She has moderate tenderness over the right side of her head but no obvious scalp lesions.

- **Most likely diagnosis:** Giant cell (temporal) arteritis (GCA).

- **Best next diagnostic step:** Erythrocyte sedimentation rate (ESR).

ANALYSIS

Objectives

1. Be familiar with the clinical features that help to distinguish a benign headache from one representing a serious underlying illness.

2. Know the clinical features and diagnostic tests for GCA.

3. Know the clinical features of migraine and cluster headaches and of subarachnoid hemorrhage.

Considerations

Although headaches are a very common complaint, this patient has features that are of greater concern: older age of onset, abrupt onset and severe intensity, and dissimilarity to previous milder headaches. The mnemonic SNOOP can be used as reminders of red flags, or danger signs of significant underlying pathology, and is outlined in Table 38–1. She is very concerned about the headaches and is worried that they indicate a brain tumor. She has no meningeal signs, and her neurologic examination is nonfocal. She has stiffness and achiness of the shoulder and hip girdles. Together these factors make the diagnosis of GCA a strong possibility. GCA usually has its onset in patients aged 50 or older (females more than males), and involves inflammation of the medium- or large-size vessels. Her low-grade fever and generalized body aches may represent polymyalgia rheumatica, which is closely associated with GCA. The diagnosis would be suggested by an elevated ESR, and then confirmed by temporal artery biopsy. Although GCA is not a common cause of headache, untreated patients often progress to permanent visual loss as a consequence of involvement of the ophthalmic artery, so a high index of suspicion is necessary to begin investigation. An elevated ESR necessitates further diagnostic testing, such as a temporal artery biopsy. In the meantime, empiric corticosteroids may help prevent complications.

Table 38-1 • RED FLAGS FOR SERIOUS HEADACHE DISORDERS
Any of these findings should prompt further investigation, including brain imaging (CT or MRI): • **S**ystemic symptoms, illness, or condition (fever, cancer, HIV or other immunocompromised state) • **N**eurologic signs or symptoms (altered mental status, loss of consciousness, focal neurologic signs, seizures, meningismus) • **O**nset is new (especially age >40) or sudden (thunderclap headache) • **O**ther associated conditions or features (head trauma, headache awakens from sleep, worse with Valsalva, exertion, or sexual activity) • **P**revious headache history with progressive symptoms, or change in frequency, severity

APPROACH TO:

Headaches

DEFINITIONS

TEMPORAL ARTERITIS: Also known as giant cell arteritis, temporal arteritis is a common form of systemic vascular inflammation affecting patients older than 50 years. Medium- and large-sized vessels, especially the superficial temporal artery, are affected.

BERRY ANEURYSM: A small saccular outpouching that looks like a berry and classically occurs at the point at which a cerebral artery departs from the circle of Willis at the base of the brain. They can rupture, causing subarachnoid hemorrhage.

CLINICAL APPROACH

Headache is one of the most common complaints of patients in medical practice. It periodically afflicts 90% of adults, and almost 25% have recurrent severe headaches. As with many common symptoms, a broad range of conditions, from trivial to life-threatening, might be responsible. The **majority of patients** presenting with **headache** have **tension-type, migraine,** or **cluster**; however, fewer than 1 in 20 have significant underlying pathology. Because headache symptoms usually are accompanied by a paucity of associated findings, including those on laboratory examination, the clinician must depend largely on a thorough history with a general and focused neurologic examination as the initial workup. Careful history and physical examination, keeping in mind the "red flags" of headaches (see Table 38–1), will serve the clinician well. Differentiating serious underlying causes of headache from more benign causes may be difficult. Table 38–2 lists some typical features of serious causes of headache.

One of the most catastrophic secondary causes of headache is **subarachnoid hemorrhage**, usually secondary to a ruptured intracerebral (berry) aneurysm. Up to 4% of patients presenting to an emergency center with severe headache, or the classic "worst ever headache," have a subarachnoid bleed. The initial hemorrhage may be fatal, may result in severe neurologic impairment, or may produce only minor symptoms such as headache. A high index of suspicion is needed because no neurologic findings may be present initially, and the patient who will

Table 38–2 • CAUSES OF HEADACHE

Disease	Clinical Features	Diagnostic Findings
Meningitis	Nuchal rigidity, headache, photophobia, and prostration; may not be febrile	Lumbar puncture is diagnostic
Intracranial hemorrhage	Nuchal rigidity and headache; may not have clouded consciousness or seizures	Hemorrhage may not be seen on CT scan; lumbar puncture shows "bloody tap" that does not clear by the last tube; a fresh hemorrhage may not be xanthochromic
Brain tumor	May present with prostrating pounding headaches that are associated with nausea and vomiting; may be associated with focal neurologic deficits, or mental status changes	CT or MRI
Temporal arteritis	May present with a unilateral pounding headache; onset generally in older patients (≤50 y) and frequently associated with visual changes	Erythrocyte sedimentation rate is the best screening test and usually is markedly elevated (ie, >50 mm/h); definitive diagnosis can be made by arterial biopsy
Acute angle-closure glaucoma	Usually consists of severe eye pain; may have nausea and vomiting; the eye usually is painful and red; the pupil may be partially dilated	Elevated intraocular pressure
Migraine headache	Unilateral throbbing headache with preceding aura, photophobia, and nausea, which is relieved with sleep	Headache *with associated features* (photophobia, nausea, aura, unilateral, throbbing, aggravation with movement)
Cluster headache	Male predominance; precipitated by alcohol; occurs with rhinorrhea and lacrimation	
Tension headache	Occipital-frontal headache; constant, "bandlike"; relieved with relaxation	Headache *without* associated features

(*Adapted with permission, from Raskin NH. Headache. In: Braunwald E, Fauci AS, Kasper KL, et al, eds.* Harrison's Principles of Internal Medicine, *16th ed. New York: McGraw-Hill, 2005:86.*)

benefit the most from intervention will often have the mildest symptoms. The first diagnostic study should be a noncontrast CT scan with thin imaging cuts at the region of the brain base. This study will be positive in more than 90% of cases on the first day, with decreasing sensitivity over the next several days. If hemorrhage is suspected but the CT is negative, lumbar puncture should be performed as soon as possible to assess for the presence of red cells or xanthochromia (yellowish discoloration of cerebrospinal fluid [CSF]); this finding indicates presence of bilirubin and differentiates subarachnoid hemorrhage from a traumatic lumbar puncture.

Giant cell arteritis, or **temporal arteritis**, is a chronic vasculitis of large- and medium-size vessels, usually involving the cranial branches of the arteries arising from the aortic arch. The clinical criteria for diagnosis include age of onset older than 50 years, new onset or type of headache pattern, tenderness or decreased pulsation of the temporal artery, elevated ESR, and abnormal findings on biopsy of the temporal artery. The presence of three or more criteria yields more than 90% sensitivity and specificity for the diagnosis. GCA is closely related to **polymyalgia rheumatica**, an inflammatory condition characterized by bilateral aching and stiffness of neck, torso, shoulders, or thighs, with a significantly elevated ESR. Both conditions probably are polygenic diseases in which various environmental and genetic factors influence susceptibility and severity. Clinical symptoms may include jaw claudication, and the most worrisome complication is permanent or partial loss of vision in one or both eyes, which can occur as an early manifestation in up to 20% of patients. Temporal artery biopsy is recommended in all patients suspected of having GCA, and long segments (>2 cm) of the artery may require excision in order to find the typical areas of segmental inflammation. Corticosteroids are the drugs of choice to treat both polymyalgia rheumatica and GCA, with daily doses of 10 to 20 mg of prednisone for polymyalgia rheumatica, and 40 to 60 mg for GCA. Steroids may prevent, but usually do not reverse, visual loss. Steroid dosage is gradually tapered, but relapse is common, as are complications of corticosteroid therapy.

Migraine headache is much more common than GCA but is more variable in its presentation. It is the most common cause of initial clinic visits for headache because of its frequency, disabling qualities, and associated symptoms. Migraine attacks are more common in women than in men. Migraine attacks may or may not have a preceding aura, may be unilateral or bilateral, and may have either throbbing or nonpulsatile pain, including the neck. Accompanying symptoms often include nausea, vomiting, photophobia or phonophobia during attacks. They may also have cranial autonomic features such as tearing or nasal congestion, leading to the misdiagnosis of sinus disease. A number of evidence-based guidelines are available for managing migraine headaches. Treatment of acute episodes involves the initial use of nonsteroidal anti-inflammatory drugs (NSAIDs), followed by triptans if symptoms persist. Preventive therapies include tricyclic antidepressants, beta-blockers, or anticonvulsants such as valproate or topiramate.

Episodic **cluster headache** is much less common, but it is more easily diagnosed by its distinctive pattern of periodic attacks of intense, unilateral, periorbital pain with nasal or ocular watering lasting only minutes to hours but recurring daily over several weeks or months. Acute attacks can be treated with oxygen or subcutaneous sumatriptan.

CASE CORRELATION

- See also Case 36 (Transient Ischemic Attacks), Case 37 (Alzheimer Dementia), Case 39 (Dizziness), and Case 43 (Meningitis).

COMPREHENSION QUESTIONS

Match the headache type (A-E) to the clinical presentation described in Questions
38.1 to 38.3.

A. Migraine headache

B. Tension headache

C. Cluster headache

D. Subarachnoid hemorrhage

E. Meningitis

38.1 A 42-year-old man with polycystic kidney disease who complained of a
sudden onset of severe headache and then lost consciousness

38.2 A 22-year-old college student with fever, headache, photophobia, and
25 white blood cells per high-power field, but no red blood cells or xanthochromia in CSF

38.3 A 31-year-old woman with a long history of intermittent severe unilateral
throbbing headache lasting hours to days associated with nausea and photophobia, but no preceding symptoms and no visual disturbance, occurring
once or twice per month

ANSWERS

38.1 **D.** The sudden onset of severe headache with diminution in level of consciousness is classic for subarachnoid hemorrhage. This patient likely had
rupture of a cerebral artery aneurysm, which is associated with polycystic
kidney disease.

38.2 **E.** The presence of white blood cells but no red blood cells in the CSF is
indicative of meningeal inflammation, likely due to viral or bacterial infection.

38.3 **A.** The patient's history is strongly suggestive of migraine, given its unilateral
and throbbing character, and the associated symptoms of nausea or photophobia. Most patients with disabling headache have migraine. Tension headache should have none of these features.

CLINICAL PEARLS

▶ Temporal arteritis usually involves one or more branches of the carotid artery and almost always occurs in patients older than 50 years. Diagnosis is suggested by an elevated ESR and confirmed by temporal artery biopsy.

▶ Visual loss is a common complication of temporal arteritis and can be prevented by initiation of high-dose corticosteroids when the diagnosis is suspected.

▶ Subarachnoid hemorrhage typically presents as a sudden onset of severe headache and is diagnosed by visualization of blood on a computed tomographic (CT) scan or by finding red blood cells or xanthochromic fluid on a lumbar puncture.

▶ Migraine is the most common type of headache for which patients seek medical attention in a clinic setting. It is an episodic headache with associated features such as nausea or photophobia.

REFERENCES

Edlow J, Caplan L. Avoiding pitfalls in the diagnosis of subarachnoid hemorrhage. *N Engl J Med.* 2000;342:29-36.

Goadsby PJ, Raskin NH. Migraine and other primary headache disorders. In: Kasper DL, Fauci AS, Hauser SL, et al. *Harrison's Principles of Internal Medicine.* 19th ed. New York, NY: McGraw-Hill; 2015:2587-2598.

Kaniecki R. Headache assessment and management. *JAMA.* 2003;289:1430-1433.

Salvarani C, Cantini F, Boiardi L, et al. Polymyalgia rheumatica and giant cell arteritis. *N Engl J Med.* 2002;347:261-278.

Snow V, Weiss K, Wall E, et al. Pharmacologic management of acute attacks of migraine and prevention of migraine headache. *Ann Intern Med.* 2002;137:840-852.

A 42-year-old Hispanic factory worker presents with complaints of dizziness. When asked to describe what "dizzy" means to her, she relates a feeling of movement, even though she is standing still. The first time it happened, she also felt a little nauseated, but she did not vomit. Since then, she has not felt nauseated. In her job, she has to look down to fold clothes coming off the line, and the dizziness occurs if she looks down too quickly. It only lasts about a minute, but it is disruptive to her work. The symptom has also occurred when she is lying down and rolls over in bed. She has no medical history or related family history. Her vital signs and heart, lung, and gastrointestinal (GI) examinations are normal. Her pupils are equal, round, and reactive to light and accommodation. Extraocular movements are intact, and no nystagmus is noted. Cranial nerve examination is normal. Strength, deep tendon reflexes, and gait are normal.

► What is your diagnosis?
► What is the best therapy for the condition?

ANSWERS TO CASE 39:
Dizziness/Benign Positional Vertigo

Summary: A previously healthy 42-year-old woman presents with intermittent positional vertigo and a normal physical examination.

- **Most likely diagnosis:** Benign positional vertigo.

- **Best treatment:** A maneuver to dislodge the loose otolith from the affected semicircular canal can be performed in the office, or medications such as meclizine can be prescribed to treat the symptoms. For severe symptoms, diazepam (Valium) or transdermal scopolamine patches can be prescribed.

ANALYSIS

Objectives

1. Understand how to categorize types of dizziness.

2. Distinguish "benign" positional vertigo from more serious central causes of vertigo.

3. Recognize the symptoms and signs related to positional vertigo.

4. Understand the treatment options for vertigo.

Considerations

This previously healthy 42-year-old woman complains of acute onset of "dizziness," especially when moving her head quickly. Upon further questioning, the symptom of vertigo is established, that is, the perception of movement when she is stationary. She has no neurologic symptoms such as cranial nerve dysfunction, headache, or history of head trauma. The normal neurologic examination similarly suggests a benign process. The patient most likely has benign positional vertigo, which is the most common cause of acute vertigo. The pathophysiology likely is debris in the semicircular canals of the middle ear. Anticholinergic medications and positional maneuvers are often useful in therapy.

APPROACH TO:
Dizziness and Vertigo

DEFINITIONS

BENIGN POSITIONAL VERTIGO: Most common cause of vertigo caused by debris in the semicircular canals of the inner ear.

DIX-HALLPIKE MANEUVER: Positional maneuver used to diagnose benign positional paroxysmal vertigo.

Table 39–1 • CHARACTERISTICS OF CENTRAL VERSUS PERIPHERAL CAUSES OF VERTIGO

	Peripheral Etiology	Central Etiology
Duration of vertigo	Intermittent (minutes, hours) but recurrent	Sudden onset, persistent symptoms
Associated tinnitus, hearing loss	Often present	Usually not present
Other neurologic deficits (cranial nerve palsies, dysarthria, extremity weakness)	Not present	Often present

VERTIGO: Illusory sensation of movement or spinning. **Peripheral vertigo** is caused by the labyrinthine apparatus or vestibular nerve, whereas **central vertigo** is caused by a brainstem or cerebellar process (Table 39–1).

CLINICAL APPROACH

The complaint of dizziness is one of the most common reasons for patients to seek medical attention, and one of the most common reasons for the clinician to throw up his or her hands in exasperation because of the vagueness of the complaint. "Dizziness" is a word that can encompass a myriad of symptoms, including light-headedness, vertigo, "feeling out of sorts," and even gait instability. **The first step in evaluating patients with this complaint is to ask open-ended questions about the sensation ("What do you mean by dizzy?")** and to listen to the patient's history. Asking leading questions ("Did you feel like the room was spinning?") can cause one to go down the wrong diagnostic path. **The majority of patients who complain of dizziness are suffering from a distinctive symptom—presyncope, dysequilibrium, or vertigo—which can be elucidated by history or physical examination.**

Presyncope is the sensation associated with near-fainting. Patients may describe feeling light-headed, a graying of vision, or "nearly blacking out." This sensation typically is brief, lasting seconds or minutes, and is self-resolving. The causes of this symptom are the same as those for syncope: most often vasovagal attacks, orthostatic hypotension, or cardiac arrhythmias. The evaluation of these patients is the same as for those with syncope (see Case 9).

Dysequilibrium is a sense of imbalance, usually while walking. It is a multifactorial disorder, commonly seen in elderly patients with impaired vision, peripheral neuropathy and decreased proprioception, and musculoskeletal problems causing gait instability. It may also be one of the presenting symptoms of patients with primary movement disorders such as parkinsonism. These symptoms may be exacerbated by medications, particularly in the elderly; examples include antihypertensives, antidepressants, and anticholinergic agents that can cause orthostatic hypotension or dizziness as a side effect.

Vertigo is the illusory sensation of movement or spinning, and usually arises from a disorder in the vestibular system. Our spatial orientation system is composed of three primary components. In the inner ear, the **semicircular canals** transduce rotational acceleration, while the **otolith organs** (utricle and saccule) sense linear acceleration. These systems send information through projections to the cerebellum, spinal cord, and cerebral cortex, cranial nerves III, IV, and VI. The **vestibular ocular reflex** maintains visual stability during head movements through these same cranial nerves, as well as projections through the medial longitudinal fasciculus. This integration of the inner ear, brain, and eyes explains why **nystagmus** is observed in patients during bouts of vertigo. It is asymmetry or discordance between the vestibular inputs from the two labyrinths or their central pathways that causes the sensation of vertigo. Physiologic vertigo includes motion sickness, or the sensation of movement that may occur when watching motion pictures.

Pathologic vertigo occurs when there are lesions in one of these systems. The first task in evaluating a patient with vertigo is to try to distinguish **peripheral** (labyrinthine apparatus or vestibular nerve) from **central** (brainstem or cerebellum) causes of vertigo. **Central causes, such as cerebellar hemorrhage or infarction, can be immediately life threatening or signify serious underlying disease and require urgent investigation.** Peripheral causes typically signify less serious diseases and can be managed comfortably on an outpatient basis. Thus, the presence of other neurologic abnormalities, headache, or evidence of increased intracranial pressure is critical to address.

The most common type of vertigo seen is termed **"benign" paroxysmal positional vertigo (BPPV)**, although the symptoms can be far from benign. Typically, this type of vertigo is precipitated by changes in head position, as in rolling over in bed, bending over, or looking upward. Patients may not have all of the typical symptoms at the same time; however, the first bout usually is abrupt in onset and associated with nausea. Subsequent occurrences may be less severe. BPPV is thought to be caused by loose, floating calcium debris in the semicircular canals that causes an increase in neurologic discharge from the vestibular system on that side.

Nystagmus during episodes of vertigo is characteristic of BPPV. To confirm the diagnosis of BPPV in the office, the **Dix-Hallpike maneuver** (Figure 39–1) can be

Figure 39–1. Dix-Hallpike maneuver. The clinician holds the patient's head and moves the patient rapidly from a sitting to a head-hanging position, first with the head facing one side and then facing the other side. Individuals with benign positional vertigo will demonstrate nystagmus after a delay of a few seconds.

performed to elicit the nystagmus and vertigo. Patients turn their head toward the examiner and lay down quickly with their head hanging somewhat lower than the body. The eyes are kept open. The typical nystagmus is a mix of rotational and vertical eye movements. There is a lag of 5 to 10 seconds for the nystagmus to occur, and it is accompanied by the sensation of vertigo. A positive **Dix-Hallpike test**, along with the absence of other otologic or neurologic findings, indicates posterior canal dysfunction in the ear that is turned downward during the exercise, and makes the diagnosis of BPPV very likely.

BPPV is a self-limited disorder that may recur at some point in the patient's future. Anticholinergic agents, such as meclizine or diphenhydramine, or benzodiazepines may help lessen symptoms. Alternatively one may attempt positional maneuvers in the office to displace the otolith from the semicircular canal back into the utricle or saccule, such as **the Epley maneuver** (Figure 39–2). Table 39–2 lists other causes of vertigo and their associated clinical features.

Other causes of peripheral vertigo include Ménière disease and acoustic neuroma. **Ménière disease** is due to idiopathic excess endolymphatic fluid. Patients may experience episodes of vertigo lasting for minutes to hours, usually associated with unilateral tinnitus, hearing loss, and ear fullness. They usually have low-frequency sensorineural hearing loss on audiometry. Treatment includes antihistamines or anticholinergics during acute attacks, and diuretics to reduce endolymphatic fluid.

Acoustic neuromas are benign slow-growing tumors of Schwann cells. Because they are slow-growing, the subtle imbalances in vestibular input are often compensated, and patients may not experience significant vertigo, only vague imbalance. Presenting symptoms typically include unilateral hearing loss and tinnitus. Treatment is usually surgical.

Finally, approximately 10% to 15% of patients have **nonspecific dizziness**, which cannot be classified as vertigo, presyncope, or dysequilibrium. Patients cannot clearly describe one of these syndromes, can report only that they feel "dizzy," have vague or unusual sensations, and have normal neurologic and vestibular examinations. The majority of these patients have some underlying **psychiatric disorder**, such as major depression, generalized anxiety, or panic disorder. Often the dizziness is associated with **hyperventilation** and can be reproduced in the office by purposeful hyperventilation. Treatment should be aimed at **reassurance** regarding the lack of pathologic causes of dizziness and at therapy for the underlying disorder with medication such as serotonin-specific reuptake inhibitors or benzodiazepines for anxiety disorders.

CASE CORRELATION

- See also Case 36 (Transient Ischemic Attacks), Case 37 (Alzheimer Dementia), and Case 38 (Headache).

Figure 39–2. Modified Epley maneuver. First the Dix-Hallpike maneuver is performed to identify the affected ear. Then the patient's head is systematically rotated so that the loose particles slide out of the posterior semicircular canal into the utricle.

Table 39–2 • COMMON CAUSES OF VERTIGO	
Benign positional paroxysmal vertigo	Nausea associated with nystagmus and vertigo with positional change, improves with time, absence of other otologic or neurologic findings, and a positive Dix-Hallpike test
Ménière disease	Intermittent attacks of severe vertigo are associated with tinnitus and hearing loss, sensation of ear fullness
Acoustic neuroma	Slow-growing tumor, so system compensates and often there is little vertigo; usually with hearing loss and tinnitus
Vertebrobasilar insufficiency	Vertigo occurs in association with brainstem symptoms such as diplopia, dysarthria, or with numbness.

COMPREHENSION QUESTIONS

39.1 A young woman presents to your office complaining of dizziness. When asked to describe the feeling, she gives a vague story of just feeling like "her head is too big" and she "feels like is not really here." The feeling is associated with palpitations, sweating, and nervousness and typically resolves in less than an hour. Her examination, including neurologic evaluation, is completely normal. Which of the following is the best next step?

A. Magnetic resonance imaging (MRI) brain scan.

B. Obtaining a thorough psychosocial history.

C. Dix-Hallpike maneuver.

D. Prescribe meclizine.

E. Referral to neurology department.

39.2 A 75-year-old man presents to the emergency room with the sudden onset of nausea and vomiting. His medical history is notable for coronary artery disease and well-controlled hypertension. On examination he refuses to open his eyes or move his head, but when finally coaxed to sit up, he immediately starts to retch and vomit. Rotational nystagmus is noted. He cannot walk because of the dizziness and nausea that walking evokes. His noncontrast brain computed tomography (CT) scan is read as normal for age. Which of the following is the best next step?

A. MRI/magnetic resonance angiography (MRA).

B. Obtain a thorough psychosocial history.

C. Dix-Hallpike maneuver.

D. Prescribe meclizine.

E. Referral to neurology.

39.3 A 65-year-old woman with a history of benign positional vertigo returns to your office for follow-up. Although manageable, the symptoms of vertigo continue to recur periodically. Between episodes she generally feels normal but occasionally somewhat "off-balance." Today, her neurologic examination is completely normal, except that the thresholds of both air and bone conduction of a vibrating 256-Hz tuning fork are elevated on the left side. Which of the following is the most likely diagnosis?

A. Intermittent benign positional vertigo

B. Otosclerosis

C. Acoustic neuroma

D. Acute basilar artery infarct

E. Panic disorder

39.4 Which of the following is the best next step for the patient described in Question 39.3?

A. Prescription for a selective serotonin reuptake inhibitor

B. Referral for a hearing aid

C. Lumbar puncture and serology for syphilis

D. Referral for an MRI

E. Reassurance

ANSWERS

39.1 **B.** This young woman is not describing vertigo. The word "dizzy" can mean several different things, so it is extremely important when obtaining the history to have the patient describe, as best he or she can, what is meant by "dizzy." Patients with vertigo often use descriptors indicating movement, such as "the room is moving around me" or "I'm on a roller coaster." Vague symptoms, or "out-of-body" experiences, or feeling disconnected from the environment, such as this young woman describes, are not typical of vertigo and indicate another problem. It would be important to know what the symptoms are associated with; for example, is there increased stress in her job or intimate relationship? Is this panic disorder or anxiety disorder?

39.2 **A.** This patient has symptoms of central vertigo. The onset of symptoms was abrupt and severe. His gait is affected. If he were able to cooperate with an examination of his cerebellar functions, it would most likely be abnormal. His age and history of hypertension and coronary artery disease place him at elevated risk for cerebellar infarction or hemorrhage. CT is not the appropriate test for examining the brainstem; MRI is much more accurate. MRA may be useful for delineating the exact vascular cause of the symptoms.

39.3 **C.** Acoustic neuromas are slow-growing tumors of the eighth cranial nerve. Because of the slow growth of the tumor, the neurologic system often is able to accommodate, so patients may have only subtle symptoms that at first may be confused with benign positional vertigo. The keys in this patient's history are the persistent low-grade feelings of dysequilibrium and the finding of probable sensorineural hearing loss on the left side. This finding indicates a possible problem with the eighth nerve, and an MRI would best delineate the anatomy.

39.4 **D.** MRI is the diagnostic test of choice. See answer to Question 39.3.

CLINICAL PEARLS

▶ Patients use the term "dizziness" to describe several sensations: vertigo, presyncope, dysequilibrium, and the nonspecific dizziness that may be associated with psychiatric disorders.

▶ Central causes of vertigo, such as cerebellar hemorrhage or infarction, can be immediately life threatening and require urgent investigation.

▶ Peripheral causes of vertigo typically produce intermittent but severe attacks of vertigo; they may have associated tinnitus or hearing loss but should not be associated with other neurologic abnormalities.

▶ Benign paroxysmal positional vertigo is the most common cause of vertigo and can be diagnosed by the history of intermittent positional symptoms, absence of other otologic or neurologic findings, and a positive Dix-Hallpike test.

▶ Benign positional vertigo can be treated with maneuvers to reposition the abnormal otolith from the semicircular canal or by anticholinergic medications such as meclizine.

REFERENCES

Balch RB. Vestibular neuritis. *N Engl J Med.* 2003;348:1027-1032.

Drachman D, Hart CW. An approach to the dizzy patient. *Neurology.* 1972;22:323-334.

Walker MF, Daroff RB. Dizziness and vertigo. In: Kasper DL, Fauci AS, Hauser SL, et al., eds. *Harrison's Principles of Internal Medicine.* 19th ed. New York, NY: McGraw-Hill; 2015:148-151.

CASE 40

A 25-year-old man comes to an outpatient clinic complaining of low-grade fever and sore throat, and he receives an injection of intramuscular penicillin for presumed streptococcal pharyngitis. He is otherwise healthy and takes no regular medications. Within 20 minutes, he begins to complain of swelling of his face and difficulty breathing. He looks dyspneic and frightened. His heart rate is 130 bpm, blood pressure is 90/47 mm Hg, and respiratory rate is 28 bpm and shallow. His face and lips are edematous, and he can barely open his eyes because of swelling. He is wheezing diffusely, and he has multiple raised urticarial lesions on his skin. An ambulance has been called.

▶ What is the most likely diagnosis?
▶ What is your next step?

ANSWERS TO CASE 40:

Anaphylaxis/Drug Reactions

Summary: A 25-year-old man develops facial edema and difficulty breathing minutes after receiving an injection of penicillin. He is tachypneic and tachycardic, with borderline hypotension. He is wheezing diffusely, his abdomen is nondistended with hyperactive bowel sounds, and his skin is warm with multiple raised urticarial lesions.

- **Most likely diagnosis:** Anaphylaxis as a result of penicillin hypersensitivity.

- **Next step:** Immediate administration of intramuscular epinephrine, along with corticosteroids and H_1 and H_2 blockers. Close observation of the patient's airway and oxygenation, with possible endotracheal intubation if he becomes compromised.

ANALYSIS

Objectives

1. Learn the clinical presentation and emergency management of anaphylaxis.

2. Understand the diagnosis and complications of serum sickness.

3. Be able to recognize and treat erythema multiforme minor and major.

Considerations

This young man developed manifestations of immediate hypersensitivity, with urticaria, facial angioedema, and bronchospasm. Penicillin is fairly allergenic and leads to an immunoglobulin (Ig)E-mediated release of histamines and other vasoactive chemicals. Epinephrine is the agent of choice in acute anaphylaxis. Antihistamines may also help. Because the airway is vulnerable to compromise as a result of severe edema, intubation to protect the airway is sometimes indicated.

APPROACH TO:

Suspected Anaphylaxis

DEFINITIONS

ANGIOEDEMA: Swelling of the lips, periorbital region, face, hands, or feet.

ANAPHYLACTOID REACTIONS: Similar clinical picture to anaphylaxis but not caused by immunologic mechanisms.

ANAPHYLAXIS: Syndrome with varied mechanisms, clinical presentations, and severity that is an acute life-threatening reaction resulting from a type I hypersensitivity reaction: **IgE-mediated activation of mast cells. Mast cell degranulation** results in release of histamine, interleukins, and other inflammatory mediators.

CLINICAL APPROACH

Common causes of anaphylaxis include drugs, hymenoptera stings (bees, wasps), radiographic contrast media (anaphylactoid), blood products, latex in medical products, allergen immunotherapy injections, and foods. **The most common cause of drug-related anaphylaxis is beta-lactam antibiotics such as penicillin.** The most common cause of food-related anaphylaxis is peanuts, partly because of the frequency with which peanut products are included in other types of foods. In fact, peanut allergy has doubled in incidence in Western countries. A recent randomized trial suggested that introducing peanut products below 1-year-old age seemed to decrease the development of peanut allergy (13.7% control vs 1.9% early exposure). It is important to note that almost any agent that can activate mast cells or basophils can cause an anaphylactic reaction. Approximately, one-third of all cases of anaphylaxis are idiopathic.

The clinical presentation of anaphylactic reactions varies greatly, but the following guidelines are a good rule of thumb. Symptoms usually develop within 5 to 60 minutes following exposure, although a delayed reaction is possible. Symptoms and signs are variable and are listed in Table 40–1. The key fact to remember is that a **true anaphylactic reaction is life threatening**. Angioedema may occur with or without urticaria but is not anaphylaxis unless the reaction is associated with other life-threatening processes, such as hypotension or laryngeal edema.

Treatment of anaphylaxis begins with first assessing the **ABCs** (airway, breathing, circulation). Intubation, if required, should not be delayed. Second, **epinephrine** should be administered to help control symptoms and blood pressure. Intramuscular epinephrine injected in the anterolateral thigh leads to more rapid and higher peak levels than does either subcutaneous or deltoid intramuscular injection. Additional treatment measures include placing the patient in a recumbent position, elevating the legs, administration of oxygen as needed, normal saline (NS) volume replacement and/or pressors as required, and administration of diphenhydramine 50 mg orally or intravenously every 4 hours as needed (Table 40–2).

Other considerations in the differential diagnosis of anaphylaxis include erythema multiforme major and minor. **Erythema multiforme minor** often occurs after herpes simplex virus (HSV) or other infections. It manifests as urticarial or bullous skin lesions. The pathognomonic finding is a **target lesion**, described as a lesion that is

Table 40–1 • CLINICAL MANIFESTATIONS OF ANAPHYLAXIS
Pruritus
Flushing, urticaria, and angioedema
Diaphoresis
Sneezing, rhinorrhea, nasal congestion
Hoarseness, stridor, laryngeal edema
Dyspnea, tachypnea, wheezing, bronchorrhea, cyanosis
Tachycardia, bradycardia, hypotension, cardiac arrest, arrhythmias
Nausea/vomiting, diarrhea, abdominal cramping
Dizziness, weakness, syncope
Sense of impending doom
Seizures

Table 40–2 • SUGGESTED TREATMENT OF ANAPHYLAXIS
Address ABCs (airway, breathing, circulation); intubate, if needed
Epinephrine either as intravenous solution (1:1000 0.1-0.3 mL in 10 mL of normal saline over several minutes) or intramuscularly (1:1000 0.3-0.5 mL every 5 min as needed)
Oxygen as needed
Place the patient in a recumbent position, elevate the legs
Normal saline volume replacement and/or pressors as required
Diphenhydramine 50 mg orally or intravenously every 4 h as needed
Other measures
• Ranitidine or other H_2 blockers
• Albuterol or levalbuterol for bronchospasm
• Glucagon if the patient is taking beta-blockers
• Systemic steroids to prevent delayed reactions

centrally inflamed but is surrounded by an area of less inflamed skin. Treatment includes management of the underlying cause when known, withdrawal of suspected causative drugs, and acyclovir if HSV involvement is suspected. **Erythema multiforme major** (Stevens-Johnson syndrome [SJS]) is similar to erythema multiforme minor but is more severe and involves two or more mucosal surfaces. It is also more likely to be induced by drugs such as sulfonamides or nonsteroidal anti-inflammatory drugs (NSAIDs) than is erythema multiforme minor. Skin findings may include petechiae, vesicles, bullae, and some desquamation of the skin. If the epidermal detachment involves less than 10% of the skin, it is considered SJS. If the epidermal detachment involves more than 30% of the skin, it is considered **toxic epidermal necrolysis** (TEN). Other symptoms include fever, headache, malaise, arthralgias, corneal ulcerations, arrhythmia, pericarditis, electrolyte abnormalities, seizures, coma, and sepsis. Treatment involves withdrawal of the suspected offending agent, treatment of concurrent infections, aggressive fluid maintenance, and supportive treatment similar to burn care. Use of corticosteroids is controversial, but they are often prescribed.

Most drug rashes are maculopapular and occur several days after starting treatment with an offending drug. They usually are not associated with other signs and symptoms, and they resolve several days after removal of the offending agent. **Serum sickness**, on the other hand, is an allergic reaction that occurs 7 to 10 days after primary administration, or 2 to 4 days after secondary administration of a foreign serum or a drug (ie, a heterologous protein or a nonprotein drug). It is characterized by fever, polyarthralgia, urticaria, lymphadenopathy, and sometimes glomerulonephritis. It is a **type III hypersensitivity reaction**, caused by the formation of **immune complexes** of IgG and the offending antigen. Treatment is based on symptomatology, as the disease usually is self-limiting. Treatment may include administration of antihistamines, aspirin, or NSAIDs, and therapy for associated disease.

Finally, several other types of drug reactions do not fit into the categories discussed. Two of the most important types are iodine allergy and anticonvulsant drug hypersensitivity. "Iodine allergy" is often associated with **radiologic contrast media**. Reactions to contrast media are the result of the hyperosmolar dye causing degranulation of mast cells and basophils rather than a true allergic reaction. These reactions can be prevented by pretreatment with diphenhydramine, H_2 blockers, and corticosteroids beginning 12 hours before the procedure. There is no evidence that a history of seafood allergy is related to adverse events from radiocontrast media. **Phenytoin** and other aromatic **anticonvulsants** have been associated with a **hypersensitivity syndrome**, characterized by a severe idiosyncratic reaction including rash and fever, often with associated hepatitis, arthralgias, lymphadenopathy, or hematologic abnormalities. The skin manifestation can range from skin rash to TEN. This is not IgE mediated, and the exact mechanism remains unclear. Treatment is supportive, and withdrawal of the offending agent.

History of Penicillin Allergy

Penicillin is the most common medication associated with anaphylaxis, reported by 10% of patients. Many reported "allergies" are adverse effects such as rashes or nausea, and not IgE-mediated immediate hypersensitivity. Also over time, individuals with true penicillin allergy may no longer have reactions. Careful history-taking is important when a patient reports a penicillin allergy, including whether there were hives, throat tightening, swelling of the lips or mouth, or difficulty breathing. When the use of penicillin is critical, and the history is unclear, then the use of skin testing may be helpful. The following are recommendations:

- When a patient reports a history highly suggestive of anaphylaxis, penicillin and cephalosporins should be avoided.

- When the history is suggestive of a non-IgE adverse effect, then a beta-lactam may be used, especially cephalosporin (since about 10% cross-reactivity).

- When the history is unclear, then penicillin skin testing may be helpful. If skin testing is unavailable, then in general penicillin should be avoided, but cephalosporins are probably acceptable given the small cross-reactivity.

CASE CORRELATION

- See also Case 41 (Urinary Tract Infection and Sepsis) and Case 42 (Neutropenic Fever/Line Sepsis).

COMPREHENSION QUESTIONS

40.1 A 55-year-old accountant complains of facial and tongue swelling. He recently started using a new bath soap. His medical problems include osteoarthritis and hypertension, for which he takes acetaminophen and lisinopril, respectively. Which of the following is the most likely etiology?

   A. Lisinopril

   B. Soap hypersensitivity

   C. Hypothyroidism

   D. Acetaminophen

   E. Food-related allergy

40.2 An 18-year-old man with epilepsy controlled with medication develops fever, lymphadenopathy, a generalized maculopapular rash, elevated transaminases, and arthralgias. He notes having been bitten by ticks while working in the yard outside. Which of the following is the most likely etiology?

A. Severe poisonivy dermatitis

B. Reaction to anticonvulsant medication

C. Acute human immunodeficiency virus (HIV) infection

D. Lyme disease

40.3 A 34-year-old man is brought into the emergency room for a severe allergic reaction caused by fire ant bites. He is treated with intramuscular epinephrine and intravenous corticosteroids. His oxygen saturation falls to 80%, and he becomes apneic. Which of the following is the best next step?

A. Intravenous diphenhydramine

B. Intravenous epinephrine

C. Oxygen by nasal cannula

D. Endotracheal intubation

E. Electrical cardioversion

40.4 A 57-year-old woman with congestive heart failure (CHF) has a positive cardiac stress test. Cardiac catheterization is required to evaluate for coronary bypass grafting. She states that she has an allergy to iodine. Which of the following is the best next step?

A. Desensitization with increasing doses of oral iodine

B. Infusion of diphenhydramine during the procedure

C. Cancel the procedure and proceed to surgery

D. Diphenhydramine and corticosteroids the night before the procedure

ANSWERS

40.1 **A.** Angiotensin-converting enzyme (ACE) inhibitors are often associated with angioedema. Angioedema secondary to ACE inhibitors can occur at any subsequent point during use, it is not isolated to their initiation.

40.2 **B.** This is a common presentation of hypersensitivity syndrome associated with aromatic anticonvulsants (phenytoin, carbamazepine, phenobarbital). Poison ivy is not associated with fever and lymphadenopathy. Lyme disease is associated with erythema migrans, an erythematous annular rash with a central clearing (target lesion) developing within days of infection. HIV is unlikely given this patient's lack of risk factors.

40.3 **D.** He has developed airway obstruction due to an anaphylactic reaction. He requires intubation and positive-pressure ventilation to maintain oxygenation. Always remember the ABC's in any clinical situation. Airway always comes first!

40.4 **D.** Pretreatment with diphenhydramine, H$_2$ blockers, and corticosteroids beginning 12 hours before the procedure greatly decreases the reaction to contrast dye.

CLINICAL PEARLS

▶ Anaphylaxis is characterized by respiratory distress caused by bronchospasm, cutaneous manifestations such as urticaria or angioedema, and gastrointestinal hypermotility. Patients may die as a consequence of airway compromise or hypotension and vascular collapse caused by widespread vasodilation.

▶ Treatment of anaphylaxis is immediate epinephrine, antihistamines, airway protection, and blood pressure support as necessary. Corticosteroids may help prevent late recurrence of symptoms.

▶ Epinephrine is the immediate drug of choice in treating anaphylaxis.

▶ Serum sickness is an immune complex-mediated disease that may include fever, cutaneous eruptions, lymphadenopathy, arthritis, and glomerulonephritis. It usually is self-limited, but treatment may be necessary for renal complications.

▶ Erythema multiforme minor is characterized by urticarial or bullous eruptions, often with target lesions, usually following herpes simplex virus infections. Erythema multiforme major (Stevens-Johnson syndrome) usually is caused by drugs and includes cutaneous and mucosal involvement.

REFERENCES

Austen KF. Allergies, anaphylaxis, and systemic mastocytosis. In: Kasper DL, Fauci AS, Hauser SL, Longo DL, Jameson JL, Loscalzo J, eds. *Harrison's Principles of Internal Medicine*. 19th ed. New York, NY: McGraw-Hill; 2015:2707-2718.

Du Toit G, Roberts G, Sayre PH, et al. Randomized trial of peanut consumption in infants at risk for peanut allergy. *N Engl J Med*. 2015;372:803-815.

Gruchalla RS, Pirmohamed M. Antibiotic allergy. *N Engl J Med*. 2006;354:601-609.

Roujeau JC, Stern RS, Wintroub BU. Cutaneous drug reactions. In: Kasper DL, Fauci AS, Hauser SL, Longo DL, Jameson JL, Loscalzo J, eds. *Harrison's Principles of Internal Medicine*. 19th ed. New York, NY: McGraw-Hill; 2015:343-349.

Sampson HA. Peanut allergy. *N Engl J Med*. 2002;346:1294-1299.

Vittorio CC, Muglia JJ. Anticonvulsant hypersensitivity syndrome. *Arch Intern Med*. 1995;155:2285-2290.

You are the intern on call in the hospital when the emergency center resident calls up a new admission. She describes an 84-year-old Alzheimer patient who was brought to the emergency room by ambulance from her long-term care facility for increased confusion, combativeness, and fever. Her medical history is significant for Alzheimer disease and well-controlled hypertension; otherwise she has been very healthy. The resident states that the patient is "confused" and combative with staff, which, per her family, is not her baseline mental status. Her temperature is 100.5°F, heart rate is 130 bpm, blood pressure is 76/32 mm Hg, respiratory rate is 24 bpm, and oxygen saturations is 95% on room air. On examination, she is lethargic but agitated when disturbed, her neck veins are flat, her lung fields are clear, and her heart rhythm is tachycardic but regular with no murmur or gallops. Abdominal examination is unremarkable and her extremities are warm and pink.

After administration of 2 L of normal saline over 30 minutes, her blood pressure is now 95/58 mm Hg, and the initial laboratory work returns. Her white blood cell count (WBC) is 14,000/mm^3, with 67% neutrophils, 3% bands, and 24% lymphocytes. No other abnormalities are noted. Chest x-rays obtained in the emergency room are normal. Urinalysis shows 2+ leukocyte esterase, negative nitrite, and trace blood. Microscopy shows 20 to 50 white blood cells per high-power field, 0 to 3 red blood cells (RBCs), and many bacteria.

▶ What is your diagnosis?
▶ What is your next step?

ANSWERS TO CASE 41:

Urinary Tract Infection with Sepsis in the Elderly

Summary: An 84-year-old woman, a nursing home resident with Alzheimer disease, is brought to the emergency room for agitation and confusion. She is found to be febrile, tachycardic, and hypotensive. Examination shows flat neck veins, clear lung fields, and no cardiac murmur or gallops; her extremities are warm and well perfused. Her hemodynamic status has improved with a fluid bolus. Laboratory examination shows evidence of a urinary tract infection (UTI).

- **Most likely diagnosis:** Septic shock, most likely as a consequence of UTI.

- **Next step:** Continued administration of blood pressure support with intravenous (IV) fluids or vasopressors as necessary. Broad-spectrum antibiotics should be started as soon as possible.

ANALYSIS

Objectives

1. Know how to diagnose a UTI.

2. Know effective treatments for UTI.

3. Recognize and know how to manage asymptomatic bacteriuria.

4. Know how to recognize and treat septic shock.

Considerations

In this patient presenting with shock, that is, hypotension leading to inadequate tissue perfusion, it is essential to try to determine the underlying cause and, thus, appropriate treatment. She has no history of hemorrhage or extreme volume losses, so hypovolemic shock is unlikely. She has flat neck veins and clear lung fields, suggesting she does not have right or left heart failure, respectively, so cardiogenic shock (eg, after a myocardial infarction) seems unlikely. Additionally, both hypovolemic and cardiogenic shock typically cause profound peripheral vasoconstriction, resulting in cold clammy extremities. This patient's extremities are warm and well perfused (inappropriately so) despite serious hypotension, suggesting a distributive form of shock. With the elevated white blood cell count with immature forms as well as the urine findings, septic shock as a consequence of UTI seems most likely.

APPROACH TO:

Suspected UTI with Sepsis

DEFINITIONS

ASYMPTOMATIC BACTERIURIA: Condition in which urine Gram stain or culture is positive, but no clinical signs or symptoms of infection are present. This condition is rarely treated unless the patient is a pregnant woman or a man with abnormal prostate or bladder dynamics.

SYSTEMIC INFLAMMATORY RESPONSE SYNDROME (SIRS): Criteria that illustrate systemic inflammation that may or may not indicate underlying infection. The criteria include temperature deviation ($>38°C$ or $<36°C$), tachypnea (respiratory rate >30 breaths per minute or $PaCO2$ <32), tachycardia (heart rate >90 bpm), and leukocyte shifts with white blood cell count $>12,000$ or <4000 or $>10\%$ immature forms (Bands).

SEPSIS: A clinical syndrome due to severe infection that includes SIRS criteria plus a known or suspected infection.

SEVERE SEPSIS: Sepsis with organ dysfunction.

SEPTIC SHOCK: Sepsis plus hypotension refractory to intravenous fluid administration or presence of hyperlactatemia despite fluid resuscitation.

CLINICAL APPROACH

UTIs are a common affliction of the elderly, affecting both debilitated and healthy adults. UTIs are second only to respiratory infections as the most common infections in patients older than 65 years. Risk factors that contribute to the high incidence of UTIs in the elderly as well as in institutionalized patients include incontinence, a history of prior UTIs, neurologic impairment, immunosuppression, poor nutrition, and comorbid disease states. These conditions may confer functional abnormalities within the urinary tract or altered defenses against infection. Furthermore, frequent hospitalizations expose these patients to nosocomial pathogens and invasive instrumentation such as indwelling catheters.

UTIs typically are diagnosed based on a combination of symptoms and urinary findings. In symptomatic patients, bacteria typically are found in high concentrations in the urine, and **10^5 colony-forming units (CFUs)/mL typically are recovered from a clean-catch** specimen. If the specimen is obtained by **catheterization, finding** more than **10^2 CFU/mL** is considered significant. In **women with symptoms of acute cystitis**, urine cultures are often not obtained, but empiric treatment can be initiated based on the **dipstick findings of leukocyte esterase** (used as a marker for pyuria) **or nitrites** (used as a marker for bacteriuria).

Most UTIs occur as one of three clinical syndromes: **acute uncomplicated cystitis** (lower tract infection), **acute uncomplicated pyelonephritis** (upper tract infection), or **catheter-associated UTI** (in hospitalized or institutionalized patients). Symptoms of cystitis reflect bladder irritation and generally include dysuria, frequency, urgency, or hematuria. **Pyelonephritis** typically presents with **systemic symptoms such as fever, chills, or nausea, flank pain**, and finding of **WBC casts** on urinalysis. Catheter-associated UTI can be diagnosed by fever, suprapubic pain, or other symptoms attributable to infection, along with a positive urine culture as defined above.

Another common clinical finding that deserves mention is **asymptomatic bacteriuria**. Asymptomatic bacteriuria is characterized by positive urine cultures without clinical symptoms. Outside of pregnancy or immunocompromised patients such as transplant recipients, no adverse clinical outcomes have been reported as a result of asymptomatic bacteriuria, and no benefits of treatment have been demonstrated.

Although in younger patients fever, dysuria, urgency, or flank pain may be presenting symptoms for a UTI, elderly and institutionalized patients often present with less obvious symptoms. These patients may be febrile or hypothermic. Common manifestations include confusion or combativeness. **Mental status or behavioral changes in the elderly** should be considered **strong indicators for serious illness**, and a thorough workup should consider etiologies beyond infections. Even with localizing symptoms suggestive of a UTI, other sources of infection should still be investigated. Both urine and blood cultures should be sent in addition to a urinalysis and complete blood count. The results of the urine and blood cultures may take 2 to 3 days to yield an organism. If the clinical picture suggests a UTI, antibiotic treatment should not await these results and should be initiated immediately.

Empiric antimicrobial therapy can be directed at the most common pathogens (Table 41–1).

For uncomplicated cystitis, oral trimethoprim-sulfamethoxazole (TMP-SMX) (Bactrim), fluoroquinolones such as ciprofloxacin, and nitrofurantoin are acceptable first-line therapy and are typically given for 3 days. Empiric therapy should be guided by knowledge of local antibiotic resistance patterns. Similar empiric treatment may be initiated for pyelonephritis, but urine cultures should be obtained. Treatment is then guided by culture results, and should be continued for 10 to 14 days. Catheter-associated UTI can only be diagnosed with positive cultures (the sample should be obtained from a new catheter, or the catheter port, but not the drainage bag), and antibiotic therapy is tailored to the identified pathogen. If possible, the catheter should be removed or replaced.

The elderly and institutionalized patients commonly acquire gram-positive and mixed infections, so broad-spectrum antibiotics pending culture results are recommended. In patients presenting with a clinical picture of sepsis, broad-spectrum antibiotic coverage against gram-positive and gram-negative organisms

---

Table 41–1 • ETIOLOGIES OF URINARY TRACT INFECTIONS

Acute uncomplicated cystitis, pyelonephritis
- *E coli* 75%-90%
- *Staphylococcus saprophyticus* 5%-15%
- *Klebsiella* spp
- *Proteus* spp
- *Enterococcus* spp

Catheter-associated UTI
- *E coli*
- *Klebsiella* spp
- *Proteus* spp
- *Citrobacter* spp
- *Morganella* spp
- *Pseudomonas aeruginosa*
- *Enterococcus* spp
- *Candida* spp

including antipseudomonal activity is recommended until cultures are available to guide therapy. The duration of therapy should be dictated by the patient's clinical status. In cases where UTIs have progressed to bacteremia, aggressive and prompt treatment is necessary to prevent the onset of septic shock. This life-threatening state may develop with little warning in elderly and institutionalized patients with multiple comorbidities, as it did in the patient in the scenario, who presents with hypotension and altered mental status because of infection, that is, in septic shock.

Shock is the clinical syndrome that results from inadequate tissue perfusion. It can be classified in a variety of ways, but one useful schema divides the causes into hypovolemic shock, cardiogenic shock, or distributive shock, usually caused by sepsis. **Hypovolemic shock** is the most common form. It results from either hemorrhage or profound vomiting or diarrhea, resulting in loss of 20% to 40% of blood volume. **Cardiogenic shock** results from a primary cardiac insult, such as a myocardial infarction, arrhythmias, or end-stage heart failure such that the heart no longer pumps effectively. Both hypovolemic and cardiogenic shocks cause a marked fall in cardiac output and may appear clinically similar with tachycardia, hypotension, and cold clammy extremities. It is essential to differentiate between the two, however, because the treatments are markedly different. Patients with **hypovolemic shock** should have **flat neck veins** and **clear lung fields;** those with **cardiogenic shock** are more likely to have markedly **elevated jugular venous pressure** and **pulmonary edema.** Treatment of hypovolemic shock is aggressive volume resuscitation, either with crystalloid solution or with blood products as necessary. Treatment of cardiogenic shock focuses on maintaining blood pressure with dopamine or norepinephrine infusions, relief of pulmonary edema with diuretics, and reducing cardiac afterload, for example, with an intra-aortic balloon pump.

Distributive shock, in contrast, is characterized by an **increase in cardiac output** but an inability to maintain systemic vascular resistance, that is, there is **inappropriate vasodilation.** Clinically, it appears different than the other forms of shock in that, despite the hypotension, the **extremities are warm and well perfused**, at least initially. If septic shock continues, cardiac output falls as a consequence of myocardial depression, multiorgan dysfunction ensues, and **intense vasoconstriction** occurs in an attempt to maintain blood pressure, the so-called "**cold phase.**" These findings portend a poor prognosis; hence, prompt recognition of septic shock in the early (warm) phase is paramount.

Although distributive shock may occur in neurogenic shock as a consequence of spinal cord injury or adrenal crisis, the most common cause is **septic shock, with the most common infectious etiologies of sepsis being urinary tract infections and pneumonia.** The initial treatment is isotonic fluid resuscitation to maintain adequate intravascular volume. Other cornerstones of therapy include broad-spectrum antibiotics targeted to the underlying infection or likely source of underlying infection and removal of the infection source. Patients often require vasopressor support (norepinephrine is the agent of choice) and mechanical ventilation to optimize tissue oxygenation. Intravenous hydrocortisone may be administered to patients with hypotension that is refractory to fluid resuscitation and vasopressors.

Septic shock is associated with high 30-day mortality rates exceeding 50%. Early diagnosis and prompt treatment are imperative because untreated shock progresses to an irreversible point that is refractory to volume expansion and other medical therapies.

CASE CORRELATION

- See also Case 40 (Anaphylaxis/Drug Reaction) and Case 42 (Neutropenic Fever).

COMPREHENSION QUESTIONS

41.1 Which of the following asymptomatic patients would most benefit from treatment of the finding of more than 10^5 CFU/mL of *Escherichia coli* on urine culture?

A. A 23-year-old asymptomatic sexually active woman

B. A 33-year-old asymptomatic pregnant woman

C. A 53-year-old asymptomatic diabetic woman

D. A 73-year-old asymptomatic woman in a nursing home

41.2 Which of the following is the best treatment for a 39-year-old woman with fever of 103°F, nausea, flank pain, and more than 10^5 CFU/mL of *E coli* in a urine culture?

A. Oral trimethoprim-sulfamethoxazole for 3 days

B. Single-dose ciprofloxacin

C. Intravenous and then oral levofloxacin for 14 days

D. Oral ampicillin for 21 to 28 days

41.3 A 57-year-old man is noted to have a blood pressure of 68/50 mm Hg, heart rate of 140 bpm, elevated jugular venous pressure, inspiratory crackles on examination, and cold clammy extremities. Which of the following is the most likely etiology?

A. Septic shock

B. Adrenal crisis

C. Cardiogenic shock

D. Hypovolemic shock

41.4   A 45-year-old man is noted to have a blood pressure of 80/40 mm Hg, heart rate of 142 bpm, and fever of 102°F. His abdomen is tender, particularly in the right lower quadrant, and acute appendicitis is diagnosed. Three liters of 0.9% saline are infused and intravenous antibiotics are administered as he is prepared for surgery. His blood pressure falls to 70/42 mm Hg. Which of the following is the most appropriate next step?

A.   Administer a beta-blocker to control his heart rate.

B.   Check a cortisol level and administer corticosteroids.

C.   Infuse fresh frozen plasma (FFP).

D.   Initiate norepinephrine intravenous infusion.

E.   IV morphine for pain control.

ANSWERS

41.1   **B.** All of these patients are asymptomatic, and no benefit from treatment in terms of reduction in symptomatic UTIs or hospitalization has been shown for any of the other cases mentioned, except for pregnancy. Treatment is undertaken to prevent upper tract infection, preterm delivery, and possible fetal loss.

41.2   **C.** The patient in this scenario has symptoms of an upper urinary tract infection, for example, pyelonephritis, and is moderately ill with nausea. She will need a 14-day course of treatment and may not be able to take oral antibiotics initially, so hospitalization and treatment with intravenous antibiotics likely will be necessary. Single-dose and 3-day regimens are useful only for acute uncomplicated cystitis in women. *E coli* is frequently resistant to ampicillin.

41.3   **C.** The patient is hypotensive with signs of left and right heart failure, that is, probably cardiogenic shock. Septic shock and adrenal crisis both are forms of distributive shock that would produce warm extremities. Hypovolemic shock should have flat neck veins and no pulmonary edema.

41.4   **D.** When septic shock is refractory to volume resuscitation with at least 30 cc isotonic fluid per kilogram ideal body weight administration, then addition of intravenous norepinephrine is the next step. Corticosteroids can be administered empirically if hypotension is refractory to vasopressors. Intravenous morphine might lower his blood pressure further. FFP is used when the patient shows evidence of coagulopathy such as disseminated intravascular coagulation.

CLINICAL PEARLS

▶ Urinary tract infections and pneumonia are the most common causes of sepsis in older patients.

▶ Urinary tract infections can be diagnosed by the presence of urinary symptoms and by more than 10^5 CFUs/mL in a clean-catch specimen and more than 10^2 CFU/mL in a catheterized specimen.

▶ In healthy women with symptoms of acute uncomplicated cystitis, cultures are not routinely sent, and treatment can be initiated based on symptoms and on a urine dipstick finding of leukocyte esterase or nitrites.

▶ Asymptomatic bacteriuria is a common finding among elderly patients and requires no treatment; it is only routinely treated in pregnancy and in transplant recipients.

▶ Sepsis is a syndrome characterized by fever, tachycardia, tachypnea, leukocytosis, and presence of a known or suspected infection. It requires early and aggressive intervention to prevent clinical deterioration.

REFERENCES

Angus DC, van der Poll T. Severe sepsis and septic shock. *N Engl J Med*. 2013;369:840-851.

Fihn SD. Acute uncomplicated urinary tract infection in women. *N Engl J Med*. 2003;349:259-266.

Hotchkiss RS, Karl IE. The pathophysiology and treatment of sepsis. *N Engl J Med*. 2003;348:138-150.

Maier RV. Approach to the patient with shock. In: Longo DL, Fauci AS, Kasper DL, et al., eds. *Harrison's Principles of Internal Medicine*. 18th ed. New York, NY: McGraw-Hill; 2012:2215-2222.

Munford RS. Severe sepsis and septic shock. In: Longo DL, Fauci AS, Kasper DL, et al., eds. *Harrison's Principles of Internal Medicine*. 18th ed. New York, NY: McGraw-Hill; 2012:2223-2232.

Shortliffe LMD, McCue JD. Urinary tract infection at the age extremes: pediatrics and geriatrics. *Am J Med*. 2002;113:S55-S66.

A 24-year-old man presents to the emergency room complaining of 24 hours of fevers with shaking chills. He is currently being treated for acute lymphoblastic leukemia (ALL). His most recent chemotherapy with hyperfractionated cyclophosphamide, vincristine, doxorubicin, and dexamethasone (CVAD) was 7 days ago. He denies any cough or dyspnea, headache, abdominal pain, or diarrhea. He has had no sick contacts or recent travel. On physical examination, he is febrile to 103°F, tachycardic with heart rate 122 bpm, blood pressure 118/65 mm Hg, and respiratory rate 22 bpm. He is ill appearing; his skin is warm and moist but without any rashes. He has no oral lesions, his chest is clear to auscultation, his heart rate is tachycardic but regular with a soft systolic murmur at the left sternal border, and his abdominal examination is benign. The perirectal area is normal, and digital rectal examination is deferred, but his stool is negative for occult blood. He has a tunneled vascular catheter at the right internal jugular vein without erythema overlying the subcutaneous tract and no purulent discharge at the catheter exit site. Of note, he reports an onset of shaking chills 30 minutes after the catheter was flushed. Laboratory studies reveal a total white blood cell (WBC) count of 1100 cells/mm^3, with a differential of 10% neutrophils, 16% band forms, 70% lymphocytes, and 4% monocytes (absolute neutrophil count [ANC] 286/mm^3). Chest radiograph and urinalysis are normal.

▶ What is the most likely diagnosis?
▶ What are your next therapeutic steps?

ANSWERS TO CASE 42:

Neutropenic Fever, Vascular Catheter Infection

Summary: A 24-year-old man with ALL is receiving immunosuppressive chemotherapy. He now presents with fever. He has no respiratory or abdominal symptoms, a clear chest x-ray, and an absolute neutrophil count of $286/mm^3$. He has a central venous catheter, with a history suggestive of possible catheter infection.

- **Most likely diagnosis:** Neutropenic fever and possible infected vascular catheter.

- **Next therapeutic step:** After drawing blood cultures, the patient should undergo broad-spectrum intravenous antibiotic administration, including coverage for gram-positive organisms such as *Staphylococcus* spp. The vascular catheter should be removed, if possible.

ANALYSIS

Objectives

1. Be familiar with the possible sources of infection in a neutropenic patient.

2. Learn the management of a patient with neutropenic fever.

3. Be able to diagnose and treat a catheter-related infection.

4. Understand the techniques to prevent infection in immunosuppressed patients, including granulocyte colony-stimulating factor (G-CSF) and vaccination of household contacts.

Considerations

This patient is being treated for a hematologic malignancy with combination chemotherapy, which has a common side effect of leukopenia and, especially, neutropenia. Generally, the nadir of the white cell count occurs 7 to 14 days after the chemotherapy. This patient has **neutropenia, defined as an absolute neutrophil count less than 500 cells/mm³**. The absolute neutrophil count is calculated by neutrophil percent multiplied by total WBC count. Infection in this immunosuppressed condition is life threatening, and immediate antibiotic coverage is paramount. Neutropenic patients are at risk for a variety of bacterial, fungal, or viral infections, but the most common sources of infection are gram-positive bacteria from the skin or oral cavity or gram-negative bacteria from the bowel. Because of the absence of white blood cells, the patient may not manifest the cardinal signs of infection: inflammation or high fever. Organisms that must be covered include the normal bacteria as well as *Pseudomonas* species and with an indwelling IV catheter also penicillin-resistant pneumococci, methicillin-resistant *Staphylococcus aureus* (MRSA). Infection of the indwelling catheter, as in this individual, is common. Rapid institution of empiric antibiotic therapy is critical while attempts to find a source of infection are in progress.

APPROACH TO:
Neutropenic Fever

DEFINITIONS

CVC: Central venous catheter.

FEVER: Single oral temperature measurement more than or equal to 101°F (38.3°C) or a temperature more than or equal to 100.4°F (38.0°C) for 1 hour or more.

MUCOSITIS: Breakdown of skin and mucosal barriers as a result of chemotherapy or radiation. Mucositis can result in bacteremia or fungemia.

NEUTROPENIA: Absolute neutrophil count less than 500 cells/mm³ or a count less than 1000 cells/mm³ with a predicted decrease to less than 500 cells/mm³.

CLINICAL APPROACH

Fever in a neutropenic patient with cancer should be considered a medical emergency. Approximately 5% to 10% of cancer patients will die of neutropenia-associated infection. Individuals with a hematologic malignancy (leukemias or lymphomas) are at even greater risk for sepsis as a result of lymphocyte or granulocyte dysfunction or because of abnormal immunoglobulin production. Chemotherapy often causes further bone marrow suppression and neutropenia. The incidence of an occult infection in a neutropenic patient increases with the **severity and duration of the neutropenia** (high risk if >7-10 days, and especially if ANC <100 cells/mm³). Some neutropenic patients (eg, the elderly or those receiving corticosteroids) may not be able to mount a febrile response to infection; thus, **any neutropenic patient showing signs of clinical deterioration should be suspected of having sepsis.**

The typical signs and symptoms of infection noted in immunocompetent patients are the result of the host's inflammatory response and may be minimal or absent in neutropenic patients. Soft tissue infections may have diminished or absent induration, erythema, or purulence; pneumonia may not show a discernible infiltrate on a chest radiograph; meningitis may not reveal cerebrospinal fluid (CSF) pleocytosis; and urinary tract infection may be present without pyuria.

Empiric antibiotic therapy should be administered promptly to all neutropenic patients at the onset of fever. Historically, gram-negative bacilli, mainly enteric flora, were the most common pathogens in these patients. Because of their frequency and high rate of mortality associated with gram-negative septicemia, empiric coverage for gram-negative bacteria, including *Pseudomonas aeruginosa*, is almost always indicated for neutropenic fever. Currently, as a consequence of frequent use of CVCs, gram-positive bacteria now account for 60% to 70% of microbiologically documented infections. Other clues that the infection is likely to be a gram-positive organism include the presence of obvious soft tissue infection, such as cellulitis or oral mucositis, which causes breaks in the mucosal barriers and allows oral flora to enter the bloodstream. If any of these factors are present, an appropriate agent, such as vancomycin, should be added to the regimen. If patients continue to be

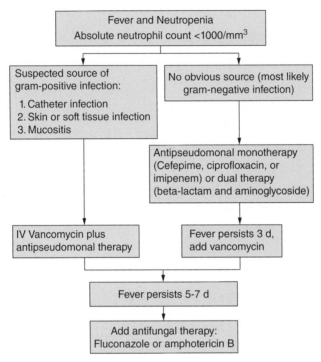

Figure 42–1. Algorithm of a suggested approach to neutropenic fever.

febrile despite antibacterial therapy, empiric antifungal therapy should be considered. Figure 42–1 shows a useful algorithm for patient management.

Central venous catheters are in widespread use and are a common site of infection in hospitalized patients and in patients receiving outpatient infusion therapy. Infection may occur as a consequence of contamination by gram-positive skin flora or by hematogenous seeding, usually by enteric gram-negative organisms or *Candida* spp. Erythema, purulent drainage, and induration are evidence of infection. The two main decisions impacting suspected catheter-related infection are (1) whether the catheter is really the source of infection and, if it is, (2) must the catheter be removed or can the infection be cleared with antibiotic therapy? **Most nontunneled or implanted catheters** should be **removed**. For the more permanent catheters, the decision to remove the catheter depends on the patient's clinical state, identification of the organism, and the presence of complications such as endocarditis or septic venous thrombosis. Infected catheters may produce several manifestations, such as infections of the subcutaneous tunnel, infection at the exit site, or catheter-related bacteremia and sepsis. Generally, **erythema overlying the subcutaneous tract** of a tunneled catheter necessitates catheter removal. Leaving the catheter in place may result in severe cellulitis and soft tissue necrosis. If there is only erythema at the exit site, it may be possible to salvage the line using antibiotics, usually vancomycin, through the CVC. Coagulase-negative staphylococci, such as *Staphylococcus epidermidis*, are the most common organisms causing line infections.

In the absence of obvious tunnel or exit-site infection, authorities recommend obtaining two or more blood cultures to try to diagnose **catheter-related bacteremia**. Catheter-related infection is suspected when a patient has two or more positive blood cultures obtained from a peripheral vein, clinical manifestation of infection (eg, fever, chills, and/or hypotension), and no apparent source for bloodstream infection except for the catheter. In some institutions, quantitative blood cultures are obtained, that is, counting colony-forming units (CFUs), with the idea that heavier colony counts will be obtained from blood drawn through an infected catheter than from blood obtained from a peripheral vein. If the catheter is removed, the tip of the catheter may be cut off and rolled across a culture plate, again using a quantitative culture method.

S aureus and **coagulase-negative *Staphylococcus* are the most common causes of catheter-associated infections.** With **coagulase-negative *Staphylococcus* bacteremia**, response to **antibiotic therapy without catheter removal** is possible up to 80% of the time; that is, one may seek to "sterilize" the CVC if it is deemed necessary. However, this is usually not advisable in critically ill or hemodynamically unstable patients in whom immediate catheter removal and rapid administration of antibiotics are essential. Bacteremia as a consequence of *S aureus*, **gram-negative organisms, and fungemia caused by *Candida* spp respond poorly to antimicrobial therapy** alone, so **prompt removal of the catheter is recommended.**

Prevention

Because of the serious complications associated with neutropenia, preventive measures are critical in cancer patients who are receiving chemotherapy. They should be **immunized against pneumococcus and influenza**, but administration of live virus vaccines, such as measles-mumps-rubella or varicella zoster, is contraindicated. G-CSF, which stimulates the bone marrow to produce neutrophils, is frequently used prophylactically in patients receiving chemotherapy to shorten the duration and depth of neutropenia, thereby reducing the risk of infection. It is sometimes used once a neutropenic patient develops a fever, but its use at that point is controversial. Prophylactic use of oral quinolones to prevent gram-negative infection or antifungal agents to prevent *Candida* infection may reduce certain types of infection but may select for resistant organisms and is not routinely used. Antifungal and antibacterial (such as an oral fluoroquinolone) prophylaxis is recommended when an ANC <100 cells/mm^3 for more than 7 days is anticipated. Other recommendations include avoiding sick contacts, overcrowded areas. Because slight trauma to mucosal surfaces can cause bacteremia, careful oral hygiene, avoidance of rectal thermometers or rectal examinations, and skin care are also important.

CASE CORRELATION

- See also Case 40 (Anaphylaxis/Drug Reaction) and Case 41 (Urine Infection Sepsis).

COMPREHENSION QUESTIONS

42.1 Which of the following infectious agents is the most likely etiology associated with an infected central venous catheter?

A. *Streptococcus pyogenes*

B. *Pseudomonas aeruginosa*

C. Coagulase-negative *Staphylococcus*

D. *Klebsiella pneumoniae*

E. *Candida albicans*

42.2 A 32-year-old man with acute myelogenous leukemia is undergoing chemotherapy. He was hospitalized 7 days ago for fever to 102°F with an absolute neutrophil count of 100 cells/mm^3, and he has been placed on intravenous imipenem and vancomycin. He continues to have fever to 103°F without an obvious source. Which of the following is the best next step?

A. Perform lumbar puncture to assess cerebrospinal fluid.

B. Continue present therapy.

C. Stop all antibiotics because he likely has drug fever.

D. Add an aminoglycoside antibiotic.

E. Add an antifungal agent.

42.3 A 68-year-old woman is diagnosed with acute leukemia and is undergoing induction of chemotherapy. Last cycle, she developed neutropenia with an absolute neutrophil count of 350 cells/mm^3, which has now resolved. Which of the following is appropriate therapy?

A. Immunization against varicella

B. Immunization against mumps

C. Use of recombinant erythropoietin before the next cycle of chemotherapy

D. Use of G-CSF after the next cycle of chemotherapy

ANSWERS

42.1 **C.** Coagulase-negative staphylococci, such as *S epidermidis*, along with *S aureus*, are the most common etiology of catheter-related infections.

42.2 **E.** Antifungal therapy should be added when the fever is persistent despite broad-spectrum antibacterial agents. Patients with neutropenia, defined as an absolute neutrophil count less than 1000 cells per uL, are a greater risk for bacterial (gram positive and gram negative) and fungal infections such as caused by Candida albicans and Aspergillus.

42.3 **D.** Granulocyte colony-stimulating factor given after chemotherapy can decrease the duration and severity of neutropenia and the subsequent risk of sepsis. Live vaccines, such as varicella and mumps, are contraindicated. Erythropoietin is not indicated because the patient is not anemic.

CLINICAL PEARLS

▶ Fever in a neutropenic patient should be considered a medical emergency and is associated with a high mortality rate.

▶ The usual sources of bacterial infection in neutropenic patients are gram-positive skin or oral flora or gram-negative enteric flora, including *Pseudomonas*.

▶ Antifungal therapy should be started in neutropenic patients who have persistent fever despite broad-spectrum antibiotic therapy and who have no obvious source of infection.

▶ Vascular catheters with evidence of infection along a subcutaneous tract or purulent discharge at the exit site should be removed; replacement over a guidewire is insufficient.

▶ If a catheter is deemed necessary but it is infected with coagulase-negative staphylococci, antibiotic treatment may sterilize the catheter, allowing it to remain in place. For *S aureus*, gram-negative rods, or fungal catheter infections, the catheter usually requires removal.

REFERENCES

Finberg R. Infections in patients with cancer. In: Kasper DL, Fauci AS, Hauser SL, et al., eds. *Harrison's Principles of Internal Medicine.* 19th ed. New York, NY: McGraw-Hill; 2015:484-492.

Hall K, Farr B. Diagnosis and management of long-term central venous catheter infections. *J Vasc Interv Radiol.* 2004;15:327.

Pizzo PA. Fever in immunocompromised patients. *N Engl J Med.* 1999;341:893-900.

Weinstein RA. Infections acquired in health care facilities. In: Kasper DL, Fauci AS, Hauser SL, et al., eds. *Harrison's Principles of Internal Medicine.* 19th ed. New York, NY: McGraw-Hill; 2015:911-918.

A 20-year-old college student is your next patient in the emergency department. When you walk into the room, he is lying on the examination table, on his side, with his arm covering his eyes. The light in the room is off. You look at his chart and see that the nurse recorded his temperature as 102.3°F, heart rate as 110 bpm, and blood pressure as 120/80 mm Hg. When you gently ask how he has been feeling, he says that for the past 3 days he has had fever, body aches, and a progressively worsening headache. The light hurts his eyes and he is nauseated, but he has not vomited. He has had some rhinorrhea, but no diarrhea, cough, or nasal congestion. He has no known ill contacts. On examination, he has no skin rash, but his pupils are difficult to assess because of photophobia. Ears and oropharynx are normal. Heart, lung, and abdomen examinations are normal. Neurologic examination reveals no focal neurologic deficits, but passive flexion of his neck worsens his headache, and he is unable to touch his chin to his chest.

▶ What condition concerns you the most?
▶ What diagnostic test would confirm the diagnosis?

ANSWERS TO CASE 43:
Bacterial Meningitis

Summary: A 20-year-old college student presents with a 3-day history of fever, headache, myalgias, and nausea. He has no respiratory or gastrointestinal symptoms, but now has developed photophobia. He is febrile to 102.3°F, tachycardic, and normotensive. His physical examination is generally unremarkable with a non-focal neurologic examination but some neck stiffness, suggesting meningeal irritation. He has no skin lesions as might be seen in meningococcemia.

- **Most concerning condition:** Meningitis (especially if bacterial).

- **Diagnostic test to confirm diagnosis:** Lumbar puncture (LP) for evaluation of the cerebrospinal fluid (CSF), possibly preceded by a computed tomographic (CT) scan of the head.

ANALYSIS

Objectives

1. Be familiar with the clinical presentations of viral and bacterial meningitis.

2. Know that LP is the diagnostic test of choice for meningitis.

3. Be familiar with the treatment for meningitis.

Considerations

This 20-year-old college student has headache, nausea, photophobia, fever, and neck pain and stiffness—all suggestive of meningitis, which could be bacterial or viral. Prompt LP and analysis of CSF are essential to establish the diagnosis. In a patient without focal neurologic signs and a normal level of consciousness, CT scan may be unnecessary prior to performing an LP. If he had a purpuric skin rash, one would be suspicious of *Neisseria meningitidis*, and appropriate antibiotics should be administered immediately. Dosing of antibiotics in suspected meningococcal infection should not await the performance of any diagnostic test because progression of the disease is rapid, and mortality and morbidity are extremely high even when antibiotics are given in a timely manner. In this patient who does not have exposures of immunosuppressed conditions suggestive of fungal or parasitic organisms, empiric therapy with IV antibiotics such as vancomycin together with cefotaxime or ceftriaxone. However, patients with HIV and low CD4 counts, immunosuppression with chemotherapy or transplant rejection agents, or chronic antibiotic therapy, or brain/spinal surgery may suggest opportunistic or unusual organisms.

APPROACH TO:
Suspected Meningitis

DEFINITIONS

MENINGITIS: Inflammation of the subarachnoid space and meninges, most often infectious, can be caused by bacteria, viruses, fungi, or protozoa.

PAPILLEDEMA: Swelling of the optic nerve caused by an increased intracranial pressure. On funduscopic examination, the optic disc margin appears hazy.

ENCEPHALITIS: Brain parenchymal injury and inflammation most often due to a virus. When focal brain parenchymal infection is caused by bacteria, it is usually termed *cerebritis* or *abscess*.

CLINICAL APPROACH

Infections of the central nervous system either involve the meninges (meningitis) or the brain parenchyma (encephalitis). The incidence is dropping due to the use of the pneumococcal and hemophilus influenza vaccines. However, the disease is still dangerous, with case fatality rate with treatment of approximately 10% to 20%, and serious morbidity such as seizures, hearing loss, or brain damage. Fatality is nearly 100% without treatment. College students are at risk due to living in closer quarters.

Bacterial meningitis is the most common pus-forming intracranial infection, with an incidence of 2.5 per 10,000 persons. The microbiology of the disease has changed somewhat since the introduction of the *Haemophilus influenzae* type B vaccine in the 1980s. Now *Streptococcus pneumoniae* **is the most common bacterial isolate**, with **N *meningitidis* a close second. Group B *Streptococcus*** or *Streptococcus agalactiae* occurs in approximately 10% of cases, more frequently in neonates or in patients older than 50 years or with chronic illnesses such as diabetes or liver disease. **Listeria monocytogenes** accounts for approximately 10% of cases and must be considered in pregnant women, the **elderly**, or patients with impaired cell-mediated immunity such as acquired immunodeficiency syndrome (AIDS) patients. *H influenzae* is responsible for less than 10% of meningitis cases. Resistance to penicillin and some cephalosporins is now of great concern in the treatment of *S pneumoniae*.

Bacteria usually seed the meninges hematogenously after colonizing and invading the nasal or oropharyngeal mucosa. Occasionally, bacteria directly invade the intracranial space from a site of abscess formation in the middle ear or sinuses. The gravity and rapidity of progression of disease depend on both host defense and organism virulence characteristics. For example, patients with defects in the complement cascade are more susceptible to invasive meningococcal disease. Patients with CSF rhinorrhea caused by trauma or postsurgical changes may also be more susceptible to bacterial invasion.

Staphylococcus aureus **and** *Staphylococcus epidermidis* are common causes of meningitis in patients following **neurologic procedures** such as placement of **ventriculoperitoneal shunts.** The brisk host inflammatory response in the subarachnoid space may cause edema, vasculitis, and coagulation of vessels, leading to severe neurologic complications including seizures, increased intracranial pressure, and stroke. Acute bacterial meningitis can progress over hours to days. **Typical symptoms include fever, neck stiffness, and headache.** Patients may also complain of photophobia, nausea and vomiting, and more nonspecific constitutional symptoms. Approximately 75% of patients will experience some confusion or altered level of consciousness. Forty percent may experience seizures during the course of their illness.

Some physical examination findings may be useful in the evaluation of a patient with suspected meningitis. **Nuchal rigidity** is demonstrated when passive or active flexion of the neck results in an inability to touch the chin to the chest. Classic tests include Kernig and Brudzinski signs. **Kernig sign** can be elicited with the patient on his or her back. The hip and knees are flexed. The knee is then passively extended, and the test is positive if this maneuver elicits pain. **Brudzinski sign** is positive if the supine patient flexes the knees and hips when the neck is passively flexed. Neither sign is very sensitive for the presence of meningeal irritation, but, if present, both are highly specific. **Papilledema**, if present, would indicate **increased intracranial pressure**, and focal neurologic signs or altered level of consciousness or seizures may reflect ischemia of the cerebral vasculature or focal suppuration.

Differential Diagnosis

The differential diagnosis of bacterial meningitis is fairly limited and can be narrowed depending on the patient's age, as discussed earlier, exposure history, and course of illness. Various viral infections may also cause meningitis. These include **enteroviruses**, which tend to be more common in the summer and fall, when patients may present with severe headache, accompanied by symptoms of gastroenteritis. The **CSF white blood cell (WBC) count will be elevated**, with a **predominance of lymphocytes**, and usually **glucose and protein levels are normal** (Table 43–1). Either herpes simplex virus (HSV)-1 or HSV-2 can cause herpes simplex meningitis. The CSF of these patients will also have a normal glucose level, whereas protein and WBC counts will be elevated with a predominance of lymphocytes. Typically, these patients have a high CSF red blood cell (RBC) count, which is not seen in bacterial meningitis in the absence of a traumatic spinal tap. In a patient with human immunodeficiency virus (HIV) infection, fungal meningitis, specifically caused by *Cryptococcus*, should be considered. Tuberculous meningitis presents subacutely and is more common in older, debilitated patients, or in patients with HIV. Rickettsial disease, specifically Rocky Mountain spotted fever, may also present with meningitis. Intracranial empyema, or brain or epidural abscess, should be considered, especially if the patient has focal neurologic findings. The one nonsuppurative diagnosis in the differential is **subarachnoid hemorrhage**. These patients present with sudden onset of the "worst headache of their lives" in the absence of other symptoms of infection. They may have photophobia, and the CSF will be grossly bloody; the supernatant will be xanthochromic, reflecting the breakdown of blood into bilirubin.

Blood cultures should be obtained in all patients with suspected meningitis. Critical to the diagnosis of meningitis is the LP and evaluation of the CSF. Table 43–1 lists typical findings in the CSF from various causes of meningitis.

Table 43-1 • CSF CHARACTERISTICS OF MENINGITIS

Causative Organism	Opening Pressure	White Blood Cell Count/Type	Glucose	Protein	Red Blood Cell Count	Special Stains/Tests
Bacteria	High	Elevated, predominantly neutrophilic	Low, <40 mg/dL	Elevated	None	Gram stain
Viral	Normal	Elevated, predominantly lymphocytic	Normal	Normal	None	Cell culture or PCR
Herpes simplex	Normal to high	As in other viral meningitis	Normal	Normal to high	High	PCR
Tuberculosis	Normal to high	Elevated, monocytes may be elevated	Very low	Very high	None	PCR, AFB smear (usually negative), and culture
Fungal	Variable	Elevated, predominantly lymphocytes	Low	Elevated	None	Fungal stains

Abbreviations: AFB, acid fast bacillus; CSF, cerebrospinal fluid; PCR, polymerase chain reaction.

The **necessity of imaging of the head and brain prior to performing an LP is controversial.** Studies show that in the patient with suspected meningitis who does not have papilledema, focal neurologic signs, or altered level of consciousness, an LP may be safely performed without preceding imaging. However, in instances in which performance of the LP may be delayed, antibiotics should be administered after blood cultures while awaiting the radiologic studies. Ideally, the CSF should be examined within 30 minutes of antibiotics, but it has been shown that if the LP is performed within 2 hours of antibiotic administration, it will not significantly alter the CSF protein, glucose, or WBC count, or Gram stain. If CSF is obtained, a culture and Gram stain should be sent. If enough fluid is available, it should also be sent for cell count and glucose and protein levels. Latex agglutination tests for *S pneumoniae* and *H influenzae* can be useful in patients pretreated with antibiotics, and, although not very sensitive, they are highly specific. If positive they can establish the infectious agent. Polymerase chain reaction (PCR) testing is available for some bacteria; however, it may be more useful in the diagnosis of herpes simplex, enteroviral, or tuberculous meningitis. In all, no more than 3.5 to 4 mL of CSF is necessary. The most critical issue in a patient with suspected bacterial meningitis, however, is the initiation of antibiotics. The CSF examination and imaging studies can be deferred in this medical emergency.

During the course of treatment, most patients will undergo some cerebral imaging studies. Computed tomographic (CT) scans are most useful in the initial presentation to exclude intracranial mass or bleeding, or to evaluate for other signs of increased intracranial pressure. However, magnetic resonance imaging (MRI) is most helpful for demonstrating any focal ischemia or infarction caused by the disease. When **HSV meningitis** is suspected, MRI should demonstrate **enhancement of the temporal lobes.** In tuberculous meningitis, enhancement of the basal region may be seen. An electroencephalogram (EEG) may be helpful in patients suspected of HSV meningitis. Within 2 to 15 days of the start of the illness, periodic sharp and slow wave complexes originating within the temporal lobes can be demonstrated at 2- to 3-second intervals. When the purpuric skin lesions are present, skin biopsy may demonstrate *N meningitidis* and can be helpful in the diagnosis. Age may give a clue regarding etiology of meningitis (Table 43–2).

Therapy

Treatment of meningitis often is empiric until specific culture data are available. Because of the growing incidence of resistant pneumococci as well as meningococci, the recommended empiric therapy in most areas is a **high-dose third-generation cephalosporin given concurrently with vancomycin.** In other areas, if the disease presentation is typical for meningococcus (with the typical rash) or the organism is identified quickly on Gram stain of the CSF, therapy with high-dose penicillin can be started if the meningococcus in that area is known to be sensitive. **Ampicillin is added when there is a suspicion of listeriosis. Acyclovir should be started for suspicion of HSV,** or four-drug antituberculosis (TB) therapy should be started if the presentation is suspicious for tuberculous meningitis.

The administration of **glucocorticoids** to reduce central nervous system (CNS) inflammation, when used, should be given just before or concurrent with the first

Table 43-2 • ETIOLOGIES OF BACTERIAL MENINGITIS BY AGE			
Age of Patient	Bacteria	Empiric Treatment	Comments
Neonate	1. Gram-negative enteric bacteria (*Escherichia coli*) and group B streptococcus 2. *L monocytogenes*	Ampicillin + cefotaxime	Vaginal organisms common
1-23 mo	1. *S pneumoniae* 2. *N meningitides* 3. *Haemophilus influenzae* type b (less common since vaccine)	Cefotaxime (or ceftriaxone) + vancomycin	Previous to vaccine, *H influenzae caused 70% of meningitis in children*
2-18 y	1. *N meningitides* 2. *S pneumoniae* 3. *H influenzae* type b (less common since vaccine)	Ampicillin + vancomycin 5 ceftriaxone	
19-59 y	1. *S pneumoniae* 2. *N meningitides* 3. *H influenzae* type b	Ampicillin + vancomycin 5 ceftriaxone	
60+ y	1. *S pneumoniae* 2. *L monocytogenes* 3. Group B streptococcus	Ampicillin + vancomycin + ceftriaxone (or cefotaxime)	*Listeria* more common

(Courtesy of Centers for Disease Control and Prevention, 2003.)

dose of antibiotics to reduce the inflammation due to the antibacterial therapy. One study in adults demonstrated decreased mortality in patients with *S pneumoniae* meningitis who were given glucocorticoids. There are stronger data supporting steroids for *H influenzae* and *S pneumoniae* meningitis in children. There is also some evidence for benefit of steroids in severe tuberculous meningitis. A Cochrane database review in 2015 concluded that corticosteroids may help reduce the incidence of hearing loss and neurologic sequelae but does not affect mortality.

Prevention of meningitis can be achieved through the administration of **vaccines and chemoprophylaxis** of close contacts. **Specific vaccinations are available for *H influenzae* type B and some strains of *S pneumoniae*** and are now routinely administered to **children. Meningococcal vaccination** is recommended for those living in dormitory situations, such as college students and military recruits, but not for the general population. **Rifampin given twice daily for 2 days** or a single dose of ciprofloxacin is recommended for **household and close contacts** of an index case of **meningococcemia or meningococcal meningitis.**

CASE CORRELATION

- See also Case 38 (Headache), Case 41 (Urine Infection Sepsis), Case 42 (Neutropenic Fever), and Case 45 (Syphilis).

COMPREHENSION QUESTIONS

43.1 An 18-year-old with a 1-week history of fever, headache, increasing confusion, and lethargy presents to the emergency room. His physical examination is normal, and he has no focal neurologic signs. The CT scan of his head is negative. An LP reveals a WBC count of 250/mm³, with 78% lymphocytes and RBCs 500/mm³ in tube 1 and 630/mm³ in tube 2, respectively. No organisms are seen on Gram stain. Which of the following is the best next step?

A. Intravenous ceftriaxone, acyclovir, and vancomycin

B. Intravenous fluconazole

C. Intravenous azithromycin

D. Careful observation with no antibiotics

43.2 A 55-year-old man with a long history of alcohol abuse presents with a 3-week history of progressive confusion and stupor. On examination he is afebrile, but he has a new right sixth cranial nerve palsy and tremulousness of all four extremities. His CSF has 250 WBCs/mm³, with 68% lymphocytes. There are 300 RBCs/mm³. Protein levels are high, and the ratio of CSF to serum glucose is very low. He is started on ceftriaxone, vancomycin, and acyclovir. A purified protein derivative (PPD) placed on admission is positive, and bacterial cultures are negative at 48 hours. Which of the following would help to confirm the diagnosis?

A. Gram stain of throat scrapings

B. CT of the head with contrast

C. MRI of the head

D. Repeat LP after 48 hours of therapy

E. Herpes simplex virus PCR

43.3 A 65-year-old man with colon cancer on chemotherapy presents with a fever and headache of 3-day duration. An LP is performed, and Gram stain reveals gram-positive rods. Which of the following therapies is most likely to treat the organism?

A. Vancomycin

B. Metronidazole

C. Ampicillin

D. Gentamicin

E. Ceftriaxone

ANSWERS

43.1 **A.** This young man most likely has viral meningitis given the modest CSF pleocytosis count with predominant lymphocytes. Given the high RBC count, it may be HSV, so acyclovir should be instituted until more specific testing can be done. However, because bacterial meningitis cannot be excluded based on the CSF analysis alone, empiric antibacterials should be given until culture results are known, usually within 48 hours.

43.2 **D.** Tuberculous meningitis is extremely difficult to diagnose, and the index of suspicion should be high in susceptible individuals. Certain clinical findings, such as nerve palsies, and CSF findings, such as an extremely low glucose and high protein levels with a fairly low WBC count, are highly suggestive but not diagnostic. Mortality is high and related to the delay in instituting therapy. The only definitive test is acid-fast bacillus (AFB) culture, but it can take 6 to 8 weeks to grow. PCR test for *Mycobacterium tuberculosis* is diagnostic if positive; however, the sensitivity is low, so a negative test does not rule out the disease. Findings such as a positive PPD, or CSF cell counts and protein levels that do not change with standard antimicrobial or antiviral therapies, can also suggest the diagnosis. Low CSF glucose is a hallmark of TB meningitis—if the glucose level falls at 48 hours, it is highly suggestive of TB. A CT scan and an MRI may demonstrate basilar meningitis in TB, but the finding is not specific.

43.3 **C.** *L monocytogenes* is a gram-positive rod that causes approximately 10% of all cases of meningitis. It is more common in the elderly and in other patients with impaired cell-mediated immunity, such as patients on chemotherapy. It is also more common in neonates. It is not sensitive to cephalosporins, and specific therapy with ampicillin must be instituted if the suspicion for this disease is high.

CLINICAL PEARLS

▶ In general, a lumbar puncture should not be delayed in a patient in whom meningitis is suspected. If lumbar puncture is contraindicated or impossible because of hemodynamic or other instability, empiric therapy should be started immediately after blood cultures are drawn.

▶ CT imaging of the brain prior to lumbar puncture is not necessary in most cases, but should be considered when the risk of brain herniation is high. These findings include new-onset seizures, signs suspicious for space-occupying lesions (such as **papilledema and focal neurologic signs**), and moderate to severe impairment in consciousness.

▶ The most common cause of bacterial meningitis in adults is *S pneumoniae*, followed by *N meningitides*. *L monocytogenes* meningitis occurs in neonates and in immunocompromised or older patients.

▶ Patients who have undergone neurosurgical procedures or who have been subject to skull trauma are at risk for staphylococcal meningitis.

▶ Hemorrhagic cerebrospinal fluid with evidence of temporal lobe involvement by imaging or EEG suggests herpes simplex virus encephalitis; acyclovir is the treatment of choice.

▶ Corticosteroid use does not affect mortality but seems to reduce hearing loss and neurologic sequelae. It should be used just before or concurrent with antibiotic therapy.

REFERENCES

Cochrane Library. Corticosteroids for bacterial meningitis. Sept 2015. http://www.cochrane.org/CD004405/ARI_corticosteroids-bacterial-meningitis. Accessed January 15, 2015.

Hasbun R, Abrahams J, Jekel J, Quagliarello VJ. Computed tomography of the head before lumbar puncture in adults with suspected meningitis. *N Engl J Med*. 2001;345:1727-1733.

Pollard AJ. Meningococcal infections. In: Kasper DL, Fauci AS, Hauser SL, Longo DL, Jameson JL, Loscalzo J, eds. *Harrison's Principles of Internal Medicine*. 19th ed. New York, NY: McGraw-Hill; 2015:1211-1219.

Roos KL, Tyler KL. Meningitis, encephalitis, brain abscess, and empyema. In: Kasper DL, Fauci AS, Hauser SL, Longo DL, Jameson JL, Loscalzo J, eds. *Harrison's Principles of Internal Medicine*. 19th ed. New York, NY: McGraw-Hill; 2015:3410-3434.

Thomas KE, Hasbun R, Jekel J, et al. The diagnostic accuracy of Kernig's sign, Brudzinski's sign, and nuchal rigidity in adults with suspected meningitis. *Clin Infect Dis*. 2002;35:46-52.

Van de Beek D, de Gans J, Spanjaard L, et al. Clinical features and prognostic factors in adults with bacterial meningitis. *N Engl J Med*. 2004;351:1849-1859.

A 62-year-old man is brought to the clinic for a 3-month history of unintentional weight loss (12 lb). His appetite has diminished, but he reports no vomiting or diarrhea. He does report some depressive symptoms since the death of his wife a year ago, at which time he moved from Hong Kong to the United States to live with his daughter. He denies a smoking history. He complains of a 3-month history of productive cough with greenish sputum. He has not felt feverish. He takes no medications regularly. On examination, his temperature is 100.4°F and respiratory rate is 16 bpm. His neck has a normal thyroid gland and no cervical or supraclavicular lymphadenopathy. His chest has few scattered crackles in the left mid-lung fields and a faint expiratory wheeze on the right. His heart rhythm is regular with no gallops or murmurs. His abdominal examination is benign, his rectal examination shows no masses, and his stool is negative for occult blood. His chest x-ray is shown in Figure 44–1.

▶ What is the most likely diagnosis?
▶ What is your next step?

Figure 44–1. Chest x-ray. (Reproduced, with permission, from Fishman AP. *Fishman's Pulmonary Diseases and Disorders*, 3rd ed. New York: McGraw-Hill, 1998:2487.)

ANSWERS TO CASE 44:
Tuberculosis (Pulmonary), Cavitary Lung Lesions

Summary: A 62-year-old man from Hong Kong has a 12-lb unintentional weight loss with diminished appetite but no vomiting or diarrhea. On examination, he has a low-grade fever, and there are a few scattered crackles in the left mid-lung fields and a faint expiratory wheeze on the right. His chest x-ray shows right upper lobe reticulonodular and left lower lobe alveolar opacities. The left lung lesion is cavitary.

- **Most likely diagnosis:** Pulmonary tuberculosis (TB).

- **Next step:** Refer him to the hospital for admission so that serial sputum samples can be collected for identification of the organism, and for culture and sensitivities to guide antimicrobial therapy.

ANALYSIS

Objectives

1. Know the natural history and the clinical and radiographic manifestations of primary and reactivation pulmonary TB and of latent TB infection.

2. Understand the methods of diagnosis of TB.

3. Learn treatment strategies for TB.

4. Know the common extrapulmonary sites of TB infection, including the pleura, lymph nodes, meninges, genitourinary tract, skeletal system, adrenal glands, and miliary.

Considerations

This elderly Asian gentleman has symptoms suggestive of TB, such as weight loss and productive cough. A chest radiograph is essential in helping to establish the diagnosis. His chest x-ray is highly suggestive of TB, but many other diseases may cause cavitary lung lesions, including other infections and malignancies. If the sputum samples do not reveal acid-fast organisms, then further testing, such as bronchoscopy, may be needed.

APPROACH TO:
Suspected Tuberculosis

DEFINITIONS

LATENT TUBERCULOSIS: Asymptomatic infection with *Mycobacterium tuberculosis.*

PRIMARY TUBERCULOSIS: Development of clinical illness immediately after infection with *M tuberculosis.*

REACTIVATION TUBERCULOSIS: Clinical illness that occurs when latent TB becomes active and infectious after a period of dormancy. The dormant period can be years after the initial infection and manifest after periods of stress or immune suppression.

CLINICAL APPROACH

Pulmonary Tuberculosis

Tuberculosis is a bacterial infection caused by the acid-fast bacillus (AFB) *M tuberculosis*, which usually is transmitted through airborne spread of droplets from infected patients with pulmonary TB. The vast majority of cases occur in developing countries, but a resurgence of cases in the United States occurred during the mid-1980s as a consequence of various factors, including human immunodeficiency virus (HIV) infection. Untreated disease can have a 1-year mortality rate of 33% and a 5-year mortality rate as high as 50%.

Often seen in children, **primary pulmonary TB usually affects the middle and lower lobes.** Lesions form in the periphery with hilar and paratracheal lymphadenopathy. Granulomatous lesions are caused by the inflammatory response of lymphocytes and macrophages. The center of the lesion may become necrotic (caseous necrosis) and liquefied, forming a cavity. Healed lesions are called **Ghon lesions.** Most patients exposed to *M tuberculosis* do not manifest clinical symptoms, but they may have a latent infection. Years later, frequently during times of stress or immunosuppression, TB may reactivate and become symptomatic. **Reactivation TB** usually involves the **apical and posterior segments of the upper lobes** or the superior segments of the lower lobes of the lungs. The course may be rapid (weeks to months), chronic and slowly progressive ("consumption"), or spontaneously remit.

Signs and symptoms are nonspecific and subacute, including **fever, night sweats, malaise, weight loss, and anorexia.** The **cough usually is productive** of purulent sputum and sometimes **streaked with blood.** A **Rasmussen aneurysm sometimes develops in proximity to a cavitary lesion as the inflammatory reaction causes thinning of the wall of an adjacent bronchial artery.** Rupture of the aneurysm can lead to massive hemoptysis. Physical findings can include fever, wasting, crackles and rhonchi, pallor, or finger clubbing. Possible laboratory abnormalities are leukocytosis, anemia, and hyponatremia secondary to the syndrome of inappropriate secretion of antidiuretic hormone (**SIADH**).

Extrapulmonary Tuberculosis

The sites of extrapulmonary spread of TB, in order of decreasing frequency of occurrence, are the **lymph nodes, pleura, genitourinary tract, bones and joints, meninges, and peritoneum.** Tuberculosis lymphadenitis is common in HIV-infected patients, children, and nonwhite women and generally is **painless adenopathy.** Pleural disease can have an exudative effusion but may require pleural biopsy for diagnosis. Tuberculosis meningitis usually has cerebrospinal fluid with high protein, a lymphocyte predominance (or neutrophils in early infection), and low glucose level. **Adjunctive glucocorticoids** may improve the treatment response in TB meningitis. Genitourinary TB can be asymptomatic or have local symptoms such as dysuria, hematuria, and urinary frequency. It is characterized by the finding of leukocytes in the urine but negative bacterial cultures—"**sterile pyuria**." Skeletal TB affects weight-bearing joints, whereas **Pott disease involves the spine**. **Miliary TB** refers to hematogenously disseminated tuberculosis, and describes the radiographic or pathologic finding of 1- to 2-mm granulomas that resemble millet seeds (hence the name). Adrenal involvement is common in military TB, and may cause **adrenal insufficiency**.

Diagnosis

The diagnosis of TB is made by combining the history and clinical picture with AFB stains or culture of a specimen (smear or tissue biopsy). When **pulmonary TB** is suspected, **three sputum samples** should be obtained while the patient is in isolation. At least one of these should be collected in the early morning. Biopsy material should not be put in formalin. Cultures may take from 4 to 8 weeks on ordinary solid media or 2 to 3 weeks on liquid media. Tuberculosis cases should be reported to the local public health department.

Purified protein derivative (PPD), or tuberculin, skin testing is useful for screening for latent TB infection but has a limited role in diagnosing active infection because of frequent false-negative results in this setting. A positive **PPD** is defined by induration of at least 5 mm after 48 to 72 hours (Table 44–1).

Interferon-gamma release assays (IGRAs) are new diagnostic tools for latent tuberculosis. They are in vitro blood tests of cell-mediated immune response to *M tuberculosis* and measure T-cell release of interferon-gamma (IFN-gamma) following stimulation by TB antigens. The Centers for Disease Control and Prevention (CDC) recommend that such tests can be used in place of tuberculin skin testing. IGRAs are preferred for patients with history of *Bacillus Calmette-Guérin* (BCG) vaccination (it is not affected by BCG). The most commonly used IGRAs are the Quantiferon TB Gold assay and the T-SPOT TB assay.

Treatment

The probable resistance pattern of the TB organism, based on the country of origin, may help to guide treatment. For individuals from areas with low drug resistance,

Table 44–1 • TUBERCULIN REACTION SIZE AND DIAGNOSIS OF LATENT *M TUBERCULOSIS* INFECTION	
Risk Group	Tuberculin Reaction Size, mm
HIV-infected persons or persons receiving immunosuppressive therapy	≥5
Close contacts of tuberculosis patients	≥5[a]
Persons with fibrotic lesions on chest radiography	≥5
Recently infected persons (≤2 y)	≥10
Persons with high-risk medical conditions[b]	≥10
Low-risk persons[c]	≥15

(Reproduced, with permission, from Longo. Harrison's Principles of Internal Medicine. 18th ed. New York: McGraw-Hill, 2012. Table 165-5.)

therapy generally starts with a **2-month course of four-drug treatment with isonia-zid (INH), rifampin, pyrazinamide, and ethambutol, followed by 4 months of INH and rifampin. Multiple drugs are used to avoid resistance.** Directly observed treatment (watching patients take the medication) should be instituted in all patients in this phase. Pyridoxine is frequently added to the regimen to prevent peripheral neuropathy caused by INH. Drug resistance or intolerable side effects may require alternate therapy. Toxicity for which patients must be monitored includes **hepatitis,** hyperuricemia, and thrombocytopenia. The World Health Organization defines treatment failure as a positive smear or culture after 5 months of therapy. **Latent TB infection** is usually treated with INH for 9 months, with the goal of preventing reactivation TB later in life.

CASE CORRELATION

- See also Case 15 (Chronic Obstructive Pulmonary Disease), Case 16 (Chronic Cough/Asthma), Case 18 (Hemoptysis), and Case 19 (Pneumonia).

COMPREHENSION QUESTIONS

44.1 A 42-year-old woman from Pakistan is being treated with infliximab for rheumatoid arthritis. After 6 months of therapy, she develops persistent fever, weight loss, and night sweats, and tuberculosis is suspected. Which of the following is the most likely location of the tuberculosis?

    A. Middle and lower lung zones

    B. Pleural space

    C. Apical segment of the upper lung lobes

    D. Cervical or supraclavicular lymph nodes

44.2 A 24-year-old man has been treated with isoniazid, rifampin, and pyrazin-amide for active pulmonary tuberculosis. After 3 months, he states that he is having numbness and tingling of both feet but no back pain. He denies taking other medications. Which of the following is the most appropriate next step?

    A. Computed tomography (CT) scan of the lumbar spine.

    B. Initiate pyridoxine.

    C. Continue the tuberculosis agents and monitor for further neurologic problems.

    D. Initiate a workup for tuberculosis adenopathy compression on the femoral nerve.

44.3 A 25-year-old woman is seen in the clinic because her father, who recently immigrated from South America, was diagnosed with and has been treated for tuberculosis. She denies a cough and her chest radiograph is normal. A PPD test shows 10 mm of induration. Her only medication is an oral contraceptive. Which of the following is the best next step?

A. Isoniazid.

B. Combination therapy including isoniazid, rifampin, and pyrazinamide.

C. Observation.

D. Induce three sputum samples.

44.4 Which of the following tests are the most important to follow for a patient receiving isoniazid and rifampin for tuberculosis treatment?

A. Renal function tests

B. Liver function tests

C. Slit-lamp examinations

D. Amylase and lipase tests

ANSWERS

44.1 **C.** Reactivation tuberculosis (in this case, likely triggered by infliximab) usually involves the apical aspects of the lungs. Primary pulmonary TB infection most often affects the middle and lower lobes. Lymphadenitis and pleural disease are the most common extrapulmonary TB infections, but they are less common than pulmonary TB.

44.2 **B.** Pyridoxine (vitamin B_6) is important for preventing the peripheral neuropathy that can complicate isoniazid therapy. If the numbness were caused by Pott disease, he should have back pain and other neurologic findings, such as lower extremity weakness.

44.3 **A.** Because this woman is a household contact of a patient with active TB, she is among the highest risk group: her skin test would be considered positive with 5-mm induration. She has latent TB infection and should be offered treatment to prevent reactivation TB later in life. INH is the treatment of choice for exposure prophylaxis.

44.4 **B.** Drug-induced liver injury is a complication of treatment with isoniazid, pyrazinamide, and rifampin. Baseline liver tests are obtained in all patients and monthly monitoring of hepatic enzymes is recommended for patients at increased risk of liver toxicity. Alcohol use, prior liver disease, pregnancy, and the first 3 months postpartum are risk factors.

CLINICAL PEARLS

▶ Reactivation pulmonary tuberculosis most commonly presents radiographically with opacities in the apical and posterior segments of the upper lobes.

▶ Tuberculin skin testing is not a diagnostic test but is a useful screening test for potential contacts of infected persons; the response cutoff for a positive test depends on the patient's level of risk. IGRAs such as TB Quantiferon Gold are also useful to diagnose latent TB.

▶ Patients with a positive tuberculin skin test and no clinical or radiographic evidence of active disease are said to have *latent tuberculosis infection*; they can be treated with isoniazid to reduce their lifetime risk of developing reactivation tuberculosis.

▶ Individuals with active tuberculosis should be initiated on multidrug therapy, such as isoniazid, rifampin, pyrazinamide, and ethambutol.

▶ Pyridoxine (vitamin B_6) is usually added to antituberculosis medications to prevent peripheral neuropathy.

REFERENCES

Blumberg HM, Burman WJ, Chaisson RE, et al. American Thoracic Society/Centers for Disease Control and Prevention/Infectious Diseases Society of America: treatment of tuberculosis. *Am J Respir Crit Care Med.* 2003;167:603-662.

Campbell IA, Bah-Sow O. Pulmonary tuberculosis: diagnosis and treatment. *BMJ.* 2006;332: 1194-1197.

Jasmer RM, Nahid P, Hopewell PC. Latent tuberculosis infection. *N Engl J Med.* 2002;347:1860-1866.

Mazurek GH, Jereb J. Updated guidelines for using interferon gamma release assays to detect *Mycobacterium tuberculosis* infection—United States, 2010. *MMWR Recomm Rep.* 2010;59(RR-5):1.

Raviglione MC, O'Brian R. Tuberculosis. In: Longo DL, Fauci AS, Kasper DL, et al., eds. *Harrison's Principles of Internal Medicine.* 18th ed. New York, NY: McGraw-Hill; 2012:1340-1359.

Zumla A, Raviglione M, Hafner R, et al. Tuberculosis. *N Engl J Med.* 2013;368:745-755.

A 23-year-old man is the next patient you see in the clinic. Under the chief complaint, the nurse has written, "Wants a general checkup." You enter the room and greet a generally healthy-appearing young, white man, who seems nervous. He finally admits that he has been worried about a lesion on his penis. He denies pain or dysuria. He has never had any sexually transmitted diseases (STDs) and has an otherwise unremarkable medical history. He is afebrile, and his examination is notable for a shallow clean ulcer without exudates or erythema on the shaft of his penis, which is nontender to palpation, and has a cartilaginous consistency. There are some small, nontender, inguinal lymph nodes bilaterally.

▶ What is the most likely diagnosis?
▶ What is the likely treatment?

ANSWERS TO CASE 45:

Syphilis

Summary: A 23-year-old healthy man reluctantly requests evaluation of a lesion on his penis. He has never had any STDs and has an otherwise unremarkable medical history. He is afebrile, and his examination is notable for a firm nontender ulcer on his penis with small, nontender inguinal lymph nodes bilaterally.

- **Most likely diagnosis:** Chancre of primary syphilis.

- **Likely treatment:** Single intramuscular injection of benzathine penicillin G.

ANALYSIS

Objectives

1. Understand the pathogenesis and natural history of *Treponema pallidum* infection.

2. Know the differential diagnosis of genital ulceration and STDs.

3. Learn the treatment of syphilis.

Considerations

This 23-year-old man reluctantly reveals his concern about a nontender ulcer of the penis. Although he has no history of STD, the most common cause of a painless ulcer of the genital area in a young, immunocompetent person is syphilis. The STDs often travel together, so he should be evaluated for other STDs such as *Chlamydia* and human immunodeficiency virus (HIV). Other causes of genital ulcers should also be considered, including chancroid and herpes virus (both usually painful), and a superficially infected skin lesion. Compliance with therapy and follow-up are crucial because syphilitic infections can progress to a chronic form that can lead to cardiovascular as well as neurologic disease. He could continue spreading the disease to others, and if he infects women of childbearing age, these women, if infected during pregnancy, could pass the infection to their newborns.

APPROACH TO:

Suspected Syphilis

DEFINITIONS

PRIMARY SYPHILIS: Initial lesion of *T pallidum* infection, usually in the form of a firm, nontender ulcer: the chancre.

SECONDARY SYPHILIS: Disseminated infection manifesting in a pruritic, maculopapular diffuse rash that classically involves the **palms and soles**, or the flat moist lesion of **condyloma lata.**

TERTIARY (LATE) SYPHILIS: Symptomatic infection involving the central nervous system, cardiovascular system, or the skin and subcutaneous tissues (gummas).

CLINICAL APPROACH

Syphilis is classically called the "great imitator" for its protean manifestations. After a decline in cases over the prior decades, the incidence of syphilis has been increasing since the 1980s. The public health consequences can be grave, so recognizing and correctly treating this disease is of great importance. An estimated 70,000 new cases of syphilis occur every year in the United States. Most occur in young adults in their twenties, and most cases are concentrated in the southern states. The number of cases reached its lowest point in the 1980s; however, these have increased since then, especially in heterosexuals, young women, and neonates. Some researchers believe this increase may be a result of cocaine use, sex for drugs trade, and perhaps the increased incidence of HIV infections.

Syphilis is caused by the spirochete *T pallidum*. The organism penetrates abraded skin or mucous membranes and then disseminates through the lymphatics and bloodstream to involve almost every organ. Within 1 week to 3 months of inoculation, a chancre usually forms at the site of entrance. Multiple ulcers may form, as in HIV-infected patients, but some patients may not notice the ulceration at all. The **chancre** of syphilis typically is **nonerythematous, with rolled borders and a clean base, with a very firm consistency on palpation**. It usually is **painless**, although it may be mildly tender if touched. Other diseases that can cause ulcerations include **chancroid**; however the ulcer in this disease usually is **painful, exudative, with ragged borders and a necrotic base**, and bleeds easily. The lymph nodes can also suppurate in chancroid, unlike in syphilis. The ulcers in **herpes simplex infections typically are painful, grouped vesicles on an erythematous base** that eventually ulcerate.

If untreated, syphilis progresses to a **second stage**, in which the disease disseminates widely, and the patient may present with a **pruritic, maculopapular diffuse rash that classically involves the palms and soles**. Patients also may have these lesions orally, called "mucous patches," and they may suffer constitutional symptoms such as fever, myalgias, and headache. Other typical skin findings include **condyloma lata**, a gray papillomatous lesion found in intertriginous areas, and patchy hair loss.

If still left untreated, the patient will pass into a quiescent, or latent, stage. Although relapses of symptoms of secondary syphilis can occur during this time, they become less frequent over years. Approximately 30% of patients will go on to develop **late-stage syphilis**. The symptoms of this stage result from the destruction of tissue caused by the chronic infection. The immune reaction to the organism causes a proliferative, obliterative endarteritis. In some organs, such as the skin, liver, and bone, these lesions are organized into **granulomas** with an amorphous or coagulated center called **gummas**. These lesions, in themselves, are benign; however, they can cause organ dysfunction through destruction of normal tissue. In the aorta, the obliterative endarteritis involves the vasa vasorum, which leads to necrosis of the media of the arterial wall. The resulting weakness of the wall leads to the formation of **saccular aneurysmal dilations of the aorta**.

Neurosyphilis is another form of tertiary disease that may occur after secondary disease or from the latent stage. The organism disseminates to the central nervous system (CNS), causing a broad range of neurologic symptoms. In the CNS, it may cause vasculitis, leading to ischemia, stroke, and focal neurologic deficits. Patients may exhibit personality changes or dementia, demyelination of the posterior column with wide-based gait and loss of proprioception (**tabes dorsalis**), or cranial nerve impairment, including the development of the Argyll Robertson pupil (accommodates but does not react to light). Lumbar puncture to exclude neurosyphilis is generally indicated when any patient with syphilis develops neurologic or ocular symptoms or if HIV-infected patients with syphilis are relatively immunosuppressed (CD4 <350) or have a high rapid plasma reagin (RPR) titer (>1:32).

The diagnosis of syphilis is always made indirectly, as the organism has not yet been cultured. Nonspecific serologic tests, such as the RPR and Venereal Disease Research Laboratory (VDRL) tests, which actually are tests for antibodies against lipid antigens that occur as part of the host reaction to *T pallidum*, are fairly sensitive for the detection of disease. However, especially at low titers, they may be nonspecific and may result in false-positive results. Therefore, **confirmatory testing** in the form of specific antibody testing for *T pallidum*, such as the **fluorescent treponemal antibody absorption (FTA-ABS) or microhemagglutination assay for *T pallidum* (MHA-TP) test**, is the next step. **Dark-field microscopy**, in which scrapings from an ulcer are placed under a phase contrast lens to actually identify the organisms, is the classic method of diagnosis but is rarely performed today. Biopsy of lesions, such as those seen in secondary syphilis with special stains, also can identify the organisms. To diagnose CNS disease, a positive cerebrospinal fluid (CSF) VDRL or RPR in the setting of increased CSF leukocytosis and protein counts, sometimes with low glucose levels, is suggestive of CNS involvement. False-negative results for VDRL in CSF are common, however, and the diagnosis is often made on clinical grounds.

Penicillin is the treatment of choice for syphilis. The most effective treatment and regimen, however, are truly unknown, because no therapeutic trials have been performed. However, current recommendations are to treat syphilis based on the stage of presentation (Table 45–1). Individuals with early disease, that is, with primary or secondary syphilis, or those with early latent syphilis (infection for <1 year) may be treated with a single intramuscular (IM) injection of benzathine penicillin G, a long-lasting IM injection. For patients with late disease, that is, latent syphilis of an unknown duration (presumed to be >1 year), or with cardiovascular manifestations or with gummas, treatment is given as three weekly IM injections of benzathine penicillin G.

Neurosyphilis is notoriously difficult to treat. Those with CNS disease or patients concurrently infected with HIV and syphilis should receive high doses of intravenous penicillin G for 10 to 14 days or longer. All patients should be followed closely to ensure that their titers fall over the year after treatment. Pregnant women who are allergic to penicillin should be desensitized and then receive penicillin, because this is the only treatment known to prevent congenital infection.

T pallidum infection usually leads to a **positive specific serologic test** (FTA-ABS or MHA-TP) for **life**, whereas an adequately treated infection will lead to a fall in

Table 45–1 • TREATMENT OF SYPHILIS BASED ON STAGE		
Stage	Clinical Manifestations	Treatment[a]
Primary disease	Chancre	Single dose of intramuscular penicillin G 2.4 mU
Secondary disease, early latent (<1 y—no symptoms)	Maculopapular rash involving palms and soles, condyloma lata	Single dose of intramuscular penicillin G 2.4 mU
Secondary disease, late latent disease (>1 y—no symptoms)	None	Intramuscular penicillin G 2.4 mU at 1-wk intervals for total of three doses
Tertiary syphilis, neurosyphilis	Various: dementia, focal neurologic deficits, cranial nerve palsies, gummas, aortitis	Intravenous penicillin for 10-14 d

[a]For patients with penicillin allergy, oral tetracycline or doxycycline for 2 weeks is acceptable treatment for patients with primary, secondary, and latent syphilis. For penicillin-allergic patients with neurosyphilis, or syphilis in pregnancy, desensitization and treatment with penicillin is required.

RPR serology. A **normal response** is considered a **fourfold drop in titers within 3 months** and a **negative or near-negative titer after 1 year.** A suboptimal response may mean inadequate treatment or undiagnosed tertiary disease.

In any patient diagnosed with an STD, the possibility that they may have other STDs should be considered.

Chlamydia is the most common bacterial STD, and can be asymptomatic, especially in women. In females, it can cause cervicitis (vaginal discharge, postcoital bleeding) and urethritis (dysuria or urinary tract infection [UTI] symptoms). It may also cause **pelvic inflammatory disease** (lower abdominal pain, vaginal discharge or dysuria, with fever and systemic symptoms), which can lead to infertility due to tubal scarring. Men with symptoms typically present with urethritis (dysuria, urethral discharge), but may also experience epididymitis (scrotal pain and fever) or proctitis (rectal pain or diarrhea). Diagnosis is usually made by antigen detection or gene probe from urethra or cervix. Treatment is usually single-dose azithromycin 1000 mg (often given under direct observation) or a 7-day course of doxycycline.

Gonorrhea due to the gram-negative diplococcus *Neisseria gonorrhoeae* can cause identical clinical syndromes as *Chlamydia* (in fact, up to 30% of patients are coinfected with both organisms), but patients are less likely to be asymptomatic, especially men. It may also cause **disseminated infection** characterized by fever, migratory polyarthritis, tenosynovitis of hands and feet, and a rash on the distal extremities. Patients with disseminated infection require hospitalization for IV antibiotics, usually ceftriaxone. Outpatients with genitourinary symptoms are treated with a single IM injection of ceftriaxone, along with a single dose of azithromycin 1000 mg or doxycycline for 7 days for *Chlamydia* coinfection.

HIV is often asymptomatic early in the course of infection, and screening should be recommended to those persons who have histories of high-risk behaviors or who have evidence of other STDs.

CASE CORRELATION

- See also Case 41 (Urine Tract Sepsis), Case 42 (Neutropenic Fever), Case 43 (Bacterial Meningitis), and Case 46 (HIV Infection).

COMPREHENSION QUESTIONS

45.1 A 25-year-old man presents to your office complaining of left knee and right great toe pain, which started 1 week ago and has not responded to over-the-counter pain relievers. He also has felt feverish and achy, has dysuria, and has developed an eye infection. Approximately 1 month ago, he was seen at an outside clinic and treated for syphilis. On examination, he is afebrile, and both eyes are injected and very sensitive to light. His left knee and the metatarsophalangeal (MTP) joint of his right great toe are swollen and tender. Which of the following is your diagnosis?

A. Gouty arthritis

B. Reactive arthritis (Reiter syndrome)

C. Infectious arthritis

D. Rheumatoid arthritis

E. Syphilis

45.2 As part of normal screening during pregnancy, a 28-year-old G2P1 has a positive RPR with a titer of 1:64 and a positive MHA-TP. She is allergic to penicillin, which causes shortness of breath and "swelling of her tongue." Which of the following treatments do you offer?

A. Erythromycin estolate.

B. Doxycycline.

C. Tetracycline.

D. Penicillin after desensitization.

E. Vancomycin.

F. Wait until delivery of the baby before treatment.

45.3 A 23-year-old man is found to have late latent syphilis (RPR 1:64) as part of a workup following his diagnosis with HIV. He is asymptomatic with a CD4 count of 150 and does not remember having lesions or rashes in the past. Prior to starting therapy with penicillin for the syphilis, the patient should undergo which of the following procedures?

A. Lumbar puncture to exclude neurosyphilis

B. Skin biopsy to confirm the diagnosis of syphilis

C. Magnetic resonance imaging (MRI) of his brain and an electroencephalogram (EEG)

D. Skin testing to exclude penicillin allergy

E. Adjustment of his HIV medications to optimize his CD4 count prior to treatment for syphilis

45.4 A 28-year-old woman is noted to have a nontender ulcer of the vulva. A herpes culture is taken of the ulcer scraping, which is negative, and the RPR titer is negative. Which of the following is the next best step?

A. Empiric treatment with doxycycline for *Chlamydia trachomatis*

B. Empiric treatment with acyclovir for herpes simplex virus (HSV)

C. Empiric treatment with azithromycin for *Haemophilus ducreyi*

D. Dark-field microscopy

E. Biopsy for possible vulvar cancer

ANSWERS

45.1 **B.** The triad of uveitis or conjunctivitis, urethritis, and arthritis is characteristic of reactive arthritis or Reiter syndrome. This poorly understood disease is thought to be caused by immune cross-reaction between antigens in infectious organisms and the host connective tissue. Organisms commonly involved include *C trachomatis*, which this patient may have contracted when he contracted syphilis but which may not have been treated. The arthritis typically involves large joints and is both progressive and additive. The uveitis can be difficult to treat; however, the dysuria of the urethritis can be transient. Patients with Reiter syndrome are often HLA-B27 positive.

45.2 **D.** This patient should be desensitized and treated with penicillin, especially because she is pregnant and may pass the disease to her child. Following treatment, her titers should be closely followed and should show at least a fourfold decrease. Treatment of the child after delivery with intravascular (IV) penicillin should be considered.

45.3 **A.** Lumbar puncture to exclude neurosyphilis is generally indicated when any patient with syphilis develops neurologic or ocular symptoms, or considered if HIV-infected patients with syphilis have a CD4 less than 350 or an RPR more than 1:32.

45.4 **D.** Approximately one-third of patients who have the primary lesion of the chancre will have negative serology and require either dark-field microscopy or biopsy with special stains to identify the spirochetes. The organism is too thin to be visualized by conventional light microscopy. Empiric treatment with penicillin is reasonable if dark-field microscopy is not available. Genital herpes and chancroid should produce painful genital ulcers, and *Chlamydia* should cause nonulcerative cervicitis or urethritis.

CLINICAL PEARLS

▶ Syphilitic chancres are generally clean, painless, ulcerative lesions and can be located anywhere on the body where inoculation occurred.

▶ The rash of secondary syphilis typically involves the palms and soles.

▶ Elevated RPR and VDRL tests are nonspecific and may be falsely positive in several normal conditions (pregnancy) and disease states (systemic lupus erythematosus). Specific treponemal antibody tests, such as the MHA-TP and the FTA-ABS test, should be performed for confirmation, but once positive, they usually stay positive for life.

▶ A declining RPR titer can be followed to test the efficacy of therapy.

▶ Central nervous system involvement can be excluded only through testing of the cerebrospinal fluid.

▶ Treatment of syphilis is based on stage: early syphilis can be treated with a single intramuscular injection of penicillin; late latent syphilis can be treated with three weekly injections; and neurosyphilis or tertiary syphilis can be treated with intravenous penicillin for 10 to 14 days.

REFERENCES

Centers for Disease Control and Prevention. 2015 Sexually transmitted diseases treatment guidelines. *Morb Mortal Wkly Rep (MMWR)*. 2015:64(RR3);1-137.

Lukehart SA. Syphilis. In: Kasper DL, Fauci AS, Hauser SL, et al., eds. *Harrison's Principles of Internal Medicine*. 19th ed. New York, NY: McGraw-Hill; 2015:1132-1140.

Marra CM, Maxwell CL, Smith SL, et al. Cerebrospinal fluid abnormalities in patients with syphilis: association with clinical and laboratory features. *J Infect Dis*. 2004;189:369-376.

A 27-year-old man infected with human immunodeficiency virus (HIV), whose last CD4 count is unknown, presents to the emergency department (ED) with a fever of 39.2°C (102.5°F). He was diagnosed with an HIV infection approximately 3 years ago when he presented to his doctor with oral thrush. He was offered highly active antiretroviral therapy (HAART) and stayed on this regimen until approximately 10 months ago, when he lost his job and insurance and could no longer pay for his medications and discontinued all treatment. He has felt more "run down" recently. For the last 3 to 4 weeks, he has had fever and a nonproductive cough, and he has felt short of breath with mild exertion, such as when walking upstairs in his house. He also noticed weight loss of approximately 5 lb in the last 2 months. On examination, he is thin with decreased muscle mass, his blood pressure is 134/82 mm Hg, pulse is 110 bpm, and respiratory rate is 28 bpm. His oxygen saturation on room air at rest is 89% but drops to 80% when he walks 100 ft, and his breathing becomes quite labored. His lungs are clear to auscultation, but white plaques cover his oral mucosa. Otherwise, his examination is unremarkable. Laboratory testing shows a leukocyte count of 2800 cells/mm³. Serum lactic (acid) dehydrogenase (LDH) is 540 U/L (normal 140-280 U/L). His chest radiograph is shown in Figure 46–1.

▶ What is the most likely diagnosis?
▶ What is your next step?
▶ What other diagnoses should be considered?

Figure 46–1. Chest radiograph. (Reproduced, with permission, from Walzer P. *Pneumocystis carinii* infection. In: Braunwald E, Fauci AS, Kasper KL, et al, eds. *Harrison's Principles of Internal Medicine*, 15th ed. New York: McGraw-Hill, 2001:1183.)

ANSWERS TO CASE 46:
HIV and Pneumocystis Pneumonia

Summary: A 27-year-old man with known HIV infection but unknown CD4 count off HAART presents with the subacute onset of fever, dry cough, weight loss, and gradually worsening dyspnea. He is not undergoing any antiretroviral therapy or taking prophylactic medications. Bilateral interstitial lung opacities are seen on chest x-ray, and he is tachypneic and hypoxemic. The presence of oral thrush suggests that he is immunosuppressed. His leukocyte count is decreased (<3500 cells/mm^3), and his LDH level is elevated.

- **Most likely diagnosis:** Acquired immunodeficiency syndrome (AIDS) and probable *Pneumocystis jirovecii* pneumonia (PJP).[1]

- **Next step:** The next step is to stabilize the patient, who is tachypneic and hypoxic but is in only mild distress and is hemodynamically stable and hypoxemia improves with supplemental oxygen. Therefore, there is time to further evaluate him without need for endotracheal intubation and mechanical ventilation. An arterial blood gas measurement can be obtained to quantify his degree of hypoxemia, as it will impact the treatment.

- **Other diagnoses to be considered:** In patients with AIDS, other opportunistic infections must be considered. Other respiratory infections, such as tuberculosis (TB), atypical mycobacteria, cryptococcosis, and disseminated histoplasmosis, must be considered. In addition, HIV-infected patients are susceptible to the usual causes of community-acquired pneumonias: *Streptococcus pneumoniae*, mycoplasma, and viruses such as influenza. AIDS patients can have coexistent community-acquired microorganisms and pneumocystis pneumonia simultaneously.

ANALYSIS

Objectives

1. Understand the natural history of HIV infection.

2. Know the types of opportunistic infections that typically affect HIV-infected patients at various levels of immunocompromise.

3. Be familiar with respiratory infections in patients with AIDS.

4. Be familiar with indications for antiretroviral therapy and for prophylactic medications against opportunistic infections.

---

[1]As of 2002, the organism has been renamed Pneumocystis jirovecii. The abbreviation PCP remains for Pneumocystis carinii pneumonia, although it should be PJP for P jirovecii pneumonia.

Considerations

This individual with HIV, currently not taking antiviral medications or any anti-biotic prophylaxis, presents with subacute dyspnea and cough. His lack of sputum production and **elevated LDH** level are suggestive of PJP. The presence of oral thrush suggests a CD4 count less than 250. If the CD4 count is less than 200 cells/mm^3, then PJP seems the most likely explanation for his symptoms and chest x-ray findings. Obtaining an arterial blood gas measurement will provide information about prognosis and help guide therapy. Arterial oxygen concentration less than 70 mm Hg or alveolar-arterial gradient (A-a) more than 35 mm Hg suggests a worse prognosis and corticosteroids may be helpful, when given concurrently with antibiotic therapy such as trimethoprim-sulfamethoxazole (TMP-SMX).

APPROACH TO:
HIV Infections

DEFINITIONS

P jirovecii (**Formerly** *P carinii*): A unicellular fungus that causes pneumonia in immunocompromised patients, especially those with HIV and CD4 counts less than 200 cells/mm^3.

AIDS: A CD4 count less than 200 cells/mm^3 or diagnosis of an AIDS-defining illness in a patient who is HIV positive.

CLINICAL APPROACH

When evaluating a patient with HIV and suspected opportunistic infection, it is essential to know or estimate the patient's level of immunodeficiency. This is reflected by the CD4 (T4) cell count. Normal CD4 levels in adults range from 600 to 1500 cells/mm^3. As levels decline to less than 500 cells/mm^3, immune function is compromised, and patients become increasingly susceptible to unusual infections or malignancies.

Approximately 30% of patients first infected with HIV will develop an **acute HIV syndrome** characterized by sudden onset of a mononucleosis-like illness with fever, headaches, lymphadenopathy, pharyngitis, and sometimes a macular rash. The rest of the patients remain asymptomatic and have a clinically **latent period** of 8 to 10 years, on average, before the clinical manifestations of immunocompromise appear. As CD4 levels decline, various opportunistic infections appear. At CD4 levels less than **500**, patients are susceptible to infections, such as recurrent pneumonias, TB, vaginal candidiasis, and herpes zoster. At CD4 levels less than **200**, patients are significantly immunocompromised and develop infections with organisms that rarely cause significant illness in immunocompetent hosts, such as *P jirovecii*, toxoplasmosis, cryptococcosis, histoplasmosis, or cryptosporidiosis. At CD4 levels less than **50**, patients are severely immunocompromised and are susceptible to disseminated infection with histoplasmosis and *Mycobacterium*

Table 46–1 • AIDS-DEFINING ILLNESSES

Bacterial infections, multiple or recurrent
Candidiasis of bronchi, trachea, or lungs
Candidiasis of esophagus
Cervical cancer, invasive
Coccidioidomycosis, disseminated or extrapulmonary
Cryptococcosis, extrapulmonary
Cryptosporidiosis, chronic intestinal (>1-mo duration)
Cytomegalovirus disease (other than liver, spleen, or nodes), onset at age >1 mo
Cytomegalovirus retinitis (with loss of vision)
Encephalopathy, HIV related
Herpes simplex: chronic ulcers (>1-mo duration) or bronchitis, pneumonitis, or esophagitis (onset at age >1 mo)
Histoplasmosis, disseminated or extrapulmonary
Isosporiasis, chronic intestinal (>1-mo duration)
Kaposi sarcoma
Lymphoid interstitial pneumonia or pulmonary lymphoid hyperplasia complex
Lymphoma, Burkitt (or equivalent term)
Lymphoma, immunoblastic (or equivalent term)
Lymphoma, primary, of brain
Mycobacterium avium complex or *Mycobacterium kansasii*, disseminated or extrapulmonary
Mycobacterium tuberculosis of any site, pulmonary, disseminated, or extrapulmonary
Mycobacterium, other species or unidentified species, disseminated or extrapulmonary
Pneumocystis jirovecii pneumonia
Pneumonia, recurrent
Progressive multifocal leukoencephalopathy
Salmonella septicemia, recurrent
Toxoplasmosis of brain, onset at age >1 mo
Wasting syndrome attributed to HIV

avium–intracellulare complex (MAC) as well as development of cytomegalovirus (CMV) retinitis, colitis, and esophagitis, or primary central nervous system (CNS) lymphoma. The Centers for Disease Control and Prevention (CDC) has published a list of clinical conditions that define progression to AIDS in a patient who is HIV positive, so-called AIDS-defining conditions (Table 46–1).

PJP remains the **most common opportunistic infection affecting AIDS patients** but often is very difficult to diagnose. The clinical presentation ranges from fever without respiratory symptoms, to mild, persistent dry cough, to significant hypoxemia and respiratory compromise. In addition, the radiographic presentation can be highly variable, ranging from a near-normal chest film to a diffuse bilateral interstitial lung opacities, lung cysts are occasionally seen. Lung opacities can progress to severe alveolar lung opacities, acute respiratory distress syndrome (ARDS) type. Pleural effusions are not part of the presentation. The cysts can rupture, causing spontaneous pneumothoraces. PJP often is suspected when patients present with subacute onset of fever and respiratory symptoms, more so, in patients with AIDS without PJP prophylaxis, but the diagnosis should usually be confirmed. **Definitive diagnosis can be established by use of Giemsa or silver stain** to visualize the organism in the induced sputum either from using aerosolized hypertonic saline to induce cough or bronchoalveolar lavage to obtain a diagnostic specimen. PCR to detect

P jirovecii DNA sequences may also be performed (direct fluorescent antibody [DFA]). **Elevated LDH** level may be used as an indirect marker for PCP, although it is nonspecific and may also be elevated in disseminated histoplasmosis or lymphoma. It is useful as a negative predictor because **patients with an LDH level** less than **220 IU/L are very unlikely to have PCP.** Similarly, if patients have a CD4 count more than 250 cells/mm^3 or if they were taking PCP prophylaxis with TMP-SMX, the diagnosis of PCP should be considered highly unlikely.

The level of oxygenation of PCP patients by arterial blood gas is useful because it may affect prognosis and therapy. Patients with arterial PO$_2$ less than **70 mm Hg or A-a gradient more than 35 mm Hg** have significant disease and have an **improved prognosis** if **prednisone is given in conjunction with antimicrobial therapy.** After prednisone is given to patients with hypoxemia, the usual treatment for PCP is TMP-SMX. Patients who are allergic to sulfa can be treated with alternative regimens, including inhaled pentamidine, clindamycin with primaquine, dapsone, or atovaquone.

Many other respiratory infections are possible and should be considered in patients with AIDS. Diagnosis can be suggested by chest radiography. Diffuse interstitial lung opacities are seen with PCP, disseminated histoplasmosis, *Mycobacterium tuberculosis*, and other mycobacterial infections. Patchy alveolar and nodular lung opacities can be seen in the mentioned infections as well in viral infections for CMV and pleural-based opacities can be seen with TB and cryptococcal lung disease. Cavitary lesions can be seen with TB, PCP, and coccidiomycosis. Clinical and travel history should also be considered. Since the **most common causes of bacterial pneumonia in AIDS patients are the same organisms that cause pneumonia in immunocompetent hosts,** acute onset of fever and productive cough, with pulmonary opacities, is most consistent with **community-acquired pneumonia**. A more indolent or chronic history of cough and weight loss, especially in a patient who has a high-risk background (ie, prisoner, homeless, recent immigrant), should raise the question of **tuberculosis.** In patients with CD4 count more than 200 cells/mm^3, the radiographic appearance of TB is likely to be similar to that of other hosts, for example, bilateral apical lung opacities with cavitation; in those with CD4 count less than 200 cells/mm^3, the radiographic appearance is extremely variable. Patients with suspected pulmonary TB should be placed in respiratory isolation until it is assured they are not spreading airborne tuberculous infection. A negative purified protein derivative (PPD) (tuberculin skin test) or interference-gamma release assays (IGRAs) does not rule out tuberculosis in an immunocompromised host. Diagnosis and treatment of TB is discussed in Case 44, but it should be noted that, TB in AIDS patients is more likely to spread hematogenously and produce extrapulmonary manifestations. In HIV patients, *Mycobacterium kansasii* can cause pulmonary disease and radiographic findings identical to those of *M tuberculosis*.

Several other opportunistic infections in AIDS deserve mention. **Cerebral toxoplasmosis** is the **most common CNS mass lesions in AIDS patients.** It typically presents with headache, seizures, or focal neurologic deficits, and it is seen on computed tomography (CT) or magnetic resonance imaging (MRI) scan, usually as multiple enhancing lesions, often located in the basal ganglia. Presumptive diagnosis often is made based on the radiologic appearance, supported by serologic evidence of infection. The major alternative diagnosis for CNS mass lesions is **CNS lymphoma**. This diagnosis is considered if there is a single mass lesion or if the lesions do not regress after 2 weeks of empiric toxoplasmosis therapy with sulfadiazine with pyrimethamine. If this is the case, historically, the next diagnostic step has been stereotactic brain biopsy. However, recent evidence indicates that examination of the cerebrospinal fluid (CSF) for **Epstein-Barr virus DNA** is a useful strategy because it is present in more than 90% of patients with **CNS lymphoma**.

Another CNS complication that requires a high index of suspicion is **cryptococcal meningitis**. It is a chronic indolent infection, which often presents with vague symptoms of mood or personality changes, headaches, or visual disturbance. If the diagnosis is considered, one can screen for evidence of cryptococcal infection by a serum cryptococcal antigen or perform a lumbar puncture. The CSF frequently shows a lack of inflammatory response (ie, normal white blood cell [WBC] count), but the patient often presents with elevated intracranial pressures. Diagnosis can be confirmed by demonstrating the yeast by India ink stain, by fungal culture, or by measuring the level of cryptococcal antigen from CSF. Treatment of cryptococcal meningitis requires induction with intravenous amphotericin B plus flucytosine, then chronic suppression with oral fluconazole. At times, frequent lumbar punctures with removal of large volumes of CSF are required to treat the intracranial hypertension, and CSF shunts may be required.

At very low CD4 counts (<50 cells/mm^3), patients with AIDS are also susceptible to **CMV** infections. This can be manifested as viremia with persistent fever and constitutional symptoms, retinitis that can lead to blindness, esophagitis that can cause severe odynophagia, colitis, and necrotizing adrenalitis, which occasionally destroys sufficient adrenal tissue to produce clinical adrenal insufficiency. Therapy for severe CMV infections includes intravenous ganciclovir, valganciclovir, foscarnet, or cidofovir.

MAC is one of the most frequent opportunistic infections occurring in patients with very low CD4 counts. The most frequent presentations are disseminated infection with persistent fevers, weight loss, and constitutional symptoms, as well as gastrointestinal (GI) symptoms such as abdominal pain or chronic watery diarrhea. It often is diagnosed by obtaining a mycobacterial blood culture. Treatment with azithromycin or clarithromycin, plus ethambutol, and rifabutin is required for weeks until CD4 count improves in an attempt to clear the bacteremia.

Because of the frequency and severity of common opportunistic infections, **antimicrobial prophylaxis** is routinely given as a patient's immune status declines. With CD4 counts less than 200 cells/mm^3, PCP prophylaxis should be given as one double-strength tablet of TMP-SMX daily. When counts fall to less than 100 cells/mm^3 and patients have a positive *Toxoplasma* serology, toxoplasmosis can be prevented with daily dosing of TMP-SMX. If CD4 levels are less than 50 cells/mm^3, MAC prophylaxis consists of clarithromycin 500 mg twice daily or azithromycin 1200 mg weekly. Prophylaxis can be discontinued if HAART is started and the patient's CD4 levels recover (usually >100 cells/mm^3 for more than 3 months).

HAART includes a combination at least three drugs often consisting of two nucleoside reverse transcriptase inhibitors, along with either a nonnucleoside reverse transcriptase inhibitor or a protease inhibitor. HAART is very potent and has dramatically revolutionized the treatment of HIV patients, producing suppression of viral replication and allowing a patient's CD4 count to recover. Initiation of antiretroviral therapy is usually indicated in any of the following circumstances: (1) acute HIV infection, (2) asymptomatic infection with CD4 count <500, (3) pregnancy, (4) symptomatic patient regardless of CD4 count, (5) history of an AIDS-defining condition, (6) HIV patients with hepatitis B and/or hepatitis C coinfection, or (7) HIV-associated nephropathy (HIVAN).

However, initiation of HAART likely is not practical in acutely ill patients because the medications are not easy to take and often cause side effects that can be confused with the underlying disease process. Additionally, within 1 to 2 months of starting HAART, improvement in the immune system can actually cause worsening symptoms as a result of host responses, termed the **"immune reconstitution inflammatory syndrome" (IRIS)**. Therefore, it may be better to wait until the acute illness has resolved and to initiate antiretroviral therapy after the patient has recovered, in consultation with an infectious diseases expert, when reliable follow-up has been assured.

CASE CORRELATION

- See also Case 15 (Chronic Obstructive Pulmonary Disease), Case 16 (Chronic Cough/Asthma), Case 18 (Hemoptysis), Case 19 (Pneumonia), Case 44 (Tuberculosis), and Case 45 (Syphilis).

COMPREHENSION QUESTIONS

46.1 A 32-year-old woman with a 5-year history of HIV infection is noted to have a CD4 count of 100 cells/mm^3. She is admitted to the hospital with a 2-week history of fever, shortness of breath, and a dry cough. Which of the following diagnostic tests would most likely confirm the diagnosis?

    A. Silver stain or DFA of the sputum

    B. Gram stain of the sputum showing gram-positive diplococci

    C. Acid-fast smear of the sputum

    D. Serum cryptococcal antigen

46.2 Which of the following is the most likely organism to cause a lobar pneumonia in a patient with AIDS?

    A. *P jirovecii*

    B. *M tuberculosis*

    C. *Histoplasmosis capsulatum*

    D. *S pneumoniae*

46.3 A 44-year-old woman infected with HIV is noted to have a CD4 count of 180 cells/mm³. Which of the following is recommended as a useful prophylactic agent in this patient at this point?

A. Fluconazole

B. Azithromycin

C. Trimethoprim-sulfamethoxazole

D. Ganciclovir

46.4 A 36-year-old woman with HIV is admitted with new-onset seizures. The CT scan of the head reveals multiple ring-enhancing lesions of the brain. Which of the following is the best therapy for the likely condition?

A. Rifampin, isoniazid, ethambutol

B. Ganciclovir

C. Penicillin

D. Sulfadiazine with pyrimethamine

ANSWERS

46.1 **A.** The fever, dry cough, and dyspnea are consistent with PJP, which is diagnosed by silver stain or DFA of the sputum, sometimes bronchoalveolar lavage is necessary to obtain adequate samples. Sputum Gram stain is useful when there is suspicion for a lobar community acquired pneumonia most commonly caused by S. pneumoniae which is more likely to have an acute onset. Acid-fast smear of the sputum would help diagnose TB and patients in question stems will often have secondary symptoms such as weight loss and night sweats. Cryptococcus is more likely to present in the CNS (i.e. meningitis) in an immunosuppressed host and unlikely in this patient.

46.2 **D.** The same organisms that cause community-acquired pneumonia in immunocompetent individuals are causative in HIV patients. Additionally, HIV patients may be more susceptible to encapsulated organisms such as *S pneumoniae* and *Haemophilus influenzae*.

46.3 **C.** When the CD4 count falls to less than 200 cells/mm³, trimethoprim-sulfamethoxazole prophylaxis is generally initiated to prevent PJP. Prophylaxis against MAC usually is started when the CD4 count is less than 50 cells/mm³, and toxoplasmosis prophylaxis usually is started when the CD4 count is less than 100 cells/mm³. Prophylaxis for toxoplasmosis is TMP-SMX and for MAC is azithromycin or clarithromycin.

46.4 **D.** The most common cause of a mass lesion of the brain in an HIV patient is toxoplasmosis, which is treated with sulfadiazine with pyrimethamine. Rifampin, isoniazid, and ethambutol are appropriate treatment for TB. Ganciclovir is used to treat CMV retinitis that often presents when the CD4 count is <50. Penicillin is the appropriate treatment for syphilis. Neurosyphilis usually presents with signs of meningitis, cranial nerve palsies, or dementia.

CLINICAL PEARLS

▶ *Pneumocystis* pneumonia typically has a subacute presentation with fever and a dry cough, in HIV patients with a CD4 count less than 200 cells/mm³ who are not on PJP prophylaxis. Patients can present with a normal chest x-ray, a discrete bilateral interstitial lung opacities or diffuse severe alveolar lung opacities (ARDS type), and typically have an elevated serum lactic acid dehydrogenase level.

▶ Pulmonary tuberculosis should always be considered in AIDS patients with respiratory symptoms and suggestive history; its radiographic presentation may be atypical.

▶ The most common causes of bacterial pneumonia in AIDS patients are the same as those in immunocompetent patients, that is, community-acquired organisms such as *S pneumoniae.*

▶ In patients with CD4 counts less than 200 cells/mm³, trimethoprim-sulfamethoxazole prophylaxis is effective in preventing *Pneumocystis* pneumonia and in preventing toxoplasmosis when the CD4 count is less than 100 cells/mm³. When the CD4 is less than 50 cells/mm³, clarithromycin or azithromycin can prevent *M avium*–intracellulare complex.

▶ Highly active antiretroviral therapy is effective in reducing viral replication, increasing CD4 counts, and restoring immunocompetence but generally should not be initiated during an acute illness due to the risk of IRIS.

REFERENCES

Fauci AS, Lane HC. HIV disease: AIDS and related disorders. In: Longo DL, Fauci AS, Kasper DL, et al., eds. *Harrison's Principles of Internal Medicine.* 18th ed. New York, NY: McGraw-Hill; 2012:1506-1587.

Gray F, Chretien F, Vallat-Decouvelaere AV, et al. The changing pattern of HIV neuropathology in the HAART era. *J Neuropathol Exp Neurol.* 2003;62:429-440.

Smulian AG, Walzer PD. Pneumocystis infection. In: Longo DL, Fauci AS, Kasper DL, et al., eds. *Harrison's Principles of Internal Medicine.* 18th ed. New York, NY: McGraw-Hill; 2012:1671-1674.

Thomas CF, Limper AH. Pneumocystis pneumonia. *N Engl J Med.* 2004;350:2487-2498.

Wolff AJ, O'Donnell AE. Pulmonary manifestations of HIV infection in the era of highly active antiretroviral therapy. *Chest.* 2001;120:1888-1893.

A 65-year-old white woman is brought to the emergency department (ED) by her family for increasing confusion and lethargy over the past week. She was recently diagnosed with limited-stage small cell lung cancer, but has not begun cancer treatment. She has not been febrile or had any other recent illnesses. She is not taking any medications. Her blood pressure is 136/82 mm Hg, heart rate is 84 bpm, and respiratory rate is 14 bpm and unlabored. She is afebrile. On examination, she is an elderly appearing woman who is difficult to arouse and reacts only to painful stimuli. She is able to move her extremities without apparent motor deficits, and her deep tendon reflexes are decreased symmetrically. The remainder of her examination is normal, with a normal jugular venous pressure and no extremity edema. You order some laboratory tests, which reveal the serum sodium level is 108 mmol/L, potassium 3.8 mmol/L, bicarbonate 24 mEq/L, blood urea nitrogen (BUN) is 5 mg/dL, and creatinine is 0.5 mg/dL. Serum osmolality is 220 mOsm/kg, and urine osmolality is 400 mOsm/kg. A computed tomographic (CT) scan of the brain shows no masses or hydrocephalus.

▶ What is the most likely diagnosis?
▶ What is your next step in therapy?
▶ What are the complications of therapy?

ANSWERS TO CASE 47:

Hyponatremia, Syndrome of Inappropriate Secretion of Antidiuretic Hormone

Summary: A 65-year-old white woman with small cell lung cancer has increasing confusion and lethargy over the past week. She is afebrile and normotensive, and she has no edema or jugular venous distention. She is lethargic but is able to move her extremities without apparent motor deficits, and her deep tendon reflexes are decreased symmetrically. Her serum sodium level is 108 mmol/L, potassium is 3.8 mmol/L, bicarbonate is 24 mEq/L, BUN is 5 mg/dL, and creatinine is 0.5 mg/dL; serum osmolality is 220 mOsm/kg, and urine osmolality is 400 mOsm/kg. A CT scan of the brain shows no masses or hydrocephalus.

- **Most likely diagnosis:** Coma/lethargy secondary to severe hyponatremia, which is most likely caused by a paraneoplastic syndrome of inappropriate secretion of antidiuretic hormone (SIADH).

- **Next therapeutic step:** Treat the hyponatremia with hypertonic saline.

- **Most serious complication of this therapy:** Osmotic cerebral demyelination, also referred to as central pontine myelinolysis.

ANALYSIS

Objectives

1. Learn the causes of hyponatremia.

2. Understand the use of laboratory testing in the diagnosis of hyponatremia.

3. Know how to treat hyponatremia, and some of the potential complications of therapy.

Considerations

This elderly woman with small cell lung cancer presents in a stuporous state with hypotonic hyponatremia. She appears euvolemic, as she does not have findings suggestive of either volume overload (jugular venous distention or peripheral edema) or volume depletion. She has no focal neurologic deficits or apparent masses on CT scan of the brain suggesting cerebral metastases. The most likely cause for her altered mental status alteration is hyponatremia. The patient does not take medications; thus, with the situation of hypotonic hyponatremia in a euvolemic state and with inappropriately concentrated urine, the most likely etiology is inappropriate antidiuretic hormone produced by the lung cancer. Therapy is guided by the severity of the hyponatremia and the symptoms. Because this individual is stuporous and the sodium level is severely decreased, hypertonic saline is required with fairly rapid partial correction. This therapy is not benign and requires monitoring in intensive care unit (ICU). Also, the target is not correction of the sodium level to normal (135 mmol/L) but rather to a level of safety, such as 120 to 125 mmol/L.

APPROACH TO:
Hyponatremia

DEFINITIONS

ANTIDIURETIC HORMONE (ADH): Also referred to as arginine vasopressin (AVP), ADH is the posterior pituitary hormone that controls excretion of free water and thus, indirectly, sodium concentration and serum tonicity.

OSMOLALITY: Concentration of osmotically active particles, which draw water into a compartment; normal range is 280 to 300 mOsm/kg.

SYNDROME OF INAPPROPRIATE SECRETION OF ANTIDIURETIC HORMONE: Nonphysiologic elevation of ADH levels as a consequence of ectopic production, as in malignancy, or stimulation of excess pituitary production by various pulmonary or central nervous system (CNS) diseases.

CLINICAL APPROACH

Hyponatremia is defined as a serum sodium level <135 mmol/L and is, by far, the **most common electrolyte disturbance among hospitalized patients.** Patients are often asymptomatic, especially if the hyponatremia develops slowly. Depending on the rapidity with which the hyponatremia develops, most patients do not have symptoms until the serum sodium level is in the low 120 mmol/L range. The clinical manifestations are related to osmotic water shifts leading to cerebral edema; thus, the symptoms are mainly neurologic. Early symptoms include headache, nausea, and vomiting; later symptoms may progress to lethargy, confusion, seizures, or coma.

Serum sodium concentrations are important because they almost always reflect tonicity, the effect of extracellular fluid on cells that will cause the cells (eg, brain cells) to swell (hypotonicity) or to shrink (hypertonicity). For purposes of this discussion, we use serum osmolality as an indicator of tonicity.

Hypotonic hyponatremia *always* occurs because there is water gain, that is, impairment of free water excretion. If one considers that the normal kidney capacity to excrete free water is approximately 18 to 20 L/d, it becomes apparent that it is very difficult to overwhelm this capacity solely through excessive water intake, as in psychogenic polydipsia. Therefore, when hyponatremia develops, the kidney is usually holding on to free water, either pathologically, as in SIADH, or physiologically, as an attempt to maintain effective circulating volume when patients are significantly volume depleted. Hyponatremia can also occur in cases of sodium loss, for example, as a consequence of diuretic use, or because of aldosterone deficiency. However, in those cases, there is then a secondary gain of free water.

To determine the cause of the hypotonic hyponatremia, the physician must clinically **assess the volume status** of the patient by history and physical examination. A useful algorithm for assessment of patients with hyponatremia is seen in Figure 47–1.

A history of vomiting, diarrhea, or other losses, such as profuse sweating, suggests **hypovolemia**, as do flat neck veins, dry oral mucous membranes, and diminished urine output. In cases of significant hypovolemia, there is a physiologic increase in

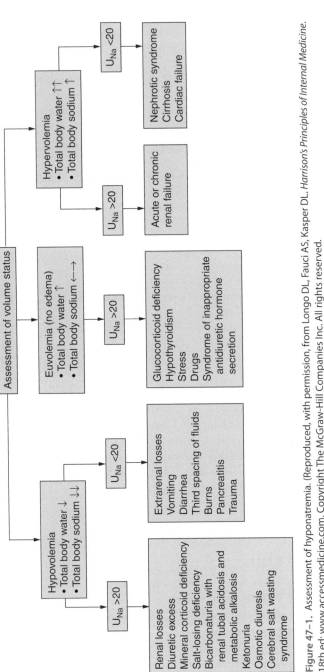

Figure 47–1. Assessment of hyponatremia. (Reproduced, with permission, from Longo DL, Fauci AS, Kasper DL. *Harrison's Principles of Internal Medicine.* 18th ed: www.accessmedicine.com. Copyright The McGraw-Hill Companies Inc. All rights reserved.

ADH in an attempt to retain free water to maintain circulating volume, even at the expense of hypotonicity. In these cases, the excess ADH is not "inappropriate" as in SIADH, but extremely appropriate. At this point, one can **check the urinary sodium levels**. In hypovolemia, the kidney should be avidly retaining sodium, so the urine sodium level should be less than 20 mmol/L. If the patient is hypovolemic, yet the urine sodium level is more than 20 mmol/L, then kidneys do not have the ability to retain sodium normally. Either kidney function is impaired by the use of diuretics, or the kidney is lacking necessary hormonal stimulation, as in adrenal insufficiency, or there is a primary renal problem, such as tubular damage from acute tubular necrosis. When patients are **hypovolemic**, treatment of the hyponatremia requires **correction of the volume status, usually replacement with isotonic (0.9%) saline.**

Hypervolemia is usually apparent as edema or elevated jugular venous pressure. It commonly occurs as a result **of congestive heart failure, cirrhosis of the liver, or the nephrotic syndrome.** In these edematous disorders, there is usually a total body excess of both sodium and water, yet arterial baroreceptors perceive hypoperfusion or a decrease in intravascular volume, which leads to an increase in the level of ADH and, therefore, retention of free water by the kidneys. Renal failure itself can lead to hypotonic hyponatremia because of an inability to excrete dilute urine. In any of these cases, the usual initial treatment of hyponatremia is administration of diuretics to reduce excess salt and water.

Thus, hypovolemic or hypervolemic hyponatremia is often apparent clinically and often does not present a diagnostic challenge. **Euvolemic hyponatremia**, however, is a frequent problem that is not so easily diagnosed. Once the clinician has diagnosed the patient with euvolemic hypotonic hyponatremia, the next step is to measure the urine osmolarity. This measurement is taken to determine whether the kidney is actually capable of excreting the free water normally (urine osmolality should be maximally dilute, <100 mOsm/kg) or whether the free water excretion is impaired (urine not maximally concentrated, >150-200 mOsm/kg). If the urine is maximally dilute, it is handling free water normally but its capacity for excretion has been overwhelmed, as in central polydipsia. More commonly, free water excretion is impaired and the urine is not maximally dilute as it should be. Two important diagnoses must be considered at this point: **hypothyroidism** and **adrenal insufficiency. Thyroid hormone and cortisol both are permissive for free water excretion, so their deficiency causes water retention.** Cortisol deficiency in secondary adrenal insufficiency can mimic SIADH. In contrast, patients with primary adrenal insufficiency (Addison disease) also lack aldosterone, so they have impaired ability to retain sodium, and often appear hypovolemic and may even present in shock.

Euvolemic hyponatremia is most commonly caused by **SIADH.** Nonphysiologic nonosmotically mediated (therefore "inappropriate") secretion can occur in the setting of pulmonary disease, CNS disease, pain, in the postoperative period, or as part of a paraneoplastic syndrome. Because of retention of free water, patients actually have mild (although clinically inapparent) volume expansion. Additionally, if they have a normal dietary sodium intake, the kidneys do not retain sodium avidly. Therefore, modest natriuresis occurs so that the urine sodium level is elevated >20 mmol/L. **SIADH is a diagnosis of exclusion**: the patient must be hypoosmolar but euvolemic, with urine that is not maximally dilute (osmolality >150-200 mOsm/L), urine sodium more than 20 mmol/L, and normal adrenal and thyroid function. Some laboratory clues to SIADH are low BUN and low uric acid levels. Unless the patient has severe neurologic symptoms, the **usual initial treatment of SIADH is free water restriction.** Patients with **severe neurologic symptoms,** such as seizures or coma, require **rapid** partial correction of the sodium level. The treatment of choice is hypertonic (eg, 3%) saline. When there is concern that the saline infusion might cause volume overload, the infusion can be administered with a loop diuretic such as furosemide. The diuretic will cause the excretion of hypotonic urine that is essentially "half-normal saline," so a greater portion of sodium than water will be retained, helping to correct the serum sodium level.

When hyponatremia occurs for any reason, especially when it occurs slowly, the brain adapts to prevent cerebral edema. Solutes leave the intracellular compartment of the brain over hours to days, so patients may have few neurologic symptoms despite very low serum sodium levels. If the serum sodium level is corrected rapidly, the brain does not have time to readjust, and it may shrink rapidly as it loses fluid to the extracellular space. It is believed that this rapid shrinkage may trigger demyelination of the cerebellar and pontine neurons. This **osmotic cerebral demyelination,** or **central pontine myelinolysis,** may cause **quadriplegia, pseudobulbar palsies, a "locked-in" syndrome, coma, or death.** Demyelination can occur even when fluid restriction is the treatment used to correct the serum sodium level. For any patient with hyponatremia, the general rule is that chronic hyponatremia should be corrected slowly, and acutely developing hyponatremia can be corrected more quickly. In chronic hyponatremia, the serum sodium concentration should correct no faster than 0.5 to 1 mEq/h.

For patients with chronic hypervolemic hyponatremia, as in heart failure or cirrhosis, vasopressin antagonists (tolvaptan and conivaptan are approved for use in the United States) are now available and are very effective in increasing free water excretion and raising serum sodium concentrations. Therapy with these agents is typically initiated in the hospital with close monitoring of sodium concentration.

> ## CASE CORRELATION
> - See also Case 18 (Hemoptysis/Lung Cancer), Case 37 (Dementia), Case 49 (Adrenal Insufficiency), and Case 50 (Hypercalcemia).

COMPREHENSION QUESTIONS

47.1 A 24-year-old man develops seizures following an emergent splenectomy after a car accident. His serum sodium level is initially 116 mEq/L and is corrected to 120 mEq/L over the next 3 hours with hypertonic saline. Which of the following factors most likely led to his hyponatremia?

A. Elevation of serum vasopressin

B. Administration of hypertonic solutions

C. Volume depletion

D. Seizure-induced hyponatremia

47.2 A 56-year-old man presents to the doctor for the first time complaining of fatigue and weight loss. He has never had any health problems, but he has smoked a pack of cigarettes per day for about 35 years. He is a day laborer and is currently homeless and living in a shelter. His physical examination is notable for a low to normal blood pressure, skin hyperpigmentation, and digital clubbing. He appears euvolemic. You tell him you are not sure of the problem as yet, but you will draw some blood tests and schedule him for follow-up in a week. The laboratory calls that night and informs you that the patient's sodium level is 126 mEq/L, potassium level is 6.7 mEq/L, creatinine level is normal, and bicarbonate and chloride levels are low. Which of the following is the likely cause of his hyponatremia given his presentation?

A. SIADH

B. Hypothyroidism

C. Gastrointestinal losses

D. Adrenal insufficiency

E. Renal insufficiency

47.3 An 83-year-old woman comes to your clinic complaining of a headache and mild confusion. Her medical history is remarkable only for hypertension, which is well controlled with hydrochlorothiazide. Her examination and laboratory tests show no signs of infection, but her serum sodium level is 119 mEq/L, and plasma osmolarity is 245 mOsm/kg. She appears to be clinically hypovolemic. Which of the following is the best initial therapy?

A. Fluid restriction

B. Infusion of 0.9% saline

C. Infusion of 3% saline

D. Infusion of 3% saline with furosemide

47.4 A 58-year-old man has undergone a lengthy colon cancer surgery. On the first postoperative day, he is noted to have significant hyponatremia with a sodium level of 128 mEq/L. You suspect that the hyponatremia is due to the intravenous infusion of hypotonic solution. Which of the following laboratory findings supports your diagnosis?

A. Urine sodium >20 mmol/L

B. Urine osmolality >200 mOsm/L

C. Serum osmolarity <280 mOsm/kg

D. Serum potassium >5 mEq/L

ANSWERS

47.1 **A.** In the postoperative state or in situations where the patient is in pain, the serum vasopressin level may rise, leading to inappropriate retention of free water, which leads to dilution of the serum. Concomitant administration of hypotonic fluids may exacerbate the situation.

47.2 **D.** Hyponatremia in the setting of hyperkalemia and acidosis (low bicarbonate level) is suspicious for adrenal insufficiency. This patient's examination is also suggestive of the diagnosis, given his complaints of fatigue, weight loss, low blood pressure, and hyperpigmentation. The diagnosis is made by an early morning cortisol test or by measuring the response to adrenocorticotropic hormone (ACTH) stimulation, showing low cortisol levels. In this case, the cause of the adrenal gland destruction is probably either tuberculosis or lung cancer.

47.3 **B.** Because the patient is hypovolemic, probably as a result of the use of diuretics, volume replacement with isotonic saline is the best initial therapy. Hyponatremia caused by thiazide diuretics can occur by several mechanisms, including volume depletion. It is most common in elderly women.

47.4 **C.** In a patient with hyponatremia due to the infusion of excessive hypotonic solution, the serum osmolarity should be low. The kidneys in responding normally should attempt to retain sodium and excrete water; hence, the urine sodium concentration should be low, and the urine osmolality should be low. When the infusion of hypotonic solution is used, the serum potassium level will also be low. This is in contrast to a situation of mineralocorticoid deficiency in which the sodium level will be decreased and potassium level may be elevated. Similarly, hyperaldosteronism can lead to hypertension and hypokalemia (Conn syndrome).

CLINICAL PEARLS

▶ Hyponatremia almost always occurs by impairment of free water excretion.

▶ SIADH is a diagnosis of exclusion. Criteria include a euvolemic patient, urine that is not maximally dilute (osmolality >150-200 mmol/L), urine sodium >20 mmol/L, and normal adrenal and thyroid function.

▶ Hypovolemic patients with hyponatremia should be treated with volume replacement, typically with isotonic (0.9%) saline.

▶ Euvolemic patients with asymptomatic hyponatremia can be treated with fluid restriction. Patients with severe symptoms, such as coma or seizures, can be treated with hypertonic (3%) saline.

▶ The rate of sodium correction generally should not exceed 0.5-1 mEq/h; otherwise central pontine myelinolysis (osmotic demyelination) can occur.

REFERENCES

Androgue H, Madias N. Hyponatremia. *N Engl J Med*. 2000;342:1581-1589.

Lin M, Liu SJ, Lim IT. Disorders of water imbalance. *Emerg Med Clin North Am*. 2005;23:749-770.

Mount DB. Fluid and electrolyte disturbances. In: Kasper DL, Fauci AS, Hauser SL, et al., eds. *Harrison's Principles of Internal Medicine*. 19th ed. New York, NY: McGraw-Hill Education; 2015: 295-312.

A 38-year-old woman presents to your clinic for evaluation of menstrual irregularity. She states that her periods started when she was 12 years old, and they have been fairly regular ever since, coming once every 28 to 30 days. She has had three previous uncomplicated pregnancies and deliveries. However, approximately 9 months ago, her cycles seemed to lengthen, and for the last 3 months she has not had a period at all. She stopped breast-feeding 3 years ago, but over the last 3 months she noticed that she could express a small amount of milky fluid from her breasts. She had a bilateral tubal ligation after her last pregnancy, and she has no other medical or surgical history. She takes no medications except multivitamins. Over the last year or so, she thinks she has gained about 10 lb, and she feels as if she has no energy despite adequate sleep. She has noticed some mild thinning of her hair and slightly more coarse skin texture. She denies headaches or visual changes. Her physical examination, including pelvic and breast examinations, are normal. She is not obese or hirsute. Slight whitish nipple discharge is elicited from her breasts. Her pregnancy test is negative.

► What is the most likely diagnosis?
► What is the most likely etiology for the condition?

ANSWERS TO CASE 48:

Oligomenorrhea Caused by Hypothyroidism and Hyperprolactinemia

Summary: A 38-year-old woman complains of oligomenorrhea and now secondary amenorrhea, along with galactorrhea. She has experienced weight gain, fatigue, mild thinning of her hair, and slightly more coarse skin. She denies headaches or visual changes, which might suggest a pituitary adenoma. Her physical examination, including pelvic and breast examinations, are normal. She is not obese or hirsute. You can elicit slight whitish nipple discharge.

- **Most likely diagnosis:** Oligomenorrhea and galactorrhea due to hypothyroidism.

- **Most likely etiology:** Primary hypothyroidism is the most likely diagnosis, most often due to autoimmune (Hashimoto) thyroiditis.

ANALYSIS

Objectives

1. Understand the differential diagnosis of secondary amenorrhea and the approach to the investigation of possible hormonal causes.

2. Understand the interactions of the hormones involved in the hypothalamic-pituitary-gonadal axis.

3. Recognize the clinical features and diagnostic evaluation of hypothyroidism.

4. Be familiar with the treatment of hypothyroidism.

Considerations

This 38-year-old woman presents with secondary amenorrhea, weight gain, fatigue, and galactorrhea despite having previously normal menses and discontinuing breast-feeding 3 years ago. Her history of fatigue, weight gain, and hair loss suggest a systemic cause of her symptoms, possibly hypothyroidism. However, her normal physical examination with lack of myxedema or bradycardia, normal reflexes, normal cognition, and nondisplaced point of maximal impulse suggest mild hypothyroidism. Lack of virilization or obesity does not exclude polycystic ovarian syndrome (PCOS), but their absence makes this diagnosis less likely. Hypothyroidism alone could attribute to galactorrhea, because hypothyroidism can be associated with hyperprolactinemia. Prolactinomas can also cause galactorrhea as well as secondary amenorrhea, however, and should be excluded.

APPROACH TO:
Oligomenorrhea

DEFINITIONS

AMENORRHEA: *Primary*—Absence of menarche by the age of 16 regardless of the presence or absence of secondary sex characteristics. *Secondary*—Absence of menstruation for 3 or more months in women with normal past menses.

GALACTORRHEA: Any discharge of milk-containing fluid from the breast, may be unilateral or bilateral, and may appear clear, milky, or bloody.

OLIGOMENORRHEA: Menses occurring at infrequent intervals of more than 40 days or fewer than nine menses per year.

POLYCYSTIC OVARIAN SYNDROME: Syndrome characterized by infertility, hirsutism, obesity, and amenorrhea or oligomenorrhea, and often clinically significant insulin resistance.

CLINICAL APPROACH

The assessment of oligomenorrhea is similar to the workup for secondary amenorrhea with the understanding that secondary amenorrhea is present when a normally menstruating woman stops having periods for 3 consecutive months or more. **The most common cause of both symptoms, and the easiest to exclude in the clinic, is pregnancy.** A negative in-clinic pregnancy test should be confirmed with a serum beta–human chorionic gonadotropin (hCG). Primary amenorrhea is present when the first menses has not appeared in a girl by the age of 16 and is generally caused by a variety of genetic or congenital defects and is commonly associated with disorders of puberty. Given this patient's age and history, primary amenorrhea is not a consideration; thus, a diagnostic pathway for secondary amenorrhea/oligomenorrhea should be undertaken.

Problems of the Hypothalamic-Pituitary-Ovarian Axis

Excluding pregnancy and problems in the genital outflow tract, disorders of the hypothalamic-pituitary-ovarian axis account for the largest number of cases of oligomenorrhea and amenorrhea. Disorders of the hypothalamus account for the largest percentage of abnormality (>45%); these include problems of nutrition (rapid weight loss/anorexia), excessive exercise, stress, and infiltrative diseases (eg, craniopharyngioma, sarcoidosis, histiocytosis).

The largest single cause of oligomenorrhea is PCOS, accounting for 30% of all cases. PCOS was once thought to be a disease originating in the ovary; however, it now is known that **PCOS is a much more complicated neuroendocrine disorder** with evidence of **estrogenization**, as well as **insulin resistance**. The diagnosis is a clinical one (anovulation, hyperandrogenism, and small follicles on the ovary on ultrasound) after ruling out other causes. These women often have glucose intolerance and may develop metabolic syndrome. They are at risk for cardiovascular disease and endometrial cancer.

Table 48–1 • DIFFERENTIAL DIAGNOSIS OF OLIGOMENORRHEA[a]

	History	Laboratory	Therapy
Polycystic ovarian syndrome	Irregular menses since menarche, obesity, hirsutism	Slightly elevated testosterone, elevated LH/FSH	Oral contraceptive agent
Hypothyroidism	Fatigue, cold intolerance	Elevated TSH	Thyroxine replacement
Hyperprolactinemia	Headache, bitemporal hemianopsia, galactorrhea, medications, hypothyroidism	Elevated prolactin level	Depends on etiology
Ovarian failure	Hot flushes, hypoestrogenemia	Elevated FSH and LH	Replacement of hormones
Sheehan syndrome	Postpartum hemorrhage, unable to breast-feed	Low pituitary hormones (FSH, TSH, ACTH)	Replacement of pituitary hormones

Abbreviations: ACTH, adrenocorticotropic hormone; FSH, follicle-stimulating hormone; LH, luteinizing hormone; TSH, thyroid-stimulating hormone.
[a]Pregnancy must always be suspected with oligomenorrhea or amenorrhea.

Other important causes of amenorrhea include diseases of the pituitary, specifically neoplasms (eg, prolactinomas, functioning or nonfunctioning adenomas), which account for 18% of cases. Empty sella syndrome, caused by cerebrospinal fluid (CSF) herniation into the pituitary fossa, and Sheehan syndrome, caused by severe obstetric hemorrhage and/or maternal hypotension at delivery, are important causes of atrophy and ischemia of the pituitary. If suspected, they should be investigated by magnetic resonance imaging (MRI). Finally, disorders such as premature ovarian failure (loss of all functional ovarian follicles before the age of 40), diseases of the thyroid, and adult-onset adrenal hyperplasia should be considered and investigated if supported by history and physical examination with the appropriate laboratory studies (Table 48–1).

The history and physical examination will narrow the range of possible causes. In this patient, the history of fatigue, weight gain, and galactorrhea, along with previously normal menses and a normal physical examination, place **hypothyroidism** at the top of the list. In primary hypothyroidism, the hypothalamus increases thyrotropin-releasing hormone (TRH), which also stimulates prolactin secretion. Measurement of both thyroid hormone and prolactin levels would be indicated in this case. **Prolactinomas** are the most common functional pituitary tumors in both men and women, and should be suspected if the prolactin level is markedly elevated, >200 μg/L. If prolactin levels are markedly elevated, pituitary imaging with MRI is indicated. Hyperprolactinemia from any cause inhibits hypothalamic gonadotropin-releasing hormone (GnRH) secretion, leading to amenorrhea in women, and infertility and diminished libido in men. In the workup of secondary amenorrhea, these two diagnoses are the easiest to start with because the tests are noninvasive and relatively inexpensive.

Hypothyroidism

Hypothyroidism is defined as the insufficient production of thyroid hormone. Secondary hypothyroidism as a result of dysfunction of hypothalamic and pituitary hormone secretion is much less common but should be suspected in a patient with a history suggestive of Sheehan syndrome or with symptoms or signs of a tumor in the region of the sella. **Ninety-five percent of cases of hypothyroidism** are caused by **primary thyroid gland failure**, resulting in insufficient thyroid hormone production. In the United States, **the most common cause of hypothyroidism is autoimmune (Hashimoto) thyroiditis**, in which cytotoxic antibodies are produced, which leads to thyroid atrophy and fibrosis. The next most common cause is surgical or radioactive iodine treatment for hyperthyroidism, or Graves disease. **Worldwide, iodine deficiency** is the **most common cause of goitrous (enlarged thyroid) hypothyroidism**, but in the United States, this is rare.

Most hypothyroid patients present with vague and nonspecific symptoms. **Elderly** individuals may be suspected of having **dementia or depression** when the cause is really hypothyroidism. In general, symptoms of fatigue, weight gain, muscle cramping, cold intolerance, hair thinning, menstrual changes, or carpal tunnel syndrome are common and should prompt an investigation of thyroid function. In severe, prolonged hypothyroidism, a syndrome termed **myxedema** may develop. These patients present with dull facies, swollen eyes, and doughy extremities from the accumulation of hydrophilic polysaccharides in the dermis, sparse hair, and a thickened tongue. They may have an enlarged heart, nonmechanical intestinal obstruction (ileus), and a delayed relaxation phase of their deep tendon reflexes. Without treatment, they may become stuporous and hypothermic, especially if challenged with an intercurrent illness. This is a life-threatening emergency with a high mortality, even when managed aggressively with intravenous levothyroxine.

When testing outpatients for hypothyroidism, measurement of the **serum thyroid-stimulating hormone (TSH)** level is the most sensitive and useful test. Because almost all cases of hypothyroidism are caused by thyroid gland failure, the normal pituitary response is to markedly increase the TSH levels in an attempt to stimulate the failing gland. Falling levels of thyroid hormone produce logarithmic increases in the TSH concentration. **Measurement of TSH alone would be insufficient in suspected cases of pituitary disease**, so measurement of the thyroid hormone level can also be performed. One should remember that almost all thyroxine (T_4) circulates bound to protein, but it is the free or unbound fraction that is able to diffuse into cells and become active. Most laboratories can now measure **free T_4** directly, or it can be estimated by using the **free thyroxine index (FTI)**. The FTI is calculated from measurements of total T_4 and the T_3 resin uptake test. When there is excess thyroid-binding globulin (TBG), as in pregnancy or oral contraceptive use, T_4 levels will be high (as a consequence of the large amount of carrier protein), but T_3 uptake will be low (value varies inversely with amount of TBG present). Conversely, when there is a low level of TBG, as in a hypoproteinemic patient with nephrotic syndrome, the T_4 level will necessarily also be low (not much carrier protein), but the T_3 uptake will be high. If both total T_4 and T_3 uptake are low, the FTI is low, and the patient is hypothyroid.

In mild cases, or **subclinical hypothyroidism**, the TSH level is mildly elevated (4-10 mU/L), but the free T_4 or FTI is within the normal range. Patients may be asymptomatic or report the vague and subtle symptoms of hypothyroidism, such as fatigue. About half of such patients will progress to overt hypothyroidism within 5 years. They often have some **derangement of cholesterol metabolism, such as elevated total and low-density lipoprotein (LDL) cholesterol.** Thyroid hormone replacement can be prescribed in an attempt to relieve symptoms or possibly to reduce cardiovascular risk, or if positive antithyroid antibodies are present.

In clinical hypothyroidism, the TSH level is markedly elevated, and the free T_4 or FTI is low. The overwhelming majority of patients with hypothyroidism can be treated with once-daily dosing of synthetic levothyroxine, which is biochemically identical to the natural hormone. **Levothyroxine is relatively inexpensive, has a long half-life (6-7 days), allowing once-daily** dosing, and gives a predictable response. Older thyroid preparations, such as desiccated thyroid extract, are available but are not favored because they have a high content of T_3, which is rapidly absorbed and can produce tachyarrhythmias, and the T_4 content is less predictable.

If there is no residual thyroid function, the daily replacement dose of levothyroxine is 1.6 μg/kg, or typically 100 to 150 μg. In **older patients and in those with known cardiovascular disease, dosing should start at a lower level,** such as 25 to 50 μg/d, and be increased at similar increments once every 4 to 6 weeks until the patient achieves a euthyroid state. Overly rapid replacement with the sudden increase in metabolic rate can overwhelm the coronary or cardiac reserve. The goal of treatment is normalized TSH, ideally in the lower half of the reference range. The **TSH level will take 6 to 8 weeks to readjust to a new dosing level,** so follow-up laboratory testing should be scheduled accordingly. Patients may not experience full relief of symptoms until 3 to 6 months after normal TSH is achieved.

CASE CORRELATION

- See also Case 49 (Adrenal Insufficiency), Case 50 (Hypercalcemia), Case 51 (Diabetes), and Case 53 (Hyperthyroidism).

COMPREHENSION QUESTIONS

48.1 A 42-year-old woman presents to your clinic for her annual physical examination. On examination, you note neck fullness. When you palpate her thyroid, it is enlarged, smooth, rubbery, and nontender. The patient is asymptomatic. You send her for thyroid function testing: her T_4, free T_4, and T_3 are normal, but her TSH is slightly elevated. Which of the following is the most likely diagnosis?

   A. Iodine deficiency

   B. Thyroid cancer

   C. Hashimoto thyroiditis

   D. Graves disease

   E. Multinodular goiter

48.2 Which of the following laboratory tests could be performed to confirm your diagnosis of the patient in Question 48.1?

A.   Repeat thyroid function tests

B.   Thyroid ultrasound

C.   Nuclear thyroid scan

D.   Anti-thyroperoxidase (TPO) antibody tests

E.   Complete blood count with differential

48.3 A 19-year-old gymnast active in national competition is brought to your clinic by her mother because the daughter's menses have ceased for the last 3 months. Prior to this, she was always regular. She denies excess dieting, although she does work out with her team 3 hours daily. Her physical examination is normal except for her body mass index (BMI) of 20 kg/m². Which of the following laboratory tests should be ordered first?

A.   Thyroid function tests

B.   Complete blood count

C.   Luteinizing hormone (LH)/follicle-stimulating hormone (FSH)

D.   Prolactin

E.   Beta-hCG

48.4 A 35-year-old woman who was diagnosed with hypothyroidism 4 weeks ago presents to your clinic complaining of persistent feelings of fatigue and sluggishness. After confirming your diagnosis with a measurement of the TSH, you started her on levothyroxine 50 μg daily. She has been reading about her diagnosis on the Internet and wants to try desiccated thyroid extract instead of the medicine you gave her. On examination, she weighs 175 lb, her heart rate is 64 bpm at rest, and her blood pressure is normal. Which of the following is the best next step?

A.   Tell her that this delay in resolution of symptoms is normal and schedule a follow-up visit with her in 2 months.

B.   Change her medication, as requested, to thyroid extract and titrate.

C.   Increase her dose of levothyroxine and have her come back in 4 weeks.

D.   Tell her to start a multivitamin with iron to take with her levothyroxine.

ANSWERS

48.1 **C.** Hashimoto thyroiditis is the most common cause of hypothyroidism with goiter in the United States. It is most commonly found in middle-aged women, although it can be seen in all age groups. Iodine deficiency is exceedingly uncommon in the United States because of iodized salt. Graves disease is a hyperthyroid condition. Patients with multinodular goiter usually are euthyroid. Patients with thyroid cancer usually are euthyroid.

48.2 **D.** Hashimoto thyroiditis is an autoimmune disease of the thyroid. Several different autoantibodies directed toward components of the thyroid gland will be present in the patient's serum; however, of these, anti- TPO antibody almost always is detectable. These antibodies are the markers, not the cause, of gland destruction. On thyroid biopsy, lymphocytic infiltration and fibrosis of the gland are pathognomonic. The presence of these autoantibodies predicts progressive gland failure and the need for hormone replacement. None of the other tests will be helpful.

48.3 **E.** In a young woman with oligomenorrhea, pregnancy should always be the first diagnosis considered. Urine pregnancy tests are easily performed in the clinic and are highly sensitive. Serum beta-hCG can be measured to confirm a negative test. In this patient, the next most likely diagnosis is hypothalamic hypogonadism, secondary to her strenuous exercise regimen. These young women are at risk for osteoporosis and should be counseled on adequate nutrition and offered combined oral contraceptives if the amenorrhea persists.

48.4 **C.** Levothyroxine is the preferred replacement hormone for hypothyroidism. The amount of hormone batch to batch and the patient dose response are believed to be more predictable than with other forms of hormone replacement, such as thyroid extract, which is made from desiccated beef or pork thyroid glands. There is no evidence that the natural hormone replacement is superior to the synthetic form. The dose of levothyroxine should be titrated to relief of symptoms, as well as to normalization of the TSH. Other medications, especially iron-containing vitamins, should be taken at different times than levothyroxine because they may interfere with absorption.

CLINICAL PEARLS

▶ The most common causes of oligomenorrhea are disorders of the hypo-thalamic-pituitary-gonadal axis, such as polycystic ovarian syndrome and hypothyroidism.

▶ Hypothyroidism may cause hyperprolactinemia. Hyperprolactinemia from any cause induces hypothalamic dysfunction, leading to menstrual irregularities in women, and diminished libido and infertility in men.

▶ The most common cause of hypothyroidism is primary thyroid gland failure as a result of Hashimoto thyroiditis.

▶ A low free T_4 or free thyroxine index and a high thyroid-stimulating hormone characterize primary hypothyroidism.

▶ Synthetic levothyroxine (T_4) replacement is the treatment of choice for hypothyroidism; in older patients, you need to "start low and go slow."

▶ The goal of therapy is to normalize the thyroid-stimulating hormone level in primary hypothyroidism and to relieve symptoms.

REFERENCES

Cooper DS. Subclinical hypothyroidism. *N Engl J Med.* 2001;345:260-265.

Jameson JL, Weetman AP. Disorders of the thyroid gland. In: Kasper DL, Fauci AS, Hauser SL, et al., eds. *Harrison's Principles of Internal Medicine.* 19th ed. New York, NY: McGraw-Hill Education; 2015:2283-2308.

Jonklaas J, Bianco AC, Bauer AJ, et al. Guidelines for the treatment of hypothyroidism: prepared by the American Thyroid Association task force on thyroid hormone replacement. *Thyroid.* 2014;24(12):1670-1751.

Melmed S, Jameson JL. Anterior pituitary tumor syndromes. In: Kasper DL, Fauci AS, Hauser SL, et al., eds. *Harrison's Principles of Internal Medicine.* 19th ed. New York, NY: McGraw-Hill Education; 2015:2261-2274.

A 58-year-old woman comes to the office after she experienced a near-fainting spell 1 day ago. She was outside playing tennis when she vomited and felt light-headed. She spent the rest of the day lying down with mild, diffuse, abdominal pain and nausea. She had no fever or diarrhea. She reports several months of worsening fatigue, mild, intermittent, generalized abdominal pain, and loss of appetite with a 10- to 15-lb unintentional weight loss. Her medical history is significant for hypothyroidism for which she takes levothyroxine. She takes no other medications. On examination, her temperature is 99.8°F, heart rate is 102 bpm, blood pressure is 89/62 mm Hg, and normal respiratory rate. She does become light-headed, and her heart rate rises to 125 bpm upon standing with a drop in systolic blood pressure to 70 mm Hg. She is alert and well tanned, with hyperpigmented creases in her hands. Her chest is clear, and her heart rhythm is tachycardic but regular. On abdominal examination, she has normal bowel sounds and mild diffuse tenderness without guarding. Her pulses are rapid and thready. She has no peripheral edema. Initial laboratory studies are significant for Na 121 mEq/L, K 5.8 mEq/L, HCO_3 16 mEq/L, glucose 52 mg/dL, and creatinine 1.0 mg/dL.

▶ What is the most likely diagnosis?
▶ What is your next step?

ANSWERS TO CASE 49:

Adrenal Insufficiency

Summary: A 58-year-old woman presents with orthostatic hypotension, intermittent chronic abdominal pain, and constitutional symptoms such as fatigue and unintentional weight loss. She also has hyponatremia, hyperkalemia, acidosis, and hypoglycemia. All of this patient's clinical features are consistent with acute adrenal insufficiency. The most common cause of adrenal insufficiency is idiopathic autoimmune destruction.

- **Most likely diagnosis:** Primary adrenal insufficiency.

- **Next step:** After drawing a cortisol level, immediate administration of intravenous saline with glucose and stress doses of corticosteroids.

ANALYSIS

Objectives

1. Know the presentation of primary and secondary adrenal insufficiency and of adrenal crisis.

2. Know the most common causes of primary and secondary adrenal insufficiency.

3. Know the treatment of adrenal insufficiency.

Considerations

This patient has a low-grade fever, which may be a feature of adrenal insufficiency, or it may signify infection, which can precipitate an adrenal crisis or produce a similar clinical picture. It is important to diagnose and treat any underlying infection. Because of the adrenal insufficiency and the aldosterone deficiency, she has volume depletion, hypoglycemia, and hypotension. Thus, immediate intravenous replacement with normal saline with 5% glucose is critical. A low serum cortisol level with the patient's clinical presentation and without other explanation confirms the diagnosis of adrenal insufficiency.

APPROACH TO:

Suspected Adrenal Insufficiency

DEFINITIONS

ADDISON DISEASE: Long-term insufficient function of the adrenal cortex leading to underproduction of corticosteroids.

ACTH STIMULATION TEST: An examination to evaluate the cortisol level after an intravascular (IV) injection of adrenocorticotropic hormone (ACTH). A normal individual should have an increase in cortisol, whereas a patient with adrenal insufficiency will have no response or a limited one.

CLINICAL APPROACH

Etiology

Primary adrenal insufficiency (**Addison disease**) refers to adrenal failure or destruction or infiltration of the adrenal glands. The **most common cause in the United States is autoimmune destruction** of the **adrenal glands**. The most common cause worldwide is tuberculous adrenalitis. Other causes include chronic granulomatous infections (histoplasmosis, coccidiomycosis), bilateral adrenal hemorrhage (usually in the setting of sepsis with disseminated intravascular coagulation [DIC]), adrenal metastases (commonly from lung, breast, or stomach cancers), or X-linked adrenoleukodystrophy, a genetic disorder with adrenal and neurologic manifestations. Patients with acquired immunodeficiency syndrome (AIDS) often develop adrenal involvement as a result of infection with cytomegalovirus (CMV) or *Mycobacterium avium–intracellulare*. In primary adrenal insufficiency, the glands themselves are destroyed so that the patient becomes deficient in cortisol and aldosterone. Primary adrenal insufficiency is a relatively uncommon disease seen in clinical practice. A **high level of suspicion**, particularly in individuals who have suggestive signs or symptoms, or who are susceptible by virtue of associated autoimmune disorders or malignancies must be maintained. The nonspecific symptoms might be otherwise missed for many years until a stressful event leads to crisis and death.

Secondary adrenal insufficiency is adrenal failure caused by a lack of ACTH stimulation from the pituitary gland. It can be caused by an autoimmune, infiltrative, metastatic disease of the pituitary. The **most common reason, however, is chronic exogenous administration of corticosteroids**, which can suppress the entire hypothalamic-pituitary-adrenal axis. Because of the widespread use of corticosteroids, secondary adrenal insufficiency is relatively common. In secondary adrenal insufficiency, the renin-angiotensin system usually is able to maintain near-normal levels of aldosterone so that the patient is deficient only in cortisol.

Clinical Features

The clinical presentation depends on the relative deficiency of glucocorticoids and mineralocorticoids, ACTH excess, and other associated disorders. **Acute adrenal insufficiency**, or addisonian crisis, may present with **weakness, nausea, vomiting, abdominal pain, fever, hypotension, and tachycardia**. Laboratory findings may **include hyponatremia, hyperkalemia, metabolic acidosis**, azotemia as a consequence of aldosterone deficiency, and hypoglycemia and eosinophilia as a consequence of cortisol deficiency. Patients with adrenal insufficiency may go into crisis when stressed by infection, trauma, or surgery. The **clinical features may appear identical to those of septic shock**; the only clues that the cause is adrenal disease may be the hypoglycemia (blood sugar is often elevated in sepsis) and profound **hypotension, which may be refractory to administration of pressors** but is reversed almost immediately when steroids are given.

Chronic adrenal insufficiency has nonspecific clinical features, such as **malaise, weight loss, chronic fatigue, and gastrointestinal symptoms such as anorexia, nausea, and vomiting.** A patient may have hypoglycemia and postural hypotension as a result of volume depletion. **Hyperpigmentation** is seen over time in primary adrenal insufficiency caused by elevated melanocyte-stimulating hormone production from the pituitary as a byproduct of high ACTH levels. It is typically seen as generalized hyperpigmentation of skin and mucous membranes. It is increased in sun-exposed areas or over pressure areas, such as elbows and knees, and may be noted in skin folds. In secondary adrenal insufficiency, patients are deficient in cortisol because of a lack of ACTH from the pituitary, but aldosterone production is maintained by the renin-angiotensin system. Therefore, volume depletion and hyperkalemia are not present and the patient will not manifest the typical hyperpigmentation.

Diagnosis

Cortisol levels show a diurnal variation. Cortisol levels are high in the morning and low as the day progresses, and levels should be elevated in stressful situations such as acute medical illness, surgery, or trauma. A **morning plasma cortisol level less than or equal to 5 μg/dL in an acutely ill patient is definitive evidence of adrenal insufficiency.** Conversely, a random cortisol level more than 20 μg/dL usually is interpreted as evidence of intact adrenal function. As in other endocrine deficiency states, the diagnostic test in this case is a stimulation test (conversely, in endocrine excess states, the diagnostic test is often a suppression test). **The ACTH stimulation test** is used to confirm primary adrenal insufficiency. Synthetic ACTH (cosyntropin) 250 μg is administered intravenously, and serum cortisol levels are measured at baseline and then at 30- and 60-minute intervals. An increase in the cortisol level of 7 μg/dL or a maximal stimulated level more than 18 μg/dL is considered normal and indicates intact adrenal function. If cosyntropin stimulation testing indicates probable adrenal insufficiency, ACTH levels can then be measured to distinguish between primary (high ACTH) and secondary (low ACTH) adrenal failure.

The insulin-glucose tolerance test is the gold standard for testing the entire hypothalamic-pituitary axis. It is based on the principle that if a stressful situation is induced (in this case, hypoglycemia), the ACTH level should rise with a consequent increase in cortisol levels. Computed tomography (CT) scan and magnetic resonance imaging (MRI) are helpful in evaluating adrenal and pituitary disease after biochemical confirmation.

Treatment

Treatment of addisonian crisis includes **intravenous 5% glucose with normal saline** to correct volume depletion and hypoglycemia and administration of **corticosteroid therapy.** Hydrocortisone usually is given intravenously at doses of 100 mg every 6 to 8 hours, or it can be given as a bolus followed by a continuous infusion. At high doses, the hydrocortisone provides both glucocorticoid and mineralocorticoid activity. A cortisol level should be drawn before treatment to confirm the diagnosis. Causes of the acute crisis should be identified and treated; in particular, there should be a **search for infection.**

Long-term treatment of patients with primary adrenal insufficiency includes replacement doses of **glucocorticoids** (eg, hydrocortisone 25-30 mg/d) and **mineralocorticoids** (eg, fludrocortisone 0.1-0.2 mg/d). Patients with secondary adrenal insufficiency still produce aldosterone, as mentioned earlier, so only glucocorticoids must be replaced. In both cases, to prevent the long-term complications of glucocorticoid excess (diabetes, hypertension, obesity, osteoporosis, cataracts), patients should not be overtreated. Stress doses of steroids should be given for intercurrent illnesses. Patients should wear a medical alert bracelet.

Stress Dose Steroids

When a patient has adrenal insufficiency or adrenal suppression due to chronic superphysiologic corticosteroid use (equivalent of prednisone 15 mg/d for 3 weeks or longer during the prior 12 months), then stress dose steroids are needed for events such as surgery, acute illness. Hydrocortisone 100 mg IV every 6 to 8 hours is a standard dose.

CASE CORRELATION

- See also Case 47 (Hyponatremia, SIADH), Case 52 (Diabetic Ketoacidosis), and Case 53 (Hyperthyroidism).

COMPREHENSION QUESTIONS

49.1 Which of the following is the most common cause of secondary adrenal insufficiency?

 A. Autoimmune process

 B. Surgical excision

 C. Hemorrhagic shock

 D. Exogenous corticosteroids

 E. ACTH failure due to panhypopituitarism

49.2 A 30-year-old woman takes prednisone 15 mg/d for systemic lupus erythematosus. She is admitted to the hospital for a cholecystectomy. Which of the following is the most important intervention for her?

 A. Hydrocortisone intravenously before surgery and every 6 hours for 24 hours.

 B. Double the prednisone the night before and hold her steroids the day of the surgery.

 C. Use of cyclophosphamide in lieu of corticosteroids for 2 weeks following surgery to promote wound healing.

 D. Cancel the surgery and use lithotripsy to break up the stones.

49.3 A 30-year-old woman who is 12 weeks' postpartum is noted to have adrenal insufficiency and a very distinct tan, although she hardly ventures outside. Which of the following is the most likely etiology?

A. Long-term steroid use

B. Sheehan syndrome (pituitary insufficiency)

C. Brain tumor

D. Autoimmune adrenal destruction

49.4 What is the best diagnostic test for a patient with suspected Cushing syndrome (ACTH-producing adenoma)?

A. Random cortisol level

B. ACTH-stimulation test

C. Overnight 1-mg dexamethasone suppression test

D. Pituitary MRI

ANSWERS

49.1 **D.** Long-term steroid use, with secondary suppression of pituitary secretion of ACTH, is the most common cause of secondary adrenal insufficiency. Autoimmune adrenalitis is the most common cause of primary adrenal insufficiency. Surgical excision of the adrenal glands would result in primary adrenal insufficiency. Hemorrhage of the adrenal glands is more common in the setting of sepsis and another cause of primary adrenal insufficiency.

49.2 **A.** A stress dose of corticosteroids is important to prevent adrenal insufficiency before surgery.

49.3 **D.** Hyperpigmentation occurs as a result of increased melanocyte-stimulating factor, a byproduct of ACTH, and occurs in primary adrenal insufficiency. Secondary causes of adrenal insufficiency such as Sheehan syndrome result in low ACTH levels and do not cause the "tanned" appearance. A brain tumor such as an ACTH producing pituitary adenoma would cause over activation of the adrenal glands resulting in a Cushingoid appearance and hyperpigmentation due to the excess ACTH.

49.4 **C.** Elevated cortisol greater than 5 μg/dL in the morning after a dose of dexamethasone at night indicates autonomous ACTH production (failure to be suppressed with dexamethasone). ACTH stimulation test is for adrenal insufficiency. Cortisol levels vary throughout the day, and are only useful when elevated to exclude adrenal insufficiency. Most ACTH-producing pituitary tumors are less than 5 mm and may not be seen on MRI.

CLINICAL PEARLS

▶ Primary adrenal insufficiency presents with weakness, fatigue, abdominal pain with vomiting, hyperpigmentation, and hyponatremia with hypotension, which may be refractory to pressors.

▶ Treatment of adrenal crisis is immediate administration of salt (saline), sugar (glucose), and steroids (hydrocortisone).

▶ The most common causes of primary adrenal insufficiency in the United States are autoimmune destruction, metastatic disease, and infectious causes (eg, cytomegalovirus in advanced acquired immunodeficiency syndrome). The most common cause worldwide is tuberculosis.

▶ Secondary adrenal insufficiency is the most common form of the illness and usually is a result of suppression of the hypothalamic-pituitary axis by exogenous corticosteroids.

REFERENCES

Arlt W. Disorders of the adrenal cortex. In: Kasper DL, Fauci AS, Hauser SL, Longo DL, Jameson JL, Loscalzo J, eds. *Harrison's Principles of Internal Medicine*. 19th ed. New York, NY: McGraw-Hill Education; 2015:2940-2961.

Carroll TB, Aron DC, Findling JW, et al. Glucocorticoids and adrenal androgens. In: Gardner DG, Shoback D, eds. *Basic and Clinical Endocrinology*. 9th ed. New York, NY: McGraw-Hill Education; 2011:334-377.

Oelkers W. Adrenal insufficiency. *N Engl J Med*. 1996;335:1206-1212.

A 63-year-old African-American woman is brought to the emergency center for upper arm pain and swelling following a fall at home. The family has noted that for approximately the past 2 months, the patient has become progressively fatigued and absentminded, and she has developed loss of appetite and weight loss. She has been getting up to urinate several times per night and complains of thirst; however, a glucose test for diabetes in her doctor's office was negative. This morning, she lost her balance because she felt "light-headed" and fell, landing on her left arm. Physical examination is notable for an elderly, thin woman in mild distress as a result of pain. She is afebrile, and her blood pressure is 110/70 mm Hg and heart rate is 80 bpm. Her thyroid gland is normal to palpation. Her mucous membranes are somewhat dry and sticky. Heart and lung examinations are normal, and carotid auscultation reveals no bruits. Examination of her extremities is significant only for deformity of the left mid-humerus with swelling. The left radial pulse is 2+ and symmetric. The radiologist calls you to confirm the fracture of the mid-left humerus but also states that there is the suggestion of some lytic lesions of the proximal humerus and recommends a skull film (Figure 50–1). Serum creatinine level is 2.1 mg/dL, with normal electrolyte and glucose concentrations, but serum calcium level is 13 mg/dL and hemoglobin level is 9.2 g/dL.

▶ What is the most likely diagnosis?
▶ What is the most likely underlying etiology in this patient?
▶ What is your next therapeutic step?

Figure 50–1. X-ray of skull showing osteolytic lesions.

ANSWERS TO CASE 50:
Hypercalcemia/Multiple Myeloma

Summary: A 63-year-old African-American woman is evaluated for a humeral fracture sustained during a fall because of light-headedness. She has a 2-month history of fatigue, absentmindedness, loss of appetite and weight, and nocturia. Her vital signs are normal, and she appears dehydrated. In addition to the fracture seen on x-ray, she also has lytic lesions of the proximal humerus. She has renal insufficiency, anemia, and hypercalcemia.

- **Most likely diagnosis:** Hypercalcemia with pathologic fracture of the left humerus.

- **Most likely underlying etiology:** Multiple myeloma.

- **Next therapeutic step:** Initial therapy of the hypercalcemia with intravenous (IV) fluids could be started in the emergency room.

ANALYSIS

Objectives

1. Know the clinical presentation and differential diagnosis of hypercalcemia.

2. Know the treatment of symptomatic hypercalcemia.

Considerations

The patient presents with acute confusion, fatigue, and lethargy, all symptoms of hypercalcemia, consistent with the calcium level of 13 mg/dL. The first step in therapy should be intravenous saline to restore volume status and facilitate urinary calcium excretion. Given the rapidity of onset of symptoms, weight loss, age, and presence of lytic bone lesions, the first concern should be for malignancy, such as multiple myeloma, or bony metastases from an undiagnosed cancer. Both serum and urine electrophoresis would help to identify the presence of a monoclonal gammopathy. Normal serum parathyroid hormone (PTH) and PTH-related protein (PTHrP) levels would exclude other causes of hypercalcemia (diagnostic algorithm is given in Figure 50–2 and causes of hypercalcemia in Table 50–1). Treatment then can be aimed at the underlying cause (Table 50–2).

APPROACH TO:
Hypercalcemia

DEFINITIONS

CORRECTED CALCIUM LEVEL: Add 0.8 mg/dL to the serum total calcium for every 1 g/dL of albumin level below 4 g/dL. Example: If the serum calcium

Figure 50–2. Algorithm for evaluation of patients with hypercalcemia. FHH, familial hypocalciuric hypercalcemia; MEN, multiple endocrine neoplasia; PTH, parathyroid hormone; PTHrP, parathyroid hormone–related protein. (Reproduced, with permission, from Potts JT. Diseases of the parathyroid gland and other hyper- and hypocalcemia disorders. In: Braunwald E, Fauci AS, Kasper DL, et al, eds. *Harrison's Principles of Internal Medicine*, 16th ed. New York: McGraw-Hill, 2005:2260.)

level is 9 mg/dL and the albumin level is 2 g/dL, the corrected calcium level is 10.6 mg/dL.

HYPERCALCEMIA: Elevated serum calcium levels after correction for albumin concentration (normal range approximately 8.8-10.4 mg/dL).

CLINICAL APPROACH

Hypercalcemia

The most common causes of hypercalcemia include malignancies or hyperparathyroidism, accounting for 90% of cases. Other causes include granulomatous disorders such as sarcoidosis and tuberculosis; less commonly, hypercalcemia may be the presentation of intoxication with vitamin A, vitamin D, or calcium-containing antacids, or may occur as a side effect of therapies with drugs such as lithium or thiazide diuretics. Genetic conditions such as familial hypocalciuric hypercalcemia and hyperparathyroidism as part of a multiple endocrine neoplasia syndrome are less common causes.

The differential diagnosis can be narrowed based on the chronicity of the patient's presentation and the presence or absence of other symptoms and signs. **Primary hyperparathyroidism,** usually caused by a **solitary parathyroid adenoma,** is the most likely cause when hypercalcemia is discovered in an otherwise **asymptomatic** patient

Table 50–1 • CAUSES OF HYPERCALCEMIA

Disease Process	Mechanism	Clinical Presentation	Diagnostic Evaluation	Treatment
Primary hyperparathyroidism	Elevated PTH leading to increased turnover of bone	Solitary adenoma or part of multiple endocrine neoplasia (MEN); nephrolithiasis, peptic ulcers, and mental changes (stones, bones, groans, etc)	Hypercalcemia, hypophosphatemia, elevated PTH	Medical therapy for mild symptoms; surgery for symptoms of hypercalciuria or osteoporosis
Malignancy	Local destruction of bone (multiple myeloma or leukemia or lymphoma) or humoral release of PTHrP (solid tumors such as breast, renal, or lung cancer)	Symptoms of hypercalcemia and of the particular cancer	Imaging of bones (either plain film or bone scan), PTHrP levels, serum protein electrophoresis,[a] bone marrow biopsy	Treatment of the tumor and control of cancer, bisphospho-nates, calcitonin
Sarcoidosis (and other granulomatous disorders)	Excess $1,25(OH)_2D$ synthesized in macrophages and lymphocytes	Pulmonary symptoms, lymphadenopathy, erythema nodosum	Low PTH levels and elevated $1,25(OH)_2D$ levels. Elevated ACE level, biopsy showing granulo-mas	Bisphosphonates or calcitonin; glucocorticoids for sarcoidosis
Excessive vitamin D intake	Increased calcium intestinal absorption and, if severe, bone resorption	Symptoms of hypercalcemia	Low PTH levels, markedly elevated levels of $25(OH)_2D$, and normal $1,25(OH)_2D$ levels	Decrease vitamin D and calcium intake
Renal insufficiency	Secondary hyperparathyroidism as a result of partial resistance to PTH effects	Bone pain, pruritus, ectopic calcification, osteomalacia	Elevated renal function tests	Limit dietary phosphate intravenous calcitriol

Abbreviations: ACE, angiotensin-converting enzyme; PTH, parathyroid hormone; PTHrP, parathyroid hormone-related protein.

Table 50–2 • TREATMENT OF SEVERE HYPERCALCEMIA		
Treatment	Onset	Adverse Effects
Hydration ± loop diuretic	Acute (effect seen in hours)	Volume overload, electrolyte disturbances
Bisphosphonates	Subacute (1-2 d)	Hypophosphatemia, hypomagnesemia, hypocalcemia, osteonecrosis of jaw
Calcitonin	Acute (hours)	Efficacy short-lived (tachyphylaxis)
Glucocorticoids (effective in cancer-induced hypercalcemia)	Lengthy (days)	Hyperglycemia, osteoporosis, immune suppression
Dialysis (renal insufficiency)	Acute (hours)	Volume shifts, electrolyte disorders, complicated procedure

on routine laboratory screening. Most patients have no symptoms with mild hypercalcemia less than 12 g/dL, except perhaps some polyuria and dehydration. With levels more than 13 mg/dL, patients begin developing increasingly severe symptoms, including central nervous system (CNS) symptoms (lethargy, stupor, coma, mental status changes, psychosis), gastrointestinal symptoms (anorexia, nausea, constipation, peptic ulcer disease), kidney problems (polyuria, nephrolithiasis, prerenal azotemia), and musculoskeletal complaints (arthralgias, myalgias, weakness). The **symptoms of hyperparathyroidism** can be remembered as **stones** (kidney), **moans** (abdominal pain), **groans** (myalgias), **bones** (bone pain), and **psychiatric overtones** (mental status changes). Diagnosis can be established by finding hypercalcemia, hypophosphatemia, and inappropriately elevated PTH levels. Patients with primary hyperparathyroidism may be treated surgically with parathyroidectomy if the patient is symptomatic, if the calcium is greater than 1 mg/dL above upper limit of normal, if less than 50 years old, or if there is significantly decreased bone mineral density (T score < −2.5).

However, a patient presenting with acute onset of **symptomatic hypercalcemia** is more likely to have a **malignancy**. Multiple myeloma, lymphoma, and leukemia all can present with hypercalcemia, as can solid tumors such as breast, lung, and kidney cancers. Some of these cancers cause elevated calcium levels by **stimulating osteoclast activity** through direct bone marrow invasion (multiple myeloma, leukemia, and breast cancer). Others produce **excess 1,25-vitamin D** (lymphomas), whereas still others secrete a **PTHrP** that binds the PTH receptor (kidney and lung). Cancer-related hypercalcemia can be differentiated from primary hyperparathyroidism by finding a suppressed PTH level.

In this case scenario, checking electrolytes to assess acid-base status and renal function are important tests to consider. A normal complete blood count (CBC) and peripheral smear would make leukemia a less likely cause. Levels of PTH and specific assays for PTHrP are generally measured. If multiple myeloma is suspected, serum and urine electrophoresis for monoclonal antibody spikes should be examined. Radiographs showing lytic or blastic lesions may be helpful; finally, a bone marrow biopsy may be considered.

Multiple Myeloma

Multiple myeloma is a neoplastic proliferation of plasma cells that usually produce monoclonal immunoglobulins. Patients typically present with **lytic bone lesions, hypercalcemia, renal insufficiency, anemia,** and an elevated globulin fraction on serum chemistries, which, if separated by electrophoresis, shows a **monoclonal proliferation** (M-spike). The **diagnosis** of multiple myeloma requires laboratory and clinical criteria: a **monoclonal antibody spike** in the serum, or light chains in the urine, and more than **10% clonal plasma cells in the bone marrow, and end-organ damage such as lytic bone lesions.**

Patients with lower-level monoclonal IgA or IgG antibody production without the signs or symptoms of multiple myeloma have what is termed a *monoclonal gammopathy of undetermined significance* (**MGUS**). MGUS is much more common than myeloma, affecting up to 1% of the population more than 50 years, or up to 10% of people older than age 75. Long-term studies demonstrate that approximately 1% per year of these patients with MGUS will progress to develop multiple myeloma. Patients with MGUS typically require no therapy. Some patients with myeloma with no bone lesions or other end-organ damage have an indolent course ("**smoldering myeloma**") and can be **observed without treatment** for many years if asymptomatic. **Therapy for symptomatic multiple myeloma** includes evaluation for autologous stem cell transplant, and induction chemotherapy with high-dose pulsed **dexamethasone**, in combination with thalidomide or lenalidomide, and bortezomib.

CASE CORRELATION

- See also Case 31 (Osteoarthritis), Case 32 (Low Back Pain), Case 35 (Osteoporosis).

COMPREHENSION QUESTIONS

50.1 On routine blood work performed for a life insurance application, a 48-year-old premenopausal woman was found to have a calcium level of 12 mg/dL (normal = 8.8-10.4 mg/dL) and a phosphate level of 2 mg/dL (normal = 3.0-4.5 mg/dL). She is not anemic and has no symptoms. Her medical history is significant for osteoporosis, discovered on a dual-energy x-ray absorptiometry (DEXA) scan performed last year. Which of the following is the most likely cause of her hypercalcemia?

A. Multiple myeloma

B. Parathyroid adenoma

C. Familial hypocalciuric hypercalcemia

D. Sarcoidosis

E. Undiagnosed breast cancer

50.2 A 62-year-old asymptomatic woman is noted to have multiple myeloma and hypercalcemia, but no bone lesions or end-organ damage. Which of the following therapies is useful for immediate treatment of the hypercalcemia?

A. Bisphosphonates.

B. Erythropoietin.

C. Dexamethasone plus thalidomide.

D. Interferon-alpha.

E. Observe without treatment since she is asymptomatic.

50.3 A 22-year-old African-American woman presents with worsening cough over 6 weeks, which did not improve with a course of antibiotics or antitussives. Her serum calcium level is found to be 12.5 mg/dL, and a chest x-ray reveals bilateral hilar lymphadenopathy. She has erythema nodosum on her legs. Which of the following is the most likely diagnosis?

A. Sarcoidosis

B. Mycoplasma pneumonia

C. Acute lymphoblastic leukemia

D. Squamous cell carcinoma of the lung

E. Pulmonary embolism

50.4 A 66-year-old man with known metastatic squamous cell carcinoma of the esophagus is brought to the emergency room for increasing lethargy and confusion. He is clinically dehydrated, his serum calcium level is 14 mg/dL, and his creatinine level is 2.5 mg/dL but 1 month ago it was 0.9 mg/dL. Which therapy for his hypercalcemia should be instituted first?

A. Intravenous bisphosphonate

B. Intravenous furosemide

C. Glucocorticoids

D. Intravenous normal saline

E. Chemotherapy for squamous cell carcinoma

ANSWERS

50.1 **B.** An asymptomatic, most likely chronically elevated calcium level is most likely caused by primary hyperparathyroidism due to a parathyroid adenoma. The hypercalcemia is presumed to be chronic because she has osteoporosis and is premenopausal. Familial hypocalciuric hypercalcemia can also lead to elevated serum calcium and low serum phosphate levels, but is usually asymptomatic and is far more rare than primary hyperparathyroidism.

50.2 **A.** Bisphosphonates are helpful in controlling hypercalcemia through inhibition of osteoclastic bone reabsorption. Dexamethasone, in combination with thalidomide, is useful in treatment of the myeloma, with a slower effect on the calcium level. Erythropoietin is inappropriate and is used to increase synthesis of red blood cells in those with renal failure. Interferon-alpha is also not an appropriate treatment for hypercalcemia. It is appropriate to treat chronic hepatitis B and as an adjuvant to surgical treatment for malignant melanoma.

50.3 **A.** Both sarcoidosis and lymphoma can present with cough, dyspnea, and hilar adenopathy on chest x-ray. In approximately 10% of cases, sarcoidosis can cause elevated calcium levels through the production of 1,25-vitamin D that occurs in the macrophages of the granulomas. This can also be seen in granulomas caused by tuberculosis and in lymphoma. Leukemia usually does not present in this manner, although it can cause hypercalcemia. Squamous cell carcinoma of the lung would be unusual in a patient of this age, and the radiographic presentation is atypical. The case scenario is consistent with Lofgren syndrome, an acute presentation of sarcoidosis, which includes hilar adenopathy, erythema nodosum, migratory polyarthralgia, and fever, seen most often in women.

50.4 **D.** Although all of the other therapies listed may be helpful in the treatment of hypercalcemia, given the clinical findings of dehydration and elevated creatinine level with a history of previously normal renal function, volume expansion with normal saline would correct the dehydration and presumed prerenal azotemia, allowing the kidneys to more efficiently excrete calcium. Other therapies can be added if the response to normal saline alone is insufficient.

CLINICAL PEARLS

► Hypercalcemia that is acutely symptomatic is most likely caused by cancer. Asymptomatic hypercalcemia is most likely caused by primary hyperparathyroidism.

► In primary hyperparathyroidism, serum parathyroid hormone and calcium levels are elevated, and phosphate levels are decreased. In malignancy-related hypercalcemia, the calcium level is high and parathyroid hormone levels are suppressed.

► Symptoms of hyperparathyroidism can be remembered as "stones, moans, groans, bones, and psychiatric overtones."

► MGUS and symptomatic multiple myeloma are on opposite ends of a spectrum of neoplastic disease of plasma cells.

► The classic triad of multiple myeloma consists of bone pain due to lytic lesions, anemia, and renal insufficiency.

REFERENCES

Bataille R, Harousseau J. Multiple myeloma. *N Engl J Med*. 1997;336:1657-1664.

Deftos LJ. Hypercalcemia in malignant and inflammatory diseases. *Endocrinol Metab Clin North Am*. 2002;31:141-158.

Munshi NC, Longo DL, Anderson KC. Plasma cell disorders. In: Kasper DL, Fauci AS, Hauser SL, et al., eds. *Harrison's Principles of Internal Medicine*. 19th ed. New York, NY: McGraw-Hill Education; 2015:710-719.

Potts JT. Diseases of the parathyroid gland and calcium homeostasis. In: Kasper DL, Fauci AS, Hauser SL, et al., eds. *Harrison's Principles of Internal Medicine*. 19th ed. New York, NY: McGraw-Hill; 2015:2466-2488.

While seeing patients in your preceptor's clinic, you have the opportunity to meet and examine one of her long-time patients, a 52-year-old woman who presents for her yearly physical examination. She has been fine and has no complaints today. Her medical history is notable only for borderline hypertension and moderate obesity. Last year her fasting lipid profile was acceptable for someone without known risk factors for coronary artery disease. Her mother and older brother have diabetes and hypertension. At prior visits, you see that your preceptor has counseled her on a low-calorie, low-fat diet and recommended that she start an exercise program. However, the patient says she has not made any of these recommended changes. With her full-time job and three children, she finds it difficult to exercise, and she admits that her family eats out frequently. Today her blood pressure is 140/92 mm Hg. Her body mass index (BMI) is 29 kg/m². Her examination is notable for acanthosis nigricans at the neck but otherwise is normal. A Papanicolaou (Pap) smear is performed, and a mammogram is offered. The patient has not eaten yet today, so on your preceptor's recommendation, a fasting plasma glucose test is performed, and the result is 140 mg/dL.

► What is your diagnosis?
► What is your next step?

ANSWERS TO CASE 51:

Type 2 Diabetes Diagnosis and Management

Summary: A 52-year-old woman presents for her yearly physical examination. Her medical history is notable only for borderline hypertension and moderate obesity. She has a family history of diabetes and hypertension. The patient has not followed the recommended lifestyle changes. Today, her blood pressure is 140/92 mm Hg, and her BMI is 29 kg/m². Her examination is notable for acanthosis nigricans at the neck, suggesting insulin resistance. A fasting plasma glucose level is 140 mg/dL, which is consistent with diabetes mellitus.

- **Most likely diagnosis:** Given her obesity, family history, and the finding of acanthosis nigricans, this patient most likely has type 2 diabetes. Diagnostic criteria for diabetes as defined by the American Diabetes Association (ADA) include (1) symptoms of diabetes and (2) fasting plasma glucose of 126 mg/dL or greater.

- **Next step:** Dietary counseling, assess for end-organ disease, and check hemoglobin A_{1C} (A_1c).

ANALYSIS

Objectives

1. Know the diagnostic criteria for type 2 diabetes.

2. Understand the initial medical management of diabetes.

3. Understand cardiovascular risk modification in diabetic patients.

4. Understand the prevention of microvascular complications of diabetes.

Considerations

This patient has a diagnosis of diabetes mellitus unless there was a laboratory error (patient not truly fasting). If this patient's diagnosis of diabetes is confirmed, she will require patient education, lifestyle modification, and medical therapy to prevent acute and chronic complications of diabetes. Strict glycemic control can reduce the incidence of microvascular complications such as retinopathy and nephropathy. In addition, patients with diabetes are among the highest at risk for cardiovascular disease, so risk factor modifications, such as smoking cessation and lowering of cholesterol, are essential. **Diabetes confers the same level of risk for coronary events, such as heart attack, as in patients with established coronary artery disease.** Thus, in this patient, the target blood pressure is less than 130/80 mm Hg, and the target low-density lipoprotein (LDL) cholesterol is less than 100 mg/dL.

APPROACH TO:
Suspected Diabetes Mellitus

DEFINITIONS

TYPE 1 DIABETES: Autoimmune destruction of the pancreatic beta-cells and complete loss of endogenous insulin production. The presentation of this type of diabetes usually is acute, with hyperglycemia and metabolic acidosis. These patients are dependent on exogenous insulin delivery.

TYPE 2 DIABETES: Heterogeneous syndrome of insulin resistance caused by genetic factors and/or obesity and relative insulin deficiency. Oral medications to enhance endogenous insulin production or improve insulin sensitivity are useful. Exogenous insulin may be used when oral medications are no longer sufficient for adequate glycemic control.

CLINICAL APPROACH

As the prevalence of obesity increases in the American population, so does the prevalence of type 2 diabetes. Ninety percent of all new cases of diabetes diagnosed in the United States are type 2, and it is estimated that this disease affects approximately 8% of the population older than 20 years. **Diabetes is the leading cause of blindness, renal failure, and nontraumatic amputations of the lower extremities.** It is a major risk factor in patients with coronary artery disease, peripheral vascular disease, and stroke.

In contrast to type 1 diabetics, patients with type 2 diabetes usually have a **prolonged asymptomatic phase.** During these years of asymptomatic hyperglycemia, however, organ damage begins to occur. Therefore, several organizations recommend screening of certain high-risk populations. The **risk factors** for diabetes include obesity or overweight (BMI >25 kg/m^2); other signs of an insulin-resistance syndrome or "metabolic" syndrome, such as hypertension or low high-density lipoproteins (HDLs) and triglycerides more than 250 mg/dL; first-degree relative with diabetes; history of gestational diabetes; or being a member of a high-risk ethnic group, including African Americans, Hispanics, American Indians, Asian Americans, or Pacific Islanders. **Screening should be performed every 3 years beginning at age 45, or earlier if overweight (BMI >25 kg/m^2).**

Most patients with type 2 diabetes mellitus are insulin resistant and hyperinsulinemic for years before developing overt diabetes. They are able to maintain normoglycemia for a long time, then develop postprandial hyperglycemia, and later develop both postprandial and fasting hyperglycemia (ie, hyperglycemia all the time). Thus, a **glucose tolerance test** to detect postprandial hyperglycemia would be the most sensitive test for diabetes mellitus but is time consuming and difficult to perform in a clinical practice. The **fasting plasma glucose** is the most specific test. **Hemoglobin A$_{1C}$ >6.5%** has now also been recognized as an acceptable diagnostic criteria (Table 51–1). If there are no clear symptoms of hyperglycemia, the diagnosis of diabetes should be confirmed on a subsequent day by repeat measurement, repeating the same test for confirmation. However, if two different tests (eg, fasting

Table 51–1 • TESTS FOR DIAGNOSING DIABETES			
Test	Normal	Impaired Fasting Glucose/Impaired Glucose Tolerance ("Prediabetes")	Diabetes
Fasting plasma glucose	<100 mg/dL	100-125 mg/dL	>126 mg/dL
Hemoglobin A$_{1C}$	<5.6%	5.75%-6.4%	>6.5%
2-h glucose tolerance test (75-g load)	<140 mg/dL	140-199 mg/dL	>200 mg/dL

glucose and A$_{1C}$) are available and are concordant for the diagnosis of diabetes, additional testing is not needed.

By using these tests, patients can be classified into one of three categories: (1) normal, (2) impaired glucose tolerance/impaired fasting glucose (ie, "prediabetic"), or (3) diabetic. Increased risk for microvascular complications of hyperglycemia is seen at a fasting glucose more than 126 mg/dL or A$_{1C}$ >6.5% (see Table 51–1). Once diabetes is diagnosed, therapy is instituted with three major goals.

1. Prevention of acute complications of hyperglycemia (eg, diabetic ketoacidosis or nonketotic hyperosmolar hyperglycemia) or hypoglycemia

2. Prevention of long-term complications of hyperglycemia, for example, microvascular disease such as retinopathy or nephropathy

3. Prevention of long-term complications of macrovascular disease, for example, cardiovascular or cerebrovascular disease

The foundation of diabetes therapy is **dietary and lifestyle modifications.** Exercise and even small amounts of weight loss can lower blood pressure and improve glucose control. Patients should be given instruction in nutrition and encouraged to change sedentary lifestyles.

However, most people with diabetes will eventually require medical therapy, and many patients will eventually require a combination of at least two medications. Because of the difficulty in achieving and sustaining glycemic targets and achieving significant weight loss, the ADA recommends that **metformin** should be initiated concurrent with lifestyle intervention at the time of diagnosis. **Glycemic goals should be an A$_{1C}$ <7%, preprandial glucose readings of 70 to 130 mg/dL, or peak postprandial glucose <180 mg/dL.** If patients fail to achieve these goals with initial therapy including lifestyle modification and metformin, therapeutic options include adding a second oral or injectable agent, including insulin, or switching to insulin monotherapy. A list of therapeutic agents for diabetes is included in Table 51–2.

When diabetes is diagnosed, other cardiovascular risk factors should be assessed. Blood pressure and lipid levels should be measured. With regard to lipid therapy, the cardiovascular risk in those with diabetes is equivalent to those with known coronary artery disease, so the desired **LDL goal is <100 mg/dL.** Those with higher LDL levels should undergo dietary modification, or be started on a statin.

The desired **blood pressure goal is <140/90 mm Hg.** Lower target BP of <130/80 mm Hg may be appropriate for younger patients, or patients with chronic kidney

Table 51-2 • MEDICATIONS AVAILABLE IN THE UNITED STATES FOR TREATMENT OF TYPE 2 DIABETES

Medication	Mechanism of Action/Indications	Special Considerations	Relative Cost
Insulin	↑ glucose utilization, ↓ hepatic glucose production	Weight gain, risk of hypoglycemia, need for frequent home glucose monitoring	$-$$$
Sulfonylureas (glimepiride, glipizide, glyburide)	Augments patient's own insulin production, works at the pancreatic beta-cells	Can cause hypoglycemia; can accumulate in renal insufficiency and cause prolonged hypoglycemia; best for young patients with fasting plasma glucose <300 mg/dL	$-$$
Metformin	Decreases gluconeogenesis in the liver; decreases insulin resistance	Risk of lactic acidosis in patients with renal insufficiency or liver dysfunction	$
α-Glucosidase inhibitors (acarbose)	Inhibits breakdown of complex carbohydrates in the GI tract, reduce postprandial hyperglycemia	Can cause GI distress, flatulence dose-dependent hepatotoxicity	$$
Thiazolidinediones (pioglitazone, rosiglitazone)	Promote skeletal muscle glucose uptake and decrease insulin resistance	Hepatotoxicity; edema, increased CHF risk	$$-$$$
GLP-1 agonists (exenatide, liraglutide)	↑ insulin, ↓ glucagon, slow gastric emptying	Injection, nausea, risk of pancreatitis	$$$$
DPP-4 inhibitors (saxagliptin, sitagliptin)	Prolong endogenous GLP-1 action	No hypoglycemia or weight gain, reduce dose in renal insufficiency	$$$$

disease. Several randomized trials have demonstrated a **benefit for angiotensin-converting enzyme (ACE) inhibitors** and **angiotensin receptor blockers (ARBs)** in preventing the progression of proteinuria and kidney disease.

Other routine care in diabetic patients includes frequent physician visits, at least every 3 to 6 months depending on their glucose control, at least yearly ophthalmologic examinations to screen for retinopathy, and yearly urine screens to detect microalbuminuria. Hemoglobin A_{1C} should be checked at least every 3 to 6 months, depending on the patient's glucose control. This test allows the physician to know the general glucose control over the preceding 2 to 3 months. Patients without neuropathy should have a foot examination yearly to detect early neuropathic changes; however, those with neuropathy should be examined every 3 months and be instructed on daily self-examination and prevention of injury.

CASE CORRELATION

- See also Case 48 (Oligomenorrhea), Case 52 (DKA), and Case 53 (Thyrotoxicosis).

COMPREHENSION QUESTIONS

51.1 A patient comes in for a fasting plasma glucose test. On two separate occasions, the result has been 115 mg/dL and 120 mg/dL. Which of the following is the most appropriate next step?

A. Reassurance that these are normal blood sugars.

B. Recommend weight loss, an ADA diet, and exercise.

C. Diagnose diabetes mellitus and start on a sulfonylurea.

D. Recommend cardiac stress testing.

E. Obtain stat arterial blood gas and serum ketone levels.

51.2 A 45-year-old obese Hispanic woman presents for follow-up of her diabetes. She currently takes metformin 1000 mg twice per day, and her fasting morning glucose runs approximately 170 to 200 mg/dL. Her last HbA_{1C} was 7.9. She states that she conscientiously follows her diet and that she walks 30 minutes to 1 hour daily. Which of the following is the best next step in her care?

A. Refer to an endocrinologist for an insulin pump.

B. Stop metformin and start on glimepiride.

C. Add once-a-day injection of insulin glargine (Lantus).

D. Hospitalize her urgently.

51.3 A 75-year-old woman with diabetes for approximately 20 years, diabetic retinopathy, and diabetic nephropathy with creatinine level 2.2 mg/dL is brought into the clinic by her daughter for follow-up. The patient currently takes a sulfonylurea for her diabetes and an ACE inhibitor for her protein-uria. Her daughter reports that, on three occasions in the past 2 weeks, her mother became sweaty, shaky, and confused, which resolved when she was given some orange juice. Which of the following conditions is most likely to be contributing to these episodes?

A. Excess caloric oral intake

B. Interaction between the ACE inhibitor and the sulfonylurea agents

C. Worsening renal function

D. Hyperglycemic amnesia

51.4 A 42-year-old woman who developed gestational diabetes with her last preg-nancy which was 10 years ago, is being screened for type 2 diabetes. Which of the following screening methods has the highest sensitivity?

A. Fasting serum glucose

B. 2-Hour glucose tolerance test

C. Hemoglobin A_1C

D. Random glucose

51.5 A 36-year-old man has been recently diagnosed with type 2 diabetes. If not vaccinated previously, which of the following immunizations is most impor-tant to administer?

A. Pneumococcal

B. Human papilloma virus

C. Hepatitis B

D. Rubella

E. Toxoplasmosis

ANSWERS

51.1 **B.** By diagnostic criteria, this patient falls into the definition of impaired fast-ing glucose. Although she does not yet meet the criteria for diabetes, she is at greater risk for developing diabetes in the future and for macrovascular disease. Intensive lifestyle changes (diet and exercise for 30 minutes per day, 5 days per week) can reduce or delay the development of diabetes. Patients should be monitored annually to screen for progression to diabetes.

51.2 **C.** When patients fail to achieve glycemic goal (A_{1C} <7%) using metformin and lifestyle modifications, the next step is to either add a once-daily basal insulin injection (a long-acting insulin such as NPH, glargine, or detemir) or a sulfonylurea to the regimen. Switching from one class of oral agent to another with similar potency would add no benefit.

51.3 **C.** Sulfonylureas have long half-lives and can cause prolonged hypoglycemia in elderly patients as well in those with **renal insufficiency**. Another method, such as insulin, may be more appropriate in this patient, as well as less-intensive control, aiming for an HbA_{1C} of 8% instead of 7%.

51.4 **B.** The 2-hour oral glucose tolerance test is used as the reference standard and has the highest sensitivity. Even with this "gold standard," there are undiagnosed diabetics though. The next best tests are hemoglobin A_{1C} of 6.5 or higher have sensitivity of about 60%. The Hbg A_{1C} has the advantage of correlating to long-term outcomes. A random glucose has only a 50% sensitivity and is usually not used as a screening test.

51.5 **C.** A patient who is diagnosed with diabetes should receive the hepatitis B vaccine as soon as feasible if not vaccinated previously. The Centers for Disease Control and Prevention (CDC) recommends hepatitis B vaccination for diabetics aged 18 to 59, and consideration for those >60 years due to the increased risk of hepatitis B case fatality rate in diabetics. Diabetes confers a 60% higher infection rate versus nondiabetics. Diabetics should receive an annual influenza vaccination as well as the pneumococcal vaccine after the age of 65 if the first dose was administered prior to the age of 65.

CLINICAL PEARLS

▶ Type 2 diabetes has a prolonged asymptomatic stage during which microvascular disease (eg, retinopathy or nephropathy) can occur. Physicians should have a high index of suspicion and screen those patients with risk factors.

▶ Lifestyle modification and metformin are the initial therapy for most patients initially diagnosed with type 2 diabetes.

▶ The major cause of morbidity and mortality in patients with type 2 diabetes mellitus is macrovascular disease, such as coronary artery disease, stroke, and peripheral vascular disease, so aggressive cardiovascular risk factor reduction is essential.

▶ Glycemic goals are A_{1C} <7%, preprandial glucose 70 to 130 mg/dL, or postprandial glucose <180 mg/dL. Blood pressure should be <140/90, and LDL cholesterol should be <100 mg/dL.

REFERENCES

American Diabetes Association. Standards of medical care in diabetes 2015. *Diabetes Care.* 2015; 38(suppl 1):S17-S69.

Powers AC. Diabetes mellitus. In: Kasper DL, Fauci AS, Hauser SL, et al., eds. *Harrison's Principles of Internal Medicine.* 19th ed. New York, NY: McGraw-Hill; 2015:2399-2430.

An 18-year-old woman is brought to the emergency department by her mother because the daughter seems confused and is behaving strangely. The mother reports the patient has always been healthy and has no significant medical history, but she has lost 20 lb recently without trying and has been complaining of fatigue for 2 or 3 weeks. The patient had attributed the fatigue to sleep disturbance, as recently she has been getting up several times at night to urinate. This morning, the mother found the patient in her room, complaining of abdominal pain, and she had vomited. She appeared confused and did not know that today was a school day.

On examination, the patient is slender, lying on a stretcher with eyes closed, but she is responsive to questions. She is afebrile, and has a heart rate of 118 bpm, blood pressure of 125/84 mm Hg, with deep and rapid respirations at the rate of 24 bpm. Upon standing, her heart rate rises to 145 bpm, and her blood pressure falls to 110/80 mm Hg. Her funduscopic examination is normal, her oral mucosa is dry, and her neck veins are flat. Her chest is clear to auscultation, and her heart is tachycardic with a regular rhythm and no murmur. Her abdomen is soft with active bowel sounds and mild diffuse tenderness, but no guarding or rebound. Her neurologic examination reveals no focal deficits.

Laboratory studies include serum Na 131 mEq/L, K 5.3 mEq/L, Cl 95 mEq/L, CO_2 9 mEq/L, blood urea nitrogen (BUN) 35 mg/dL, creatinine 1.3 mg/dL, and glucose 475 mg/dL. Arterial blood gas reveals pH 7.12 with PCO_2 24 mm Hg and PO_2 95 mm Hg. Urine drug screen and urine pregnancy test are negative, and urinalysis shows no hematuria or pyuria, but 3+ glucose and 3+ ketones. Chest radiograph is read as normal, and plain film of the abdomen has nonspecific gas pattern but no signs of obstruction.

▶ What is the most likely diagnosis?
▶ What is your next step?

ANSWERS TO CASE 52:
Diabetic Ketoacidosis

Summary: An 18-year-old woman presents with unintentional weight loss, nocturia, and polyuria, with hyperglycemia that likely represents new-onset diabetes mellitus, probably type 1. She is hypovolemic as a result of osmotic diuresis and has an anion gap metabolic acidosis, which is primarily caused by ketoacids. Her mental status and abdominal pain probably are manifestations of the metabolic acidosis and hyperosmolarity.

- **Most likely diagnosis:** Diabetic ketoacidosis (DKA).

- **Next step:** Aggressive hydration to improve her volume status and insulin therapy to resolve the ketoacidosis.

ANALYSIS

Objectives

1. Know how to diagnose patients with anion gap metabolic acidosis.

2. Be able to differentiate DKA, nonketotic hyperosmolar hyperglycemia, and alcoholic ketoacidosis.

3. Understand the principles of DKA management: restoration of volume, electrolyte replacement, resolution of ketosis, and control of hyperglycemia.

4. Learn the complications of DKA and of improper management.

Considerations

DKA occurs as a result of severe insulin deficiency and may be the initial presentation of diabetes mellitus, as in this patient. In all patients with DKA, one must be alert for precipitating factors, such as infection, pregnancy, or severe physiologic stressors, such as myocardial infarction. The diagnosis is based on arterial pH <7.3 with an anion gap, glucose >250 mg/dL, and elevated serum ketones (>5 mEq/L). A DKA patient is significantly volume depleted. The treatment goals include fluid resuscitation, reversal of acidosis, reduction of plasma glucose, correction of electrolyte abnormalities, and identification of the underlying cause. The serum potassium level may be initially elevated due to the acidotic state, but upon fluid correction, fall; the total body potassium is almost always low. Careful management and close monitoring will be required to correct fluid and electrolyte deficits and to prevent complications such as hypokalemia and cerebral edema. The patient in this scenario has significant DKA based on the pH of 7.11. The bicarbonate of 9 mEq/L confirms metabolic acidosis. This patient needs immediate fluid repletion with normal saline and insulin infusion. Initial laboratory work should include serum glucose, serum electrolytes, magnesium, phosphorus, amylase and lipase, urine dipstick, serum ketones, arterial blood gas (ABG), complete blood count (CBC), blood urea nitrogen (BUN) and creatinine, urine and/or blood cultures, and electrocardiography (ECG).

APPROACH TO:

Suspected Diabetic Ketoacidosis

DEFINITIONS

DIABETIC KETOACIDOSIS: A syndrome of hyperglycemia, anion gap metabolic acidosis, and ketone bodies in the serum, caused by insufficient insulin levels.

KUSSMAUL RESPIRATIONS: Deep and rapid breathing that represents hyperventilation in an attempt to generate a respiratory alkalosis to compensate for the metabolic acidosis.

CLINICAL APPROACH

Diabetic ketoacidosis is a clinical syndrome that results when the **triad of anion gap metabolic acidosis, hyperglycemia, and ketosis** is present and is caused by a significant insulin deficiency. It is a medical emergency, with an overall mortality rate less than 5% if patients receive prompt and appropriate medical treatment. The majority of episodes are preventable, and many of the deaths also are preventable with proper attention to detail during management.

Pathophysiology

In the normal physiologic state, there is a fine balance between anabolic and catabolic hormones. In the fed state, anabolic actions of insulin predominate. Glycogenesis, lipogenesis, and protein synthesis all are increased. This results in storage of energy reserves in the form of triglycerides and glycogen.

In the fasting state, insulin serves to inhibit lipolysis, ketogenesis, gluconeogenesis, glycogenolysis, and proteolysis. These effects are critical in controlling the rate of breakdown of energy stores under the influence of catabolic hormones. **Glucagon is the most important catabolic hormone.** In the fasting state, it maintains normal glucose levels by stimulating hepatic gluconeogenesis and glycogenolysis.

Diabetes is the condition of relative or absolute insulin deficiency. When there is a severe insulin deficiency and a relative excess of glucagon, lipolysis is enhanced, causing release of free fatty acids. Oxidation of the fatty acids produces ketones, such as acetoacetate and beta-hydroxybutyrate, which are organic acids and often referred to as **ketoacids.** The excess of these ketoacids can produce a life-threatening metabolic acidosis. In addition, hyperglycemia produces an osmotic diuresis, which causes severe volume depletion, and electrolyte deficiencies by washing extracellular sodium, potassium, magnesium, phosphate, and water out of the body. The combination of acidosis, hypovolemia, and electrolyte deficiencies can lead to **cardiovascular collapse, the most common cause of death in DKA.**

Clinical Presentation

Patients with diabetes have an underlying impairment in glucose metabolism and, when challenged by a stress, an increase in insulin requirements. If they are unable to meet these insulin requirements, DKA may result. **The most common precipitating events are infections** such as **pneumonia or urinary tract infection, vascular**

disorders such as myocardial infarction, or other stressors such as trauma. Diabetic ketoacidosis may be the presentation of new-onset diabetes, or it can occur in patients with established diabetes because of failure to use insulin for whatever reason or because of use of other medications (eg, glucocorticoids) that interfere with insulin action.

An episode of DKA evolves over a short period of time, typically less than 24 hours. The patient with DKA has the signs and symptoms of hyperglycemia, acidosis, and dehydration. Polyuria, polydipsia, weight loss, visual blurring, and decreased mental status are related to hyperglycemia and osmotic diuresis. Nausea, vomiting, abdominal pain, fatigue, malaise, and shortness of breath may be related to the acidosis.

Typical signs include reduced skin elasticity, dry mucous membranes, hypotension, and tachycardia related to volume depletion. **Kussmaul respirations**, deep and rapid breathing, represent hyperventilation in an attempt to generate a respiratory alkalosis to compensate for the metabolic acidosis. One may also note the **fruity breath odor** typical of ketosis.

Laboratory Diagnosis

Laboratory values show hyperglycemia (usually >250 mg/dL), acidosis (pH <7.3), anion gap (usually >15 mmol/L), and ketonemia. The most important laboratory parameters are the degree of acidosis, the anion gap, and the serum potassium level.

Patients with a very low pH (<7.0) are severely acidotic and have a worse prognosis. The lower pH is a result of the higher concentration of ketoacids, which are estimated using the anion gap. The first step in evaluating any patient with metabolic acidosis should be calculation of the **anion gap**. This concept is based on the principle of electrical neutrality, that is, all the cations must equal all the anions. The anion gap estimates those negatively charged particles that are not routinely measured and can be calculated using the following calculation:

$$\text{Anion Gap} = [\text{Na}] - [\text{Cl} + \text{HCO}_3]$$

The normal anion gap is 10 to 12 mmol/L. When it is elevated, there is an excess of unmeasured anions, which typically occurs because of one of the four causes, which are listed in Table 52–1.

Table 52–1 • CAUSES OF HIGH ANION GAP METABOLIC ACIDOSIS
Lactic acidosis
Ketoacidosis
• Diabetic
• Alcoholic
• Starvation
Toxins
• Ethylene glycol
• Methanol
• Salicylates
Renal failure (acute or chronic)

(Reproduced with permission from DuBose TD. Acidosis and alkalosis. In: Braunwald E, Fauci AS, Kasper KL, et al, eds. Harrison's Principles of Internal Medicine, 16th ed. New York: McGraw-Hill, 2005:265.)

Lactic acidosis can be a result of severe tissue hypoxia, as in septic shock or carbon monoxide poisoning, or a result of hepatic failure and subsequent inability to metabolize lactate. Ketoacidosis most commonly occurs as an acute complication of uncontrolled diabetes, but it also can be seen in starvation and alcoholism (discussed later). The ingested toxins may be organic acids themselves, such as salicylic acid, or have acidic metabolites, such as formic acid from methanol. Renal failure leads to an inability to excrete organic acids as well as inorganic acids such as phosphates (often without an anion gap).

In patients with DKA, total body potassium stores are depleted because of urinary losses, and potassium replacement will always be necessary. Initially, the measured serum potassium levels may be high despite the total body potassium deficit because of acidosis resulting in movement of potassium from the intracellular to the extracellular compartment. As the acidosis is corrected and with the administration of insulin, which drives potassium intracellularly, **serum potassium levels will fall rapidly.**

The serum sodium level can be variable. Hyperglycemia causes water to move extracellularly, which can lead to hyponatremia. Similarly, phosphate levels can be variable in the presence of body store deficits with the extracellular movement of phosphate caused by catabolic state. BUN and creatinine levels are elevated, reflecting dehydration. Serum acetoacetate may cause a false elevation in serum creatinine level because of interference with the assay.

Management

The goal of treatment is restoration of metabolic homeostasis with correction of precipitating events and biochemical deficits, which consists of the following:

1. Replacement of fluid losses with improvement of circulatory volume

2. Correction of hyperglycemia and, in turn, plasma osmolality

3. Replacement of electrolyte losses

4. Clearance of serum ketones

5. Identification and treatment of precipitating cause and complications

Close monitoring of the patient is important. A flow sheet recording vital signs, input and output, insulin dosage, and metabolic progress is important. Serum glucose concentration should be measured every 1 hour, and levels of serum electrolytes and phosphate must be assessed every 3 to 5 hours. Urinalysis, urine and blood cultures, ECG, and chest x-ray should be obtained to identify precipitating factors and complications. Other investigations should be pursued as symptoms and signs warrant.

Fluids

All patients with DKA are volume depleted as a consequence of osmotic diuresis as well as from other ongoing losses, such as vomiting. Hydration improves renal perfusion and cardiac output, facilitating glucose excretion. Rehydration may also diminish insulin resistance by decreasing levels of counterregulatory hormones and hyperglycemia. Sudden reduction in hyperglycemia can lead to vascular collapse with shift of water intracellularly. To avoid this, initial replacement fluid should be isotonic normal saline (NS) to correct circulatory volume deficit. **Over the first hour, 1 to 2 L of NS should be infused.** Following this, total body water deficit is corrected at the rate of 250 to 500 mL/h, depending on the state of hydration. The composition of fluid should be tailored according to serum sodium and chloride measurements.

Hydration should be gentler in patients with congestive heart failure or end-stage renal disease because such patients can easily get fluid overload.

Insulin

The goal of therapy is a glucose reduction of 80 to 100 mg/dL/h. Use of continuous low-dose intravenous infusion of insulin is recommended because it reduces episodes of hypoglycemia and hypokalemia, and it allows a more controlled reduction of serum glucose and osmolality. Intramuscular and subcutaneous routes can be used if tissue perfusion is adequate.

Insulin treatment may be initiated as an **intravenous bolus** of 0.1 to 0.15 U/kg. This should be followed by a **continuous infusion of 0.1 U/kg/h with hourly serum glucose determinations.** If blood glucose fails to decline at the desired rate, volume status should be reassessed, and insulin infusion should be titrated. The rate of infusion should be decreased to 0.05 U/kg/h when the blood glucose level decreases to 250 to 300 mg/dL. **Glucose levels fall more quickly than ketosis resolves.** Insulin is necessary for resolution of the ketoacidosis and can be coadministered with a glucose infusion until the anion gap is resolved. A 5% to 10% dextrose solution should be added to the hydrating solution when plasma glucose is less than 300 mg/dL. One can judge the resolution of ketoacidosis when the bicarbonate is more than 18 mEq/L, the anion gap is less than 12, the patient feels better, and the vital signs are stabilized. **Serial determination of serum ketone levels is not clinically useful** in measuring response to therapy. Laboratory tests measure acetoacetate and acetone, but not beta-hydroxybutyrate. With the administration of insulin, beta-hydroxybutyrate is first oxidized to acetoacetate, so measured ketone levels may actually increase with effective therapy. Instead, one should be guided by normalizing the anion gap when making decisions about the rate of insulin infusion. Subcutaneous insulin should be given approximately 30 minutes before stopping insulin infusion to avoid rebound acidosis.

Bicarbonate

Bicarbonate therapy is controversial and should not be given to ketoacidotic patients unless their **arterial pH is less than 7** or other indications, such as cardiac instability or severe hyperkalemia, are present. Bicarbonate therapy can cause worsening hypokalemia, paradoxical central nervous system acidosis, and delay in ketone clearance.

Electrolytes

In DKA, there is **deficit of total body potassium, phosphate, and magnesium.** Patients frequently have hyperkalemia as a result of acidosis, insulin deficiency, and hypertonicity that cause a shift of potassium extracellularly. During treatment, plasma potassium concentration will fall as the metabolic abnormalities are corrected. Potassium should be added to initial intravenous fluids once the concentration is less than 5 mEq/L. Once adequate urine output is established, 20 to 40 mEq of potassium should be added to each liter of fluid. The goal is to maintain potassium in the range of 4 to 5 mEq/L. Cardiac monitoring is recommended in the presence of hypokalemia or hyperkalemia.

Phosphate replacement should be given to patients with serum phosphate concentrations less than 1 mg/dL and to patients with moderate hypophosphatemia with concomitant hypoxia, anemia, or cardiorespiratory compromise. Careful monitoring of the serum calcium level is necessary with phosphate administration.

Magnesium and calcium can be supplemented as needed.

Precipitating Causes

It is important to correct precipitating factors in order to restore metabolic balance. Identifiable sources of infection should be treated aggressively. Possible presence of ischemia and infarction should be evaluated and treated appropriately with help from specialists as needed.

Complications

Cerebral edema, acute respiratory distress syndrome, thromboembolism, fluid overload, and acute gastric dilatation are rare, but serious, complications of DKA.

Prevention

The major precipitating factors in the development of DKA are inadequate insulin treatment and infection. These events can be prevented by patient education and effective communication with a health care team. Sick-day management regarding dosing of insulin, blood glucose monitoring, avoiding prolonged fasting, and preventing dehydration should be addressed. Socioeconomic barriers contribute to the high rates of admission for DKA. Appropriate allocation of health care resources toward preventive strategies is needed.

Other metabolic complications of deranged carbohydrate metabolism deserve mention at this point. The first is **hyperosmolar nonketotic diabetic coma**. This condition occurs mainly in patients with type 2 diabetes who become profoundly dehydrated because of osmotic diuresis. However, these patients have sufficient insulin action to prevent the development of ketoacidosis. They may present with glucose levels more than 1000 mg/dL, serum osmolarity more than 320 to 370 Osm, and neurologic symptoms ranging from confusion to seizures to coma. Compared to patients with DKA, they have a much larger fluid deficit, and therapy is primarily volume resuscitation with NS. Insulin is also used to reverse hyperglycemia but usually is given in lesser doses than is required for clearance of ketosis in DKA.

Alcoholic ketoacidosis develops in chronic alcoholics who are malnourished and have depleted glycogen stores, and is often seen in the setting of binge drinking, which may shift the ratio of the reduced form of nicotinamide adenine dinucleotide (NADH) to nicotinamide adenine dinucleotide (NAD), inhibiting gluconeogenesis. They develop an anion gap metabolic acidosis as a result of ketoacidosis and lactic acidosis. They present with the same symptoms of acidosis as do DKA patients, for example, abdominal pain, nausea, and vomiting, but with low, normal, or slightly elevated glucose levels (in contrast to DKA, in which the glucose level usually is markedly elevated). Treatment is administration of volume in the form of NS and glucose solution. Insulin administration typically is unnecessary.

> ## CASE CORRELATION
> - See also Case 41 (Urosepsis), Case 53 (Thyrotoxicosis), Case 59 (Delirium and Alcohol Withdrawal), and Case 60 (Alcohol Ketoacidosis).

COMPREHENSION QUESTIONS

52.1 Which of the following most likely will lead to a nonanion gap acidosis?
   A. Diarrhea
   B. Lactic acidosis
   C. Diabetic ketoacidosis
   D. Ethylene glycol ingestions

52.2 An 18-year-old man is noted to be in diabetic ketoacidosis with pH 7.20 and serum glucose level 400 mg/dL. Which of the following is the most accurate statement regarding this patient's potassium status?
   A. Likely to have a potassium level less than 3 mEq/L.
   B. Likely to have a potassium level more than 5 mEq/L.
   C. Likely to have a total body potassium deficit regardless of the serum level.
   D. Serum level is likely to increase with correction of the acidosis.

52.3 Which of the following is the most important first step in the treatment of diabetic ketoacidosis?
   A. Replacement of potassium
   B. Intravenous fluid replacement
   C. Replacement of phosphorus
   D. Antibiotic therapy

52.4   A 59-year-old man with a long history of diabetes with chronic renal insufficiency due to diabetic nephropathy is seen in clinic for routine laboratory
work. He is asymptomatic, but his glucose is elevated at 258 mg/dL, and his
other chemistries are as follows: sodium 135 mEq/L, potassium 5.4 mEq/L,
chloride 108 mEq/L, and bicarbonate 18 mEq/L. His creatinine is stable at
2.1 mg/dL. What is the most likely cause of his acidosis?

A.   Diabetic ketoacidosis

B.   Lactic acidosis

C.   Type 4 renal tubular acidosis

D.   Accidental salicylate overdose

ANSWERS

52.1 **A.** Diarrhea leads to bicarbonate loss and usually does not affect the anion gap.
All other choices- lactic acidosis, DKA, and ethylene glycol ingestion are causes
of a high anion gap metabolic acidosis. Common causes can be remembered
with the MUDPILES mneumonic. (Methanol, Uremia, Diabetic ketoacidosis, Propylene glycol, Iron/Isoniazid/Infection, Lactic acidosis, Ethylene glycol,
Salicylates).

52.2 **C.** Total body potassium usually is depleted regardless of the serum level, due
to the extracellular shift of potassium.

52.3 **B.** The basic tenets of treating DKA include intravenous fluid, insulin to control the glucose level, correction of metabolic disturbances (such as repletion
of potassium), and identification of the underlying etiology.

52.4 **C.** The laboratories are consistent with a nonanion gap metabolic acidosis.
Patients with chronic kidney disease due to diabetes are prone to subtle volume expansion and low plasma renin activity, leading to hypoaldosteronism.
Since aldosterone is the major hormone that promotes potassium excretion,
hyperkalemia is the primary electrolyte abnormality. The disorder is typically
associated with a mild metabolic acidosis (bicarbonate usually >17 mEq/L).
The other illnesses cause anion gap acidosis.

CLINICAL PEARLS

▶ All patients with diabetic ketoacidosis are volume depleted and require significant replacement of salt solution and, later, free water in the form of glucose solutions.

▶ Despite sometimes elevated potassium concentrations, all patients with diabetic ketoacidosis have a total body potassium deficit and will require substantial potassium replacement.

▶ Glucose levels fall more quickly than ketones resolve. Continuous insulin therapy is necessary for resolution of the ketoacidosis and can be coadministered with a glucose infusion until the anion gap is resolved.

▶ Cerebral edema can result from overly rapid correction of hyperglycemia or possibly from rapid administration of hypotonic fluids.

▶ Occurrence of diabetic ketoacidosis requires a precipitating cause, either insulin deficiency or a physiologic stressor such as infection.

REFERENCES

Delaney MF. Diabetic ketoacidosis and hyperglycemic hyperosmolar nonketotic syndrome. *Endocrinol Metab Clin North Am.* 2000;129:683-705.

Kitabchi AE. Management of hyperglycemic crises in patients with diabetes. *Diabetes Care.* 2001;24:131-153.

Magee MF. Management of decompensated diabetes. *Crit Care Clin.* 2001;117:75-107.

Powers AC. Diabetes mellitus. In: Kasper DL, Fauci AS, Hauser SL, Longo DL, Jameson JL, Loscalzo J, eds. *Harrison's Principles of Internal Medicine.* 19th ed. New York, NY: McGraw-Hill; 2015:2968-3003.

Quinn L. Diabetes emergencies in the patient with type 2 diabetes. *Nurs Clin North Am.* 2001;136:341-359.

CASE 53

A 37-year-old previously healthy woman presents to your clinic for unintentional weight loss. Over the past 3 months, she has lost approximately 15 lb without changing her diet or activity level. Otherwise, she feels great. She has an excellent appetite, no gastrointestinal complaints except for occasional loose stools, a good energy level, and no complaints of fatigue. She denies heat or cold intolerance. On examination, her heart rate is 108 bpm, blood pressure 142/82 mm Hg, and she is afebrile. When she looks at you, she seems to stare, and her eyes are somewhat protuberant. You note a large, smooth, nontender thyroid gland and a 2/6 systolic ejection murmur on cardiac examination, and her skin is warm and dry. There is a fine resting tremor.

▶ What is the most likely diagnosis?
▶ How could you confirm the diagnosis?
▶ What are the options for treatment?

ANSWERS TO CASE 53:

Thyrotoxicosis/Graves Disease

Summary: A 37-year-old woman presents with weight loss without anorexia, tachycardia, borderline hypertension, exophthalmos, and a smooth, nontender goiter.

- **Most likely diagnosis:** Thyrotoxicosis/Graves disease.

- **Confirming the diagnosis:** A low serum thyroid-stimulating hormone (TSH) level and an increased free thyroxine (T_4) level with this clinical presentation would be confirmatory of hyperthyroidism. However, other tests that would define the etiology would be thyroid-stimulating immunoglobulins or diffusely elevated uptake of radioactive iodine on thyroid scan.

- **Treatment options:** Antithyroid drugs, radioactive iodine ablation, or less commonly, surgical removal of the thyroid.

ANALYSIS

Objectives

1. Understand the clinical presentation of thyrotoxicosis.
2. Be able to discuss the causes of hyperthyroidism, including Graves disease and toxic nodule.
3. Learn the complications of thyrotoxicosis, including thyroid storm.
4. Understand the evaluation of a patient with a thyroid nodule.
5. Know the available treatment options for Graves disease and outcomes of treatment.

Considerations

This 37-year-old woman has unintentional weight loss, loose stools, and warm skin, all symptoms of hyperthyroidism. Her thyroid gland is diffusely enlarged and nontender, and she has exophthalmus (protuberant eyes), which is consistent with Graves disease. This is a systemic disease with many complications that affect the entire body, including osteoporosis and heart failure. Treatment can include elimination of the excess thyroid hormone, but definitive therapy may include radioactive (or, less commonly, surgical) ablative therapy.

APPROACH TO:

Hyperthyroidism

DEFINITIONS

HYPERTHYROIDISM: Hypermetabolic condition that results from the effect of excessive amounts of thyroid hormones produced by the thyroid gland itself.

Because almost all cases of thyrotoxicosis are caused by thyroid overproduction, these terms are often used synonymously.

THYROTOXICOSIS: Usually used as a general term for the state of thyroid hormone excess from any source, for example, exogenous ingestion.

CLINICAL APPROACH

Hyperthyroidism affects numerous body systems.

Neuromuscular system: Nervousness, tremors, and brisk reflexes are common. Inability to concentrate, proximal muscle weakness, emotional lability, and insomnia might be present.

Cardiac system: Wide pulse pressure, flow heart murmurs, and tachycardia usually are present. Atrial fibrillation is present in 10% to 20% of patients. Long-standing thyrotoxicosis can cause cardiomegaly and result in high-output heart failure.

Gastrointestinal system: Despite increased food intake, weight loss is common. Hyperdefecation usually is present as a result of increased gastrointestinal motility, but diarrhea is rare.

Eyes: Retraction of the upper eyelid as a consequence of increased sympathetic tone gives some patients a wide-eyed stare. Lid lag might be found on physical examination (sclera can be seen above the iris as the patient looks downward). Exophthalmos is distinctive of Graves disease.

Skin: The skin is warm, moist, and velvety, with fine hair texture and alopecia. Sweating usually is present as a consequence of vasodilation and heat dissipation.

Reproductive system: Hyperthyroidism impairs fertility in women and may cause oligomenorrhea. The sperm count in men is reduced. Impotence and gynecomastia might be present.

Metabolism: Weight loss is a common finding, especially in older patients who develop anorexia. Many patients develop an aversion to heat and a preference for cold temperatures.

Apathetic hyperthyroidism: Older patients with hyperthyroidism may lack typical adrenergic features and present instead with depression or apathy, weight loss, atrial fibrillation, worsening angina pectoris, or congestive heart failure.

Thyroid Storm

Thyroid storm is a dangerous condition of decompensated thyrotoxicosis. The patient has **tachycardia** (>140 bpm), **fever** (104°F-106°F), **agitation, delirium, restlessness or psychosis, vomiting, and/or diarrhea**. It usually results from untreated hyperthyroidism to which a complicating event (intercurrent illness: infection, surgery, trauma, or iodine load) is added. Treatment includes supportive care with fluids, antibiotics if needed, and specific treatment directed at the hyperthyroidism.

- Antithyroid medications to block new hormone synthesis
- Iodine solution to block the release of thyroid hormone

- Propranolol to control the symptoms induced by the increased adrenergic tone

- Glucocorticoids to decrease T_4 to triiodothyronine (T_3) conversion

Etiology of Thyrotoxicosis

Graves disease is the most common cause of hyperthyroidism (80%) and usually is seen in women, especially between the ages of 30 and 50 years. It is an autoimmune disease caused by autoantibodies that activate the TSH receptor of the thyroid follicular cell, stimulating thyroid hormone synthesis and secretion as well as thyroid gland growth. In the pregnant patient, these antibodies cross the placenta and can cause neonatal thyrotoxicosis. The disease might follow a relapsing and remitting course.

Graves disease is marked by **goiter** (enlarged thyroid gland), thyroid bruit, **hyperthyroidism, ophthalmopathy, and dermopathy.** These features are variably present. Ophthalmopathy is characterized by inflammation of extraocular muscles, orbital fat, and connective tissue, resulting in proptosis (exophthalmos), sometimes with impairment of eye muscle function (diplopia), and periorbital edema. Ophthalmopathy can progress even after treatment of thyrotoxicosis. Graves dermopathy is characterized by raised hyperpigmented orange peel texture papules. The most common site is the skin overlying the shins (pretibial myxedema). A low serum TSH will confirm the diagnosis. The degree of elevation of serum-free T_4 and free T_3 levels can give an estimate of the severity of the disease. Tests that might be helpful in determining the etiology of thyrotoxicosis are the levels of thyroid-stimulating immunoglobulin (TSI), which is elevated in Graves; thyroid peroxidase (TPO) antibodies, which are markers of autoimmunity in both Graves and Hashimoto thyroiditis; and a **thyroid uptake and scan, which will reveal a diffusely elevated iodine uptake in our patient.**

Treatment options for Graves disease are medications, radioactive iodine, or surgery. Medications include **beta-blockers** such as propranolol (which are used for symptom relief) and **antithyroid drugs** such as **methimazole** and **propylthiouracil (PTU).** The antithyroid drugs work mainly by decreasing the production of thyroid hormone. They can be used for short-term (prior to treatment with radioactive iodine or surgery) or long-term (1-2 years) treatment, after which the chance for remission is 20% to 30%. Possible side effects are rash, allergic reactions, arthritis, hepatitis, and agranulocytosis. **Radioactive iodine** is usually the treatment of choice in the United States for nonpregnant patients. It is administered as an oral solution of sodium ^{131}I that is rapidly concentrated in thyroid tissue, inducing damage that results in ablation of the thyroid, depending on the dose, within 6 to 18 weeks. At least 30% of patients will become hypothyroid in the first year after treatment and 3% each year after that, requiring thyroid hormone supplementation. Radioactive iodine is contraindicated in pregnancy, and women of reproductive age are advised to postpone pregnancy for 6 to 12 months after treatment. Pregnant women with Graves can be managed with PTU, as it has a low transplacental transfer. Graves ophthalmopathy might be exacerbated by radioactive iodine treatment, so glucocorticoids can be used to prevent this in selected patients.

Subtotal thyroidectomy usually is reserved for large goiters with obstructive symptoms (dyspnea, dysphagia). Possible complications include laryngeal nerve injury and hypoparathyroidism (due to removal of parathyroids or compromise of the vascular supply to them).

For our patient, treatment with radioactive iodine or antithyroid medications seems the most reasonable way to proceed, and a discussion regarding her options and our recommendations should take place after the diagnosis is confirmed, and nonpregnant status is confirmed.

Other causes of thyrotoxicosis include the following:

Toxic multinodular goiter: Found mainly in elderly and middle-age patients. Treatment consists of radioactive iodine or surgery. Radioactive iodine uptake is normal to increased, and the scan reveals irregular thyroid lobes and a heterogeneous pattern.

Autonomous hyperfunctioning adenoma ("hot nodule" or Plummer disease): Hyperthyroidism usually is not present unless the nodule is more than 3 cm. The iodine scan looks like the flag of Japan: it demonstrates the hot nodule as having increased uptake (dark) and the rest of the gland with suppressed uptake (white). **Hot nodules are almost never malignant.** Cold nodules (no increased thyroid hormone production and no demonstration of local uptake if thyroid scan is performed) have a 5% to 10% risk of malignancy, so fine-needle aspiration, surgical removal, or ultrasonographic follow-up is needed for these nodules.

Thyroiditis: Caused by destruction of thyroid tissue and release of preformed hormone from the colloid space. Subacute (de Quervain) thyroiditis is an inflammatory viral illness with thyroid pain and tenderness. The hyperthyroid phase lasts for several weeks to months, followed by recovery, but some patients will then develop hypothyroidism. Treatment with nonsteroidal anti-inflammatory medications and beta-blockers usually is sufficient, but in severe cases, glucocorticoids might be used. Other forms include postradiation, postpartum, subacute (painless thyroiditis), and amiodarone-induced thyroiditis. In thyroiditis, the radioactive iodine uptake is decreased.

Medications: Excessive ingestion of thyroid hormone (factitious or iatrogenic), amiodarone, and iodine load.

CASE CORRELATION

- See also Case 41 (Urosepsis), Case 52 (Diabetic Ketoacidosis), and Case 59 (Delirium and Alcohol Withdrawal),

COMPREHENSION QUESTIONS

53.1 A 44-year-old woman is noted to be nervous and has heat intolerance. Her thyroid gland is diffusely enlarged, nontender, with an audible bruit. Her TSH level is very low. Which of the following is the most likely etiology?

A. Lymphocytic thyroiditis

B. Hashimoto thyroiditis

C. Graves disease

D. Multinodular toxic goiter

53.2 Which of the following distinguishes hyperthyroidism from thyroid storm?

A. Tachycardia to heart rate 120 bpm

B. Weight loss

C. Fever and delirium

D. Large goiter

53.3 A 58-year-old woman is noted to have Graves disease and has a small goiter. Which of the following is the best therapy?

A. Long-term propranolol

B. Lifelong oral propylthiouracil (PTU)

C. Radioactive iodine ablation

D. Surgical thyroidectomy

ANSWERS

53.1 **C.** Graves disease is the most common cause of hyperthyroidism in the United States. It often includes the thyroid gland features described, as well as the distinctive eye findings.

53.2 **C.** Thyroid storm is an exaggeration of hyperthyroid features with extreme tachycardia (heart rate >140 bpm), fever, and central nervous system dysfunction, such as confusion or coma. It is a medical emergency with a high mortality.

53.3 **C.** Radioactive iodine is a definitive treatment for Graves disease. Surgery is indicated for obstructive symptoms, or for women during pregnancy. Propranolol is a good initial option to control tachycardia but not a long term option. PTU is a second line option due to the risk of hepatocellular necrosis.

CLINICAL PEARLS

▶ The most common cause of thyrotoxicosis is Graves disease. No other diagnosis is likely if the patient has bilateral proptosis and a goiter.

▶ In patients with Graves disease, thyrotoxic symptoms may be treated with antithyroid medication or by thyroid gland ablation with radioactive iodine or surgery, but the ophthalmopathy may not improve.

▶ Graves disease may remit and relapse; in patients treated medically, one-third to half will become asymptomatic within 1-2 years.

▶ After radioactive iodine ablation, most patients with Graves disease become hypothyroid and will require thyroid hormone supplementation.

▶ Hyperfunctioning thyroid nodules (excessive thyroid hormone production, suppressed thyroid-stimulating hormone, "hot" on radionuclide scan) almost never are malignant.

▶ Most "cold" thyroid nodules are not malignant, but fine-needle aspiration should be used to evaluate the need for surgical excision.

REFERENCES

Davies DF, Larsen TF. Thyrotoxicosis. In: Wilson JD, Foster DW, Kronenberg HM, et al., eds. *Williams Textbook of Endocrinology*. 9th ed. Philadelphia, PA: WB Saunders; 2003:372-421.

Hershman JM. Hypothyroidism and hyperthyroidism. In: Lavin N, ed. *Manual of Endocrinology and Metabolism*. 4th ed. Boston, MA: Little Brown; 2009:435-448.

Jameson LJ, Weetman AP. Disorders of the thyroid gland. In: Kasper DL, Fauci AS, Hauser SL, et al., eds. *Harrison's Principles of Internal Medicine*. 19th ed. New York, NY: McGraw-Hill; 2015: 2283-2308.

McDermott MT. Thyroid emergencies. In: *Endocrine Secrets*. 6th ed. Philadelphia, PA: Hanley and Belfus; 2013:309-313.

Singer PA. Thyroiditis. In: Lavin N, ed. *Manual of Endocrinology and Metabolism*. Boston, MA: Little Brown; 2002:386-395.

A healthy 52-year-old man presents to the doctor's office complaining of increasing fatigue for the past 4 to 5 months. He exercises every day, but lately he has noticed becoming short of breath while jogging. He denies orthopnea, paroxysmal nocturnal dyspnea (PND), or swelling in his ankles. The patient reports occasional joint pain, for which he uses over-the-counter ibuprofen. He denies bowel changes, melena, or bright red blood per rectum, but he reports vague left-sided abdominal pain for a few months off and on, not related to food intake. The patient denies fever, chills, nausea, or vomiting. He has lost a few pounds intentionally with diet and exercise.

On examination, he weighs 205 lb, and he is afebrile. There is slight pallor of the conjunctiva, skin, and palms. No lymphadenopathy is noted. Chest is clear to auscultation bilaterally. Examination of the cardiovascular system reveals a regular rate and rhythm, with no rub or gallop. There is a systolic ejection murmur. His abdomen is soft, nontender, with no hepatosplenomegaly. Bowel sounds are present. He has no extremity edema, cyanosis, or clubbing. His peripheral pulses are palpable and symmetric. Hemoglobin level is 8.2 g/dL.

► What is the most likely diagnosis?
► What is your next diagnostic step?

ANSWERS TO CASE 54:

Iron Deficiency Anemia

Summary: A healthy 52-year-old man complains of a 4- to 5-month history of increasing exercise intolerance, but he denies orthopnea, PND, edema, or other indications of heart failure. The patient uses a nonsteroidal anti-inflammatory drug (NSAID) regularly. He has not had any overt gastrointestinal (GI) blood loss. On examination, he has slight pallor of the conjunctiva, skin, and palms. He is anemic, with a hemoglobin level of 8.2 g/dL.

- **Most likely diagnosis:** Iron deficiency anemia as a result of chronic blood loss.

- **Next diagnostic step:** Analyze the complete blood count (CBC), particularly the mean corpuscular volume (MCV), to determine if the anemia is microcytic, normocytic, or macrocytic; assess the leukocyte count and platelet count.

ANALYSIS

Objectives

1. Understand that iron deficiency anemia is the most common cause of anemia.

2. Know the diagnostic approach to anemia.

3. Be familiar with the treatment of iron deficiency anemia.

Considerations

This 52-year-old man presents to the doctor's office with complaints of fatigue and dyspnea on exertion for the few months prior to the office visit. His physical examination is significant only for pallor. The serum hemoglobin level confirms anemia. The next step would be to characterize the anemia as microcytic, which would be consistent with iron deficiency, and confirm with further testing for total iron-binding capacity (TIBC) and ferritin. The most likely source of blood loss in male patients is the GI tract; therefore, finding iron deficiency anemia should suggest the presence of a possible GI source of bleeding, with colon cancer the most serious possibility. This patient is using an NSAID, which may predispose to erosive gastritis. Once iron deficiency anemia is confirmed, a thorough evaluation of the GI tract, including upper and lower endoscopy, is needed.

APPROACH TO:

Suspected Iron Deficiency Anemia

DEFINITIONS

ANEMIA: Decreased red blood cell (RBC) mass, leading to less oxygen-carrying capacity. Anemia is defined as a hemoglobin levels less than 13 g/dL in men, and less than 12 g/dL in women.

IRON STUDIES: Ferritin is a marker of iron stores, but it also is an acute-phase reactant, which is decreased in iron deficiency, but increased with inflammatory chronic diseases. The TIBC is an indirect measure of transferrin saturation levels and is increased in iron deficiency.

MEAN CORPUSCULAR VOLUME (MCV): Average RBC volume. This offers a method of categorizing anemias as microcytic (MCV <80 fL), normocytic (MCV 80-100 fL), and macrocytic (MCV >100 fL).

RETICULOCYTE: New RBC that usually is 1 to 1.5 days old.

RETICULOCYTE COUNT: Fraction of RBCs consisting of reticulocytes that indirectly indicates the bone marrow activity of the erythrocyte line. It usually is expressed as a percentage and normally is 1%; corrected reticulocyte count accounts for anemia.

CLINICAL APPROACH

Iron Deficiency

Although anemia may be caused by disorders of bone marrow production, red cell maturation, or increased destruction, iron deficiency is the most common cause of anemia in the United States, affecting all ages and both genders. Iron is essential to the synthesis of hemoglobin. The normal daily intake of elemental iron is approximately 15 mg, of which only 1 to 2 mg is absorbed. The daily iron losses are about the same, but menstruation adds approximately 30 mg of iron lost each month. The primary etiology for iron deficiency anemia is blood loss (Table 54–1). **In men, the most frequent cause is chronic GI tract occult bleeding.** In women, menstrual loss may be the main mechanism, but other sites must be considered. Supplemental iron is especially necessary during pregnancy because of iron transfer from the mother to the developing fetus. Iron deficiency may also be a result of increased iron requirements, diminished iron absorption, or both. Iron deficiency can develop during the first 2 years of life if dietary iron is inadequate for the demands of rapid growth. Adolescent girls may become iron deficient from inadequate diet plus the added loss from menstruation. The growth spurt in adolescent boys may also produce a significant increase in demand for iron. Other possible causes of anemia are decreased iron absorption after gastrectomy or malabsorption syndromes, such as celiac disease, but such mechanisms are less common than blood loss.

When iron loss exceeds intake, iron deposits are progressively depleted. Hemoglobin and serum iron levels may remain normal in the initial stages, but the **serum ferritin** level (iron stores) will start to fall. As serum iron levels fall, the percent of transferrin saturation falls and the **TIBC will increase,** leading to a progressive decrease in iron available for RBC formation. At this point, anemia will develop initially with normal-appearing RBCs. As the iron deficiency becomes more severe, microcytosis and hypochromia will develop. Later in the disease process, iron deficiency will affect other tissues, resulting in a variety of symptoms and signs.

Anemia is most often diagnosed on a routine laboratory test, and patients are often asymptomatic. More severe anemia may produce symptoms such as fatigue, shortness of breath, dizziness, headache, palpitations, and impaired concentration.

Table 54–1 • COMMON CAUSES OF IRON-DEFICIENCY ANEMIA
BLOOD LOSS
Gastrointestinal blood loss
• Esophageal varices
• Peptic ulcer disease
• Gastritis, eg, NSAID induced
• Small bowel polyp or carcinoma
• Colonic angiodysplasia
• Colon cancer
• Inflammatory bowel disease, eg, ulcerative colitis
• Hookworm infestation
Uterine blood loss
• Menstruation/menorrhagia
• Uterine fibroids
Other blood loss
• Chronic hemodialysis
• Surgical blood loss
• Repeated blood donation or phlebotomy
• Paroxysmal nocturnal hemoglobinuria
MALABSORPTION
• Gastrectomy
• Celiac disease
• Inflammatory bowel disease, eg, Crohn disease
INADEQUATE DIETARY INTAKE/INCREASED PHYSIOLOGIC DEMANDS
• Infancy/adolescence
• Pregnancy
• Vegetarian diet

Additionally, patients with chronic severe iron deficiency may develop **cravings for dirt, paint (pica), or ice (pagophagia), and is also linked to restless legs syndrome.** Glossitis, cheilosis, or koilonychia may develop, and in rare cases, dysphagia associated with a postcricoid **esophageal web (Plummer-Vinson syndrome)** may occur. When the anemia develops over a long period, the typical symptoms of fatigue and shortness of breath may not be evident. Many patients with iron deficiency anemia may be asymptomatic. The lack of symptoms reflects the very slow development of iron deficiency and the ability of the body to adapt to lower iron reserves and anemia.

Evaluation of Anemia

Once anemia is discovered, a CBC with differential, platelets, and RBC indices are helpful in narrowing the differential diagnosis. The first step is to look at the **MCV** to classify the common causes of anemia (Table 54–2). Iron deficiency usually leads to a microcytic anemia. The red blood cell distribution width (RDW) is a calculated index that quantitates the variation in the size of RBCs. RDW is a quantitative measure of anisocytosis (variation in cell size) that helps to distinguish uncomplicated iron deficiencies from uncomplicated thalassemia. An increased RDW associated with microcytic anemia is suggestive of iron deficiency anemia, because the bone marrow produces new erythrocytes of various sizes. A normal

Table 54–2 • CLASSIFICATION OF ANEMIA BY MCV
Microcytic (low MCV) • Iron deficiency • Thalassemia • Sideroblastic anemia • Lead poisoning
Normocytic (normal MCV) • Acute blood loss • Hemolysis • Anemia of chronic disease • Anemia of renal failure • Myelodysplastic syndromes
Macrocytic anemia (high MCV) • Folate deficiency • Vitamin B_{12} deficiency • Drug toxicity, eg, zidovudine • Alcoholism/chronic liver disease

RDW in the presence of microcytic anemia may be more suggestive of chronic disease, thalassemia, or even iron deficiency with concomitant anemia of chronic disease. A detailed history, physical examination, and further laboratory data may be necessary to achieve a final diagnosis.

The **reticulocyte count** is another important parameter to help in the differential diagnosis of anemia. A new RBC can be stained as a reticulocyte for 24 to 36 hours, after which the RBC circulates for approximately 120 days. The blood normally contains about 1 reticulocyte per 100 RBCs. The reticulocyte count, usually reported as a percentage of reticulocytes per 100 RBCs, may be falsely elevated in the presence of anemia. Therefore, a corrected reticulocyte percentage is calculated by multiplying the reported reticulocyte count by the patient's hematocrit divided by 45 (normal hematocrit). The reticulocyte may also be converted to an absolute number by multiplying the reported reticulocyte count by the RBC count and dividing by 100. The absolute reticulocyte count is normally 50,000 to 70,000 reticulocytes/mm^3. If the **reticulocyte count is low,** causes of **hypoproliferative bone marrow** disorders should be suspected. A **high reticulocyte count** may reflect **acute blood losses, hemolysis,** or a response to therapy for anemia.

Iron studies are very helpful to confirm a diagnosis of iron deficiency anemia and to help in the differential diagnosis with other types of anemia, such as anemia of chronic disease and sideroblastic anemia (Table 54–3). A low **serum ferritin concentration is a reliable indication of iron deficiency.** Serum **ferritin values are increased with chronic inflammatory disease,** malignancy, or liver injury; therefore, serum ferritin concentration may be above normal when iron deficiency exists with chronic diseases, such as rheumatoid arthritis, Hodgkin disease, or hepatitis, among many other disorders. Measurement of serum iron concentration, serum TIBC, and calculation of percent saturation of transferrin have been widely used for diagnosis of iron deficiency. **True iron deficiency** is strongly suspected on the basis of **low serum iron level** and **normal or high binding capacity,** which will result in a low calculated

Table 54-3 • CHARACTERISTICS OF MICROCYTIC ANEMIAS

Tests	Iron Deficiency	Chronic Disease	Thalassemia	Sideroblastic Anemia
Smear	Microcytic/ hypochromic	Normal microcytic/ hypochromic	Microcytic/ hypochromic with targeting	Variable
Serum iron (µg/dL)	<30	<50	Normal to high	Normal to high
TIBC (µg/dL)	>360	<300	Normal	Normal
Percent saturation (%)	<10	10-20	30-80	30-80
Ferritin (µg/L)	<15	30-200	50-300	50-300
Hemoglobin electrophoresis	Normal	Normal	Abnormal	Normal

Abbreviations: SI, serum iron; TIBC, total iron-binding capacity.
(Reproduced, with permission, from Adamson JW. Iron deficiency and other hypoproliferative anemias. In: Braunwald E, Fauci AS, Kasper KL, et al, Harrison's Principles of Internal Medicine, 17th ed. New York: McGraw-Hill, 2008:632.)

transferrin saturation. In anemia of **chronic disease, serum iron concentration is low, but the TIBC is usually also reduced**; therefore, percent transferrin saturation is typically normal. **Chronic inflammatory diseases typically cause elevation in serum ferritin concentration.** When chronic disease and iron deficiency anemia coexist, serum ferritin concentration may be normal. Sideroblastic anemia is a disease where the bone marrow produces abnormal RBCs, commonly microcytic and hypochromic. The iron studies in **sideroblastic anemia** include **increases in serum iron and serum ferritin concentration and saturation of transferrin.** An important clue to the presence of sideroblastic anemia is the presence of **stippled RBCs** in the peripheral blood smear. Iron stain in the bone marrow reveals the pathognomonic feature of engorged mitochondria in the developing RBCs called **ringed sideroblasts.**

Evaluating the peripheral blood smear for specific abnormalities in RBC morphology may be very useful for determining the etiology of anemia. In iron deficiency anemia, the peripheral blood smear shows RBCs smaller than normal (microcytes) and hypochromia.

Although the treatment of iron deficiency is straightforward, finding the underlying etiology is paramount. Treatment of iron deficiency anemia consists of iron replacement therapy, typically with **oral ferrous sulfate 325 mg two or three times daily, which provides 150 to 200 mg elemental iron.** Other iron preparations such as ferrous fumarate or ferrous gluconate can also be used, and are equally effective. Correction of anemia usually occurs **within 6 weeks**, but therapy should continue for at least 6 months to replenish the iron stores. Oral iron therapy may cause GI side effects, such as constipation, nausea, and abdominal cramping. Taking the iron with meals may help with tolerance but can reduce absorption. Failure of iron deficiency anemia to improve with oral iron supplementation suggests nonadherence to therapy, possible coexisting disease interfering with marrow response (eg, coexisting folate or B_{12} deficiency), or malabsorption of iron (celiac sprue, atrophic gastritis).

Parenteral iron therapy is indicated in rare instances, such as in patients with a poor absorption state (occurs in celiac disease, chronic kidney disease) or with excessive intolerance to oral therapy. Caution must be taken with parenteral high-molecular weight iron dextran because **anaphylaxis** may occur, but newer parenteral iron compounds are now available with lower rates of adverse events.

It should be emphasized that after diagnosis of iron deficiency is established, the cause of the iron loss should be identified. Except in menstruating women, the most common site of blood loss is the GI tract, and **most patients will require endoscopic evaluation**. Gastritis, peptic ulcers, and angiodysplasia are all common sources of blood loss, but the most serious diagnosis to exclude would be the possibility of an occult GI malignancy. Fecal occult blood testing (FOBT), such as stool guaiac tests, should not substitute for endoscopic evaluation, as even high-sensitivity FOBT have only 50% to 80% sensitivity for colorectal cancer.

CASE CORRELATION

- See Case 55 (Transfusion Medicine), Case 56 (ITP), Case 57 (Lymphocytosis), and Case 58 (Sickle Cell Anemia).

COMPREHENSION QUESTIONS

54.1 A 25-year-old man with a history of a duodenal ulcer is noted to have a hemoglobin level of 10 g/dL. He does not report any visible GI blood loss. Which of the following most likely will be seen on laboratory investigation?

A. Reticulocyte count of 4%

B. Elevated total iron-binding capacity

C. Normal serum ferritin

D. Mean corpuscular volume of 105 fL

54.2 A 22-year-old woman is pregnant and at 14-week gestation. Her hemoglobin level is 9 g/dL. She asks why she could have iron deficiency when she is no longer menstruating. Which of the following is the best explanation?

A. Occult gastrointestinal blood loss

B. Expanded blood volume and transport to the fetus

C. Hemolysis

D. Iron losses as a result of relative alkalosis of pregnancy

54.3 A 35-year-old man has undertaken a strict fad diet for 3 months. He previously had been healthy but now complains of fatigue. His hemoglobin level is 10 g/dL, and his MCV is 105 fL. Which of the following is the most likely etiology of his anemia?

A. Iron deficiency

B. Folate deficiency

C. Vitamin B_{12} deficiency

D. Thalassemia

E. Sideroblastic anemia

For the following questions (54.4-54.6) choose the laboratory parameter (A-E) that matches the clinical picture.

MCV	Ferritin	TIBC	RDW
A. Increased	Decreased	Increased	Decreased
B. Decreased	Decreased	Increased	Increased
C. Normal	Increased	Normal	Normal
D. Decreased	Increased	Normal	Normal
E. Increased	Increased	Decreased	Increased

54.4 A 20-year-old woman with heavy menses

54.5 A 34-year-old man of Mediterranean descent with a family history of anemia

54.6 A 50-year-old man with severe rheumatoid arthritis

ANSWERS

54.1 **B.** Chronic gastrointestinal blood loss leads to low ferritin levels reflecting diminished iron stores, elevated TIBC, and low iron saturation. There is a microcytic anemia (low MCV) with a low reticulocyte count. The reticulocyte count would be elevated with acute blood loss, but the patient has not experienced this.

54.2 **B.** Iron deficiency occurs in pregnancy as a result of the expanded blood volume and active transport of iron to the fetus.

54.3 **B.** Macrocytic anemia is usually a result of folate or vitamin B_{12} deficiency. Because vitamin B_{12} stores last for nearly 10 years, a dietary change of several months would more likely cause folate deficiency. Also vitamin B_{12} deficiency can lead to neurologic symptoms. Folate is found in green leafy vegetables. Iron deficiency, thalassemias, and sideroblastic anemias will likely be microcytic with a MCV <80.

54.4 **B.** This laboratory finding is diagnostic of iron deficiency anemia (microcytic, low ferritin, high TIBC, high RDW).

54.5 **D.** Thalassemia usually leads to a microcytic anemia with uniform red cell size (normal RDW) and excess iron stores.

54.6 **C.** Chronic disease generally leads to a normocytic anemia with elevated ferritin level (acute-phase reactant); although a microcytic anemia can also be seen, a normocytic anemia is more common.

CLINICAL PEARLS

▶ Anemia is a clinical finding, not a diagnosis, and requires some investigation to determine the underlying etiology.

▶ Iron deficiency anemia in men or postmenopausal women is primarily a result of gastrointestinal blood losses; therefore, finding iron deficiency anemia in this patient population warrants a thorough gastrointestinal workup.

▶ Iron deficiency anemia in women of reproductive age is most often caused by menstrual blood loss.

▶ Fecal occult blood testing is negative in approximately 20% to 50% of patients with colorectal cancer. Therefore, a negative fecal occult blood test in the presence of iron deficiency anemia should not discourage you from pursuing a thorough gastrointestinal workup.

▶ The mean corpuscular volume, red blood cell distribution width, and reticulocyte index are important parameters in the evaluation of anemia.

REFERENCES

Adamson JW. Iron deficiency and other hypoproliferative anemias. In: Kasper DL, Fauci AS, Hauser SL, et al., eds. *Harrison's Principles of Internal Medicine.* 19th ed. New York, NY: McGraw-Hill; 2015:625-631.

Adamson JW, Longo DL. Anemia and polycythemia. In: Kasper DL, Fauci AS, Hauser SL, et al., eds. *Harrison's Principles of Internal Medicine.* 19th ed. New York, NY: McGraw-Hill; 2015:392-400.

Cook JD, Skikne BS. Iron deficiency: definition and diagnosis. *J Intern Med.* 1989;226:349-355.

Weiss G, Goodnough LT. Anemia of chronic disease. *N Engl J Med.* 2005;352:1011-1023.

A 62-year-old man presents to the emergency center with the sudden onset of abdominal discomfort and passage of several large, black, tarry stools. He became diaphoretic and began to experience chest pain, similar to that of his recent myocardial infarction. Three weeks ago, he suffered an uncomplicated non-ST-elevation myocardial infarction (NSTEMI). Coronary angiography performed prior to discharge revealed no significant coronary artery stenosis. He was discharged home with aspirin, clopidogrel, atorvastatin, and metoprolol. On examination, his heart rate is 104 bpm. His blood pressure is 124/92 mm Hg while lying down but drops to 95/70 mm Hg upon standing. He appears pale and uncomfortable, and he is covered with a fine layer of sweat. His neck veins are flat, his chest is clear to auscultation, and his heart rhythm is tachycardic but regular, with a soft systolic murmur at the right sternal border and an S_4 gallop. His apical impulse is focal and nondisplaced. His abdomen is soft with active bowel sounds and mild epigastric tenderness, but there is no guarding or rebound tenderness, and no masses or organomegaly are appreciated. Rectal examination shows black, sticky stool, which is strongly positive for occult blood. His hemoglobin level is 5.9 g/dL, prothrombin time (PT) and partial thromboplastin time (PTT) both are normal, and he has normal renal function and liver function tests. Electrocardiogram (ECG) reveals sinus tachycardia with no ST-segment changes, T-wave inversion in the anterior precordial leads and no ventricular ectopy. Creatine kinase (CK) is 127 U/L with a normal CK-MB (myocardial) fraction, and troponin I levels are normal.

▶ What is the most likely diagnosis?
▶ What is your next step?

ANSWERS TO CASE 55:
Transfusion Medicine

Summary: A man with a recent myocardial infarction but no critical coronary artery stenosis on a coronary angiogram is admitted with angina pectoris at rest and ECG changes consistent with recurrent cardiac ischemia. In addition, he has melena and epigastric tenderness, indicating an upper gastrointestinal (GI) hemorrhage, likely caused by his use of antiplatelet agents. He is tachycardic and has orthostatic hypotension, likely indicating significant hypovolemia as a result of blood loss.

- **Most likely diagnosis:** Unstable angina (UA), which has been precipitated by anemia because of acute GI blood loss.

- **Next step:** Transfusion with packed red blood cells (PRBCs).

ANALYSIS
Objectives

1. Understand the indications for transfusion of red blood cells.
2. Know the complications of transfusions.
3. Be aware of alternatives to transfusion.
4. Know the indications for transfusion of platelets and of fresh frozen plasma (FFP).

Considerations

This patient has two urgent problems. He has suffered an upper GI hemorrhage with enough blood loss to cause hemodynamic compromise. In addition, he has unstable angina, given his severe prolonged chest pain at rest but lack of definitive ECG or cardiac biomarker evidence of myocardial infarction. Rather than being a primary problem with his coronary arteries, such as thrombosis or vasospasm, the cardiac ischemia is likely secondary to his acute blood loss and consequent tachycardia and loss of hemoglobin and its oxygen-carrying capacity. He should be treated with urgent replacement of blood volume.

APPROACH TO:
Symptomatic Anemia

DEFINITIONS

UNSTABLE ANGINA: Angina pectoris or equivalent ischemic discomfort occurring at rest, or severe and new onset, or in a crescendo pattern.

NON-ST-ELEVATION MYOCARDIAL INFARCTION: Clinical features of unstable angina, but with evidence of myocardial necrosis, seen in elevated cardiac biomarkers.

TRALI: Transfusion-related acute lung injury, due to an immune-mediated lung injury.

ACUTE HEMOLYTIC REACTION: Transfusion reaction due to antibody lysis of transfused red blood cells.

CLINICAL APPROACH

Symptoms attributable to anemia are manifold and depend primarily on the patient's underlying cardiopulmonary status and the chronicity with which the anemia developed. For a slowly developing, chronic anemia in patients with good cardiopulmonary reserve, symptoms may not be noted until the hemoglobin level falls very low, for example, to 3 or 4 g/dL. For patients with serious underlying cardiopulmonary disease who depend on adequate oxygen-carrying capacity, smaller declines in hemoglobin level can be devastating. Such is the case with the man in this clinical scenario, who is suffering a cardiac complication as a consequence of his anemia, in this case, unstable angina.

Unstable angina is characterized by ischemic chest pain at rest, of new onset, or occurring at a lower level of activity. Unstable angina is distinguished from NSTEMI or STEMI in that UA does not cause elevated levels of cardiac biomarkers or ST-segment elevation on ECG. Patients who present with UA or NSTEMI vary widely in their risk of death or recurrent infarction at 30 days, so they benefit from a risk-stratification assessment to guide their initial treatment and evaluation. Data from the Thrombolysis in Myocardial Infarction (TIMI) trials provided a simple and useful clinical risk scoring system. Seven independent risk factors are assessed: age >65, three or more risk factors for coronary artery disease (CAD), >50% coronary stenosis on angiography, ST deviation, two or more anginal episodes in 24 hours, symptoms despite the use of aspirin, or elevated cardiac biomarkers. Patients with higher TIMI risk scores are often treated with more aggressive antithrombotic therapy or with early coronary angiography within 48 hours of admission, and possible revascularization, if the coronary anatomy is suitable. - not sure with comma placement if revascularization is treatment with antithrombotics or with coronary angiography or both.

For this patient who had suffered a recent NSTEMI, no apparent critical coronary artery stenosis was found on angiography, which is the case in 10% of patients with UA or NSTEMI. He had been treated with medical management, including dual antiplatelet therapy with aspirin and clopidogrel. In this case, it is more likely that his angina is secondary to the acute drop in hemoglobin rather than new cardiac disease.

In this case of secondary angina, the anemia must be corrected, which requires an understanding of transfusion medicine. Anemia is generally considered to be a hemoglobin level less than 12 g/dL in women or less than 13 g/dL in men. Although lower values often can be tolerated or underlying etiologies treated, blood transfusions have been both necessary and lifesaving at times. In addition to PRBCs, there are other components of whole blood, including platelets, FFP, cryoprecipitate, and intravenous immunoglobulin (IVIg). Indications for use of each of these blood components are described below.

Indications for transfusion of PRBCs are acute surgical or nonsurgical blood loss, anemia with end-organ effects (eg, syncope, angina pectoris) or hemodynamic compromise, and in critical illness to improve oxygen-carrying capacity or delivery to tissues. However, there are no absolute guidelines or thresholds for transfusion. Many believe that a hemoglobin level of 7 g/dL is adequate in the absence of a clearly defined increased need, such as cardiac ischemia, for which a hematocrit level of at least 30% may be desired. In the absence of ongoing bleeding or destruction of red cells, we typically expect that **each unit of PRBC will result in an increase of 1 g/dL in the hemoglobin level or 3% in the hematocrit level.**

Transfusion carries a small but definite risk, including transmission of infection, reactions, and consequences. Viruses that are screened for but that can be passed include hepatitis C virus (1 in 103,000 units), human T-cell lymphocyte virus types I and II, human immunodeficiency virus (1 in 700,000), hepatitis B virus (1 in 66,000), and parvovirus B19. Rarely, bacterial contamination (eg, *Yersinia enterocolitica*) causes fevers, sepsis, and even death during or soon after transfusion. Parasites (eg, malaria) are screened for by questioning a donor's medical and travel history.

There are also noninfectious concerns, both immune and nonimmune mediated. With respect to immune mechanisms, it is possible that a recipient has preformed natural antibodies that lyse foreign donor erythrocytes, which can be associated with the major A and/or B or O blood types or with other antigens (eg, D, Duffy, Kidd). Because hemolysis can ensue, a "type and cross" is first performed, in which blood samples are tested for compatibility prior to transfusion. The most common cause of this reaction actually is clerical (ie, mislabeling). **Acute hemolytic reactions** may present with **hypotension, fever, chills, hemoglobinuria,** and **flank pain.** The transfusion must be halted immediately, and fluid and diuretics (or even dialysis) should be given to protect the kidney from failure via immune-complex deposits. Laboratory work for intravascular hemolysis should be checked (lactate dehydrogenase [LDH], indirect bilirubin, haptoglobin), as well as coagulation tests for disseminated intravascular coagulopathy (DIC). Less predictably, milder, delayed hemolytic reactions involving amnestic responses from the recipient can occur. Febrile nonhemolytic transfusion reactions can occur and may be helped by antipyretics. Reactions range from urticaria treated with diphenhydramine and transfusion interruption to anaphylaxis, in which case the transfusion must be stopped, and epinephrine and steroids are needed. Sometimes seen is transfusion-related acute lung injury (TRALI), in which the appearance of bilateral interstitial infiltrates in the lung represents noncardiogenic pulmonary edema.

Considering nonimmune consequences, the transfusion itself supplies 300 mL per unit of PRBC intravascularly, so patients can easily become volume overloaded. Adjusting the volume and rate and using diuretics will prevent this complication. Each unit of blood also provides 250 mg of iron. Multiple and frequent transfusions can cause iron overload and deposition (hemosiderosis), leading to cirrhosis, cardiac problems (eg, arrhythmia, heart failure), or diabetes.

Alternatives to transfusion have shown a role for **erythropoietin**, a hormone that promotes red cell production. It is often used in the treatment of patients with **renal failure**-related anemia. It also can be used in patients who are banking a pre-surgical autologous transfusion to encourage quicker recovery of their hemoglobin levels prior to surgery. Cell savers salvage some intraoperative blood losses, which are then transfused back into the patient. Some patients may not wish to have foreign blood products transfused based on religious convictions. In these cases, we can increase the baseline hemoglobin level by using erythropoietin and iron before planned surgery, minimize phlebotomy for laboratory testing, and use cell savers during surgery. Ultimately, however, a competent patient's wishes are to be respected.

Thrombocytopenia can frequently be treated with platelet transfusion. When a patient has a platelet count of less than $50,000/mm^3$ and has significant bleeding, or when a patient is at risk for spontaneous bleeding with a level of less than $10,000/mm^3$, platelets can be transfused. Each unit increases the platelet count from 5000 to $10,000/mm^3$. In cases such as immune thrombocytopenic purpura (ITP), in which platelets are being destroyed, however, transfusion is generally not helpful unless active bleeding is occurring. Platelet transfusion is contraindicated in patients with thrombotic thrombocytopenic purpura (TTP), as it may worsen microvascular thrombosis and cause worsening neurologic symptoms or renal failure.

FFP replaces clotting factors and is often given to reverse **warfarin (Coumadin)** **anticoagulation**. Cryoprecipitate from FFP replaces fibrinogen and some clotting factors, making it useful in patients with hemophilia A and von Willebrand disease (vWD).

IVIg (pooled polyvalent IgG) is administered to patients with immune deficiencies with low antibody levels, as well as to patients with antibody-mediated autoimmunity, such as immune (idiopathic) thrombocytopenic purpura, or as an immunomodulatory agent in Kawasaki disease. One caution is that in patients with IgA deficiency (1 in 600 individuals of European origin), transfusion with IVIg or FFP can cause anaphylaxis because of the presence of anti-IgA antibodies.

CASE CORRELATION

- See also Case 3 (Myocardial Infarction), Case 54 (Iron Deficiency Anemia), Case 56 (ITP), Case 57 (Lymphocytosis), and Case 58 (Sickle Cell Anemia).

COMPREHENSION QUESTIONS

55.1 A 32-year-old man is brought into the emergency room after a motor vehicle accident. He is noted to be in hypovolemic shock with a blood pressure of 60/40 mm Hg. He is actively bleeding from a femur fracture. The patient's hemoglobin level is 7 g/dL. His wife is positive that the patient's blood type is A positive. Which of the following is the most appropriate type of blood to be transfused?

A. Give AB-positive blood, uncross-matched.

B. Await cross-matched A-positive blood.

C. Give type-specific A-positive blood, uncross-matched.

D. Give O-negative blood, uncross-matched.

55.2 A 45-year-old woman is noted to have severe menorrhagia over 6 months and a hemoglobin level of 6 g/dL. She feels dizzy, weak, and fatigued. She receives 3 units of packed erythrocytes intravenously. Two hours into the transfusion, she develops fever to 103°F and shaking chills. Which of the following laboratory tests would most likely confirm an acute transfusion reaction?

A. LDH level

B. Leukocyte count

C. Direct bilirubin level

D. Glucose level

55.3 A 57-year-old man has a prosthetic aortic valve for which he takes warfarin (Coumadin) 10 mg/d. He is noted to have an international normalized ratio (INR) of 7 and is actively bleeding large clots from his gums, rectum, and when urinating. Which of the following is the best management for this patient?

A. Administer vitamin D.

B. Transfuse with fresh frozen plasma.

C. Administer IVIg.

D. Discontinue the warfarin (Coumadin) and observe.

ANSWERS

55.1 **D.** This patient needs a blood transfusion immediately, as evidenced by his dangerously low blood pressure. He does not have the 45 minutes required for cross-matching his blood. Even though the patient's wife is "absolutely sure" about the blood type, history is not completely reliable, and in an emergent situation such that uncross-matched blood must be given, O-negative blood (universal donor) usually is administered.

55.2 **A.** This patient is suffering from acute hemolytic transfusion reaction characterized by fever, evidence of hypotension and hemolysis. Elevated LDH and indirect bilirubin levels or decreased haptoglobin levels would be consistent with hemolysis.

55.3 **B.** When life-threatening acute bleeding occurs in the face of coagulopathy due to warfarin (Coumadin) use, the treatment is fresh frozen plasma. The INR is extremely high, consistent with a severe coagulopathy. Sometimes vitamin K administration can be helpful if the bleeding is not severe.

CLINICAL PEARLS

▶ The symptoms of anemia are related to the rapidity or chronicity with which the anemia developed as well as the patients' underlying cardio-pulmonary status.

▶ Myocardial ischemia or infarction may be precipitated by factors not related to the coronary arteries, such as tachycardia or severe anemia, with loss of oxygen-carrying capacity.

▶ Transfusion of blood carries certain risks, such as hemolytic reaction, infection (eg, human immunodeficiency virus [HIV] or hepatitis C), and transfusion-related lung injury.

▶ Platelet transfusions are indicated for severe thrombocytopenia with bleeding symptoms, but they may have limited benefit in ITP, and are definitely contraindicated in TTP.

▶ Fresh frozen plasma is used to correct coagulopathy by providing clotting factors.

REFERENCES

Cannon CP, Braunwald E. Unstable angina and non-ST-elevation myocardial infarction. In: Longo DL, Fauci AS, Kasper DL, et al., eds. *Harrison's Principles of Internal Medicine.* 18th ed. New York, NY: McGraw-Hill; 2012:2015-2021.

Dzieczkowski JS, Anderson KC. Transfusion biology and therapy. In: Longo DL, Fauci AS, Kasper DL, et al., eds. *Harrison's Principles of Internal Medicine.* 18th ed. New York, NY: McGraw-Hill; 2012:951-957.

Goodnough LT, Brecher ME, Kanter MH, et al. Transfusion medicine (part 1). *N Engl J Med.* 1999;340:438-447.

A 26-year-old woman presents to the emergency center on a Saturday afternoon complaining of bleeding from her nose and mouth since the previous night. She also noticed small, reddish spots on her lower extremities when she got out of the bed this morning. She denies fever, chills, nausea, vomiting, abdominal pain, or joint pain. The patient reports she had developed an upper respiratory infection 2 weeks prior to the emergency room visit, but the infection has now resolved. She denies significant medical problems. Her menses have been normal, and her last menstrual period was approximately 2 weeks ago. She denies excessive bleeding in the past, even after delivering her baby. Prior to this episode, she never had epistaxis, easy bruisability, or bleeding into her joints. There is no family history of abnormal bleeding. The patient does not take any medications.

On examination she is alert, oriented, and somewhat anxious. Her blood pressure is 110/70 mm Hg, her heart rate is 90 bpm, and she is afebrile. No pallor or jaundice is noted. There is bright red oozing from the nose and the gingiva. Skin examination reveals multiple 1-mm flat reddish spots on her lower extremities. The rest of the examination is normal. There is no lymphadenopathy or hepatosplenomegaly. Her complete blood cell count (CBC) is normal except for a platelet count of 18,000/mm^3. Prothrombin time (PT) and partial thromboplastin time (PTT) are normal.

▶ What is your most likely diagnosis?
▶ What is the best initial treatment?

ANSWERS TO CASE 56:

Immune Thrombocytopenic Purpura

Summary: A 26-year-old woman is seen in the emergency room because of persistent epistaxis. She denies excessive bleeding with menses or childbirth, easy bruisability, or bleeding into her joints. There is no family history of abnormal bleeding. The patient does not take any medications. Physical examination is significant only for the blood oozing from her nose and for the petechiae on her legs. There is no lymphadenopathy or hepatosplenomegaly. Her CBC shows thrombocytopenia (18,000/μL), but the other cell lines are normal.

- **Most likely diagnosis:** Immune thrombocytopenic purpura (ITP).

- **Best initial treatment:** Oral corticosteroids.

ANALYSIS

Objectives

1. Learn the clinical approach to bleeding disorders, specifically platelet disorders versus coagulation disorders.

2. Learn about the differential diagnosis of thrombocytopenia, specifically thrombocytopenic purpura versus other platelet disorders, such as thrombotic thrombocytopenic purpura (TTP), hemolytic uremic syndrome (HUS), and disseminated intravascular coagulation (DIC).

3. Learn about the treatment of ITP.

Considerations

This patient presents with mucosal bleeding, petechiae, and thrombocytopenia. She has no other history, symptoms, or physical examination findings of any systemic disease, so her problem appears to an isolated hematologic problem. Review of her CBC is important to ensure that other cell lines (white blood cell count [WBC] and red blood cell count [RBC]) are normal; if they are abnormal, conditions such as acute leukemia or a bone marrow infiltrative process must be considered. Her coagulation studies (PT and PTT) are also normal; if they were deranged, we would suspect a consumptive coagulopathy causing the thrombocytopenia and a serious underlying disorder. Her current level of thrombocytopenia does not pose a risk for spontaneous hemorrhage, but platelet counts less than 10,000/μL might place her at risk for serious or life-threatening bleeding.

> # APPROACH TO:
> ## The Patient With Abnormal Bleeding

DEFINITIONS

THROMBOCYTOPENIA: Platelet count of less than 150,000/µL.

IMMUNE THROMBOCYTOPENIC PURPURA: A hematologic disorder characterized by the destruction of blood platelets due to the presence of antiplatelet autoantibodies.

THROMBOTIC THROMBOCYTOPENIC PURPURA: A life-threatening syndrome characterized by a pentad of microangiopathic hemolytic anemia, thrombocytopenia, neurologic abnormalities, fever, and renal dysfunction.

HEMOLYTIC UREMIC SYNDROME: A clinical complex consisting of progressive renal failure that is associated with microangiopathic hemolytic anemia and thrombocytopenia.

CLINICAL APPROACH

A careful history is the most effective way to determine the presence and significance of a bleeding disorder. For a patient with abnormal bleeding, the most important history relates to any prior history of bleeding. One should inquire about history of epistaxis, menorrhagia, excessive prolonged bleeding from minor cuts, bruising, prolonged or profuse bleeding after dental extraction, excessive bleeding after major surgery or obstetric delivery, or trauma. Excessive mucosal bleeding (eg, gum and nose bleeding) and petechiae are suggestive of thrombocytopenia, or abnormal platelet function such as von Willebrand disease (vWD). On the other hand, hemarthrosis, deep hematomas, and retroperitoneal bleeding more likely reflect a severe coagulation abnormality, such as hemophilia, or deficiencies of factors VIII or IX.

Thrombocytopenia is defined as a platelet count of less than 150,000/µL, although spontaneous bleeding usually occurs at much lower platelet counts. The causes of thrombocytopenia can be divided into (1) decreased platelet production, (2) decreased platelet survival, (3) sequestration (hypersplenism), and (4) dilutional. **Impaired platelet production** is caused by a **bone marrow abnormality**, such as infiltration caused by malignancy or myelofibrosis, marrow suppression as a result of chemicals, drugs, radiation, or viruses. In bone marrow diseases, thrombocytopenia is often accompanied by abnormalities in the other cell lines. **Decreased platelet survival** is another cause of thrombocytopenia. Mild thrombocytopenia may be seen in pregnancy, and much more significant thrombocytopenia is seen with hemolysis, elevated liver enzymes, low platelets (HELLP) syndrome. Decreased platelet survival can be a result of **immune-mediated platelet destruction** triggered by medications or various infections, in autoimmune diseases like systemic lupus erythematosus (SLE) in ITP. Decreased platelet survival can also be due to **splenic sequestration** in patients with splenomegaly for various reasons (eg, portal hypertension, myelofibrosis).

ITP: Acute ITP is most common in early childhood, often following an antecedent upper respiratory infection, and usually is self-limiting. ITP in children is a distinct condition from that in adults, with a higher likelihood of spontaneous remission. **ITP in adults** is more likely to have an insidious or subacute presentation, is most likely to occur in women ages 20 to 40, and is more likely to persist for months to years, with **uncommon spontaneous remission.** The patient will present with the clinical manifestations of thrombocytopenia, such as petechiae and mucosal bleeding, but with no systemic toxicity, no lymphadenopathy or splenomegaly, normal white and red blood cell counts, and normal peripheral blood smear except for thrombocytopenia. Laboratory testing is usually focused on a search for secondary causes of thrombocytopenia such as human immunodeficiency virus (HIV), hepatitis C, antinuclear antibody (ANA) (for SLE), and a direct Coombs test to evaluate for autoimmune hemolytic anemia with ITP (Evans syndrome). Bone marrow biopsy is generally performed in patients older than 60 years to exclude myelodysplastic syndrome, and often reveals increased megakaryocytes but otherwise normal findings.

Adults with ITP and platelet count >30,000/μL and no bleeding may be observed without treatment. For those with lower platelet counts or bleeding symptoms can be treated with **oral glucocorticoids,** such as prednisone 1 mg/kg of body weight. Platelet transfusions usually are unnecessary and should be reserved for rare life-threatening situations because survival of transfused platelets in ITP may be as short as a few minutes. **Intravenous immunoglobulin (IVIg)** is often used when platelet counts are less than 10,000/mm^3 and can raise platelet counts rapidly. Anti-D is an anti-Rh(D) immune globulin for patients who have an Rh+ blood type, but it may be ineffective in patients who have had a splenectomy. Rituximab is an anti-CD20 monoclonal antibody that targets autoantibody-producing lymphocytes, and is a second-line therapy for patients with chronic ITP.

Because the spleen removes the antibody-bound platelets, patients with chronic ITP who do not respond to medical therapy may be candidates for **splenectomy.** Patients being considered for splenectomy should receive immunizations for encapsulated organisms such as *Pneumococcus* prior to surgery.

Drug-induced thrombocytopenia: When a patient presents with thrombocytopenia, any drug that the patient is using should be considered a possible cause. Common drugs known to cause thrombocytopenia include H$_2$ blockers, quinine, and sulfonamides. In general, the diagnosis is made by clinical observation of the response to drug withdrawal. Discontinuation of the offending medication should lead to improvement in the platelet count within a time frame consistent with the drug's metabolism, almost always within 7 to 10 days.

Heparin-induced thrombocytopenia (HIT): HIT is an immune-mediated disorder caused by the formation of antibodies against the heparin-platelet factor 4 complex, with the **fall in platelet count usually occurring 5 to 10 days after heparin is begun, and sooner if the patient had been sensitized by prior heparin use.** HIT can cause serious consequences. HIT differs from other drug-induced causes of thrombocytopenia in that it is **not associated with bleeding, but rather with increased risk of thrombosis.**

The four Ts are a useful mnemonic of the diagnostic criteria for HIT:

- Thrombocytopenia (nadir rarely <20,000/μL).

- Timing of platelet count drop (usually 5-10 days).

- Thrombosis.

- Other causes of thrombocytopenia are not likely.

Diagnosis depends on clinical suspicion, and utilization of an enzyme-linked immunosorbent assay (ELISA) for the HIT antibodies. Treatment includes discontinuation of the heparin (one cannot switch from unfractionated heparin to low-molecular-weight heparin because HIT antibodies will cross-react), and instead use a nonheparin anticoagulant such as argatroban, fondaparinux, or bivalirudin to treat thrombosis.

Thrombocytopenia may also be caused by consumptive coagulopathy, the most common of which is **DIC**. DIC usually is triggered by serious underlying conditions such as bacterial sepsis, malignancy such as acute promyelocytic leukemia, or obstetric catastrophes such as abruptio placentae. Any of these disease processes can produce blood exposure to pathologic levels of tissue factor, triggering uncontrolled thrombin generation with systemic fibrin deposition in the microcirculation. This uncontrolled activation of coagulation results in consumption of platelets and clotting factors, leading secondarily to bleeding. Laboratory findings include thrombocytopenia and elevated PT and PTT (reflecting the consumptive coagulopathy), and decreased fibrinogen and elevated fibrin-split products and D-dimer (reflecting uncontrolled fibrin deposition). Usually, the cause of DIC is obvious, and treatment should be directed toward correcting the underlying cause, as well as replacement of platelets and coagulation factors if there is clinically significant bleeding.

Thrombotic thrombocytopenic purpura: A less common disease process that may be confused with DIC is **TTP**. TTP may be triggered by infection such as HIV or medications such as clopidogrel, or it may be idiopathic. TTP is caused by deficiency of the ADAMTS13 protease, which cleaves ultralarge von Willebrand factor (vWF) multimers on the endothelial surface, due to the presence of an inhibitory autoantibody. As originally described, TTP has a pentad of findings: (**1**) **thrombocytopenia;** (**2**) **microangiopathic hemolytic** anemia with elevated lactate dehydrogenase (LDH) level and schistocytosis in the peripheral blood smear; (**3**) **fever;** (**4**) **fluctuating central nervous system (CNS) deficits with altered mental status;** and (**5**) **renal failure.** Patients may be acutely ill, and differentiation from DIC may be challenging, except that the PT and PTT are typically normal in TTP, but elevated in DIC. Plasma exchange is the standard treatment and has reduced the mortality of this condition greatly. Table 56–1 compares DIC, TTP, and ITP.

Hemolytic uremic syndrome: **HUS** presents very similarly to TTP, with acute renal failure, microangiopathic hemolytic anemia, and thrombocytopenia. Clinically, it may appear to be "TTP limited to the kidney," but the pathogenetic mechanisms and treatment differ from TTP. HUS occurs most often in children after a diarrheal illness, often with the hemorrhagic strain of *Escherichia coli* O157:H7. Treatment is supportive, and plasma exchange for HUS has not shown to be useful.

Table 56–1 • COMPARISON OF DIC, TTP, AND ITP			
Condition	**Etiology**	**Clinical Course**	**Treatment**
Disseminated intravascular coagulopathy (DIC)	Secondary to some other process: sepsis, trauma, metastatic malignancy, obstetric causes.	Can be relatively mild indolent course or severe life-threatening process; ongoing coagulation and fibrinolysis can cause thrombosis or hemorrhage; consumption of coagulation factors is seen as prolonged PT and PTT.	Treatment aimed at underlying cause. No proven specific treatment for the coagulation problem: if bleeding, replace factors and fibrinogen with fresh frozen plasma (FFP) or cryoprecipitate; if clotting, consider anticoagulate with heparin.
Thrombocytopenic thrombotic purpura (TTP)	Autoantibody with inhibition of ADAMTS13 protease (<10% activity) release of von Willebrand factor (vWF), triggering formation of microvascular thrombi.	May present as septic-appearing patient with fever, altered mental status, thrombocytopenia, microangiopathic hemolytic anemia, and renal failure. Normal PT and PTT. Mortality, mainly due to CNS involvement.	Plasmapheresis (removal of the excess/abnormal vWF), most patients recover. Corticosteroids.
Immune thrombocytopenic purpura (ITP)	Antiplatelet antibody leading to platelet destruction.	Children: following a viral illness with resolution; in adults, a more indolent course with progression and rarely spontaneous resolution. Isolated thrombocytopenia, normal PT, PTT.	Oral corticosteroids; intravenous immunoglobulin (IVIg); splenectomy if refractory.

von Willebrand disease: vWD patients present clinically with impaired primary hemostasis (ie, petechiae, easy bruising, mucosal bleeding, menorrhagia) with normal platelet counts, but impaired platelet function. vWD is the **most common inherited bleeding disorder.** It may occur as often as 1 in 1000 individuals. It may be acquired, or inherited as an **autosomal dominant disorder**, but is often not recognized because of relatively mild bleeding symptoms or because of excessive bleeding attributed to other causes, for example, menorrhagia attributed to uterine fibroids. von Willebrand factor (vWF) is a large complex multimeric protein that has two major functions: it allows for platelet adhesion to endothelium at sites of vascular injury, and it is the carrier protein for coagulation factor VIII, which stabilizes the molecule. vWD is a heterogenous group of disorders, but a common feature is **deficiency in the amount** or **function of vWF.** Clinical features are those of primary hemostatic defects as discussed. Typical laboratory features are reduced levels of vWF, reduced vWF activity as measured by ristocetin cofactor assay, and reduced factor VIII activity. The platelet count is usually normal, bleeding time is increased, and PTT may or may not be prolonged. Treatment is **desmopressin acetate (DDAVP)**, which causes release of vWF from endothelial stores, or use of factor VIII concentrate, which contains a large amount of vWF.

> ## CASE CORRELATION
> - See also Case 54 (Iron Deficiency Anemia), Case 57 (Lymphocytosis), and Case 58 (Sickle Cell Anemia).

COMPREHENSION QUESTIONS

56.1 A 28-year-old woman complains of excessive bleeding from her gums and has petechiae. Her CBC shows a platelet count of 22,000/mm^3 with a hemoglobin of 8.9 g/dL and a WBC count of 87,000/mm^3. Which of the following is the most likely etiology of her low platelet count?

A. Immune thrombocytopenia purpura

B. Systemic lupus erythematosus

C. Drug-induced thrombocytopenia

D. Acute leukemia

56.2 A 50-year-old man has been treated for rheumatoid arthritis for many years. He currently is taking corticosteroids for the disease. On examination, he has stigmata of rheumatoid arthritis and some fullness on his left upper abdomen. His platelet count is slightly low at 105,000/mm^3. His white blood cell count is 3100/mm^3 with neutropenia, and hemoglobin level is 9 g/dL. Which of the following is the most likely etiology of the thrombocytopenia?

A. Steroid induced

B. Splenic sequestration

C. Autoimmune destruction

D. Prior gold therapy

56.3 A 30-year-old woman with ITP has been taking maximum corticosteroid doses and still has a platelet count of 20,000/mm^3 and frequent bleeding episodes. Which of the following should she receive before her splenectomy?

A. Washed leukocyte transfusion

B. Intravenous interferon therapy

C. Pneumococcal vaccine

D. Bone marrow radiotherapy

56.4 A 65-year-old man who has a prosthetic heart valve is hospitalized for a knee replacement surgery, and placed on intravenous (IV) heparin for anticoagulation before the procedure. He drinks one glass of wine each weekend and has been diagnosed with osteoarthritis for which he takes acetaminophen. His platelet count was normal, but now is 32,000/mm³. Which of the following is the most likely cause of the thrombocytopenia?

A. Prosthetic heart valve

B. Alcohol intake

C. Acetaminophen

D. Heparin

ANSWERS

56.1 **D.** The thrombocytopenia is seen with other hematologic abnormalities, the most abnormal of which is a markedly elevated WBC count, suggesting acute leukemia.

56.2 **B.** This patient is likely suffering from Felty's syndrome characterized by rheumatoid arthritis, neutropenia, and splenomegaly. Splenomegaly from any etiology may cause sequestration of platelets, leading to thrombocytopenia.

56.3 **C.** Patients who undergo splenectomy are at risk for infections of encapsulated organisms such as *Streptococcus pneumoniae* and thus should receive the pneumococcal vaccine. It usually is given at least 2 weeks prior to splenectomy so that the spleen can help in forming a better immune response.

56.4 **D.** The patient likely has heparin-induced thrombocytopenia, which may be confirmed by assay for HIT antibodies, including IgG against platelet factor 4. Treatment consists of stopping the heparin, and starting a direct Xa inhibitor such as argatroban or bivalirudin.

CLINICAL PEARLS

▶ Disorders of primary hemostasis (thrombocytopenia or von Willebrand disease) are characterized by mucosal bleeding and the appearance of petechiae or superficial ecchymoses.

▶ Disorders of secondary hemostasis (coagulation factor deficiencies such as hemophilia) usually are characterized by the development of superficial ecchymoses as well as deep hematomas and hemarthroses.

▶ Immune thrombocytopenic purpura is a diagnosis of exclusion. Patients have isolated thrombocytopenia (ie, no red or white blood cell abnormalities); no apparent secondary causes such as systemic lupus erythematosus, HIV, or medication-induced thrombocytopenia; and normal to increased numbers of megakaryocytes in the bone marrow.

▶ Spontaneous hemorrhage may occur with platelet counts of less than $10,000/mm^3$.

▶ Platelet transfusion in immune thrombocytopenic purpura is often ineffective and is used only when there is severe life-threatening bleeding.

▶ Corticosteroids are the initial treatment of immune thrombocytopenic purpura. Patients with more severe disease can be treated with intravenous immunoglobulin; chronic refractory cases are treated with rituximab or splenectomy.

REFERENCES

Cines DB, Blanchette VS. Immune thrombocytopenic purpura. *N Engl J Med*. 2002;346:995-1008.

George JN, Raskob GE, Shah SR, et al. Drug-induced thrombocytopenia: a systematic review of published case reports. *Ann Intern Med*. 1998;129:886-890.

Konkle BA. Bleeding and thrombosis. In: Kasper DL, Fauci AS, Hauser SL, et al., eds. *Harrison's Principles of Internal Medicine*. 19th ed. New York, NY: McGraw-Hill; 2015:400-407.

Konkle BA. Disorders of platelets and vessel wall. In: Kasper DL, Fauci AS, Hauser SL, et al., eds. *Harrison's Principles of Internal Medicine*. 19th ed. New York, NY: McGraw-Hill; 2015:725-732.

A 65-year-old man with benign prostatic hypertrophy had been experiencing difficulty with urination, and so he saw his urologist to be evaluated for a transure-
thral resection of the prostate. As part of the routine preoperative evaluation, he
had a complete blood count, but that was found to be abnormal. The procedure
was cancelled and he is now referred to the internal medicine clinic for additional
evaluation.

Aside from his prostate symptoms, the patient is asymptomatic. He has not
experienced any recent fevers, chills, night sweats, arthralgias, or myalgias. His
appetite is good and his weight has been stable. He is moderately physically active,
plays golf regularly, and has not noted any fatigue or exertional dyspnea.

On examination, he is afebrile and normotensive. His conjunctivae are anicteric, and his skin and oral mucosa show no pallor. His chest is clear to auscultation, and his heart is regular without any murmurs. On abdominal examination,
his liver span seems normal, and there is no palpable spleen. He does not have any
palpable cervical, axillary, or inguinal adenopathy.

Laboratories show the following results: white blood cell (WBC) count is 56,000
with 90% mature lymphocytes and 10% neutrophils, hemoglobin is 14.8 g/dL,
hematocrit is 45%, and platelet count is 189,000/uL. Other laboratories including
electrolytes, creatinine, and transaminases are all within normal limits.

▶ What is the most likely diagnosis?
▶ What is the most appropriate next step?

ANSWERS TO CASE 57:

Lymphocytosis/CLL

Summary: A 65-year-old man has been in generally good health, and is incidentally noted to have a marked lymphocytosis (50,000/μL) on a routine laboratory test. He has had no recent fevers or other symptoms of infection. He is asymptomatic, and his physical examination is normal, without any pallor, petechiae, peripheral adenopathy, or splenomegaly. He has an elevated lymphocyte count on his CBC, but the other cell lines are normal.

- **Most likely diagnosis:** Chronic lymphocytic leukemia (CLL).

- **Most appropriate next step:** Flow cytometry of peripheral blood to demonstrate a monoclonal B-cell population, and confirm the diagnosis.

ANALYSIS

Objectives

1. Be able to evaluate a patient with leukocytosis to distinguish between acute and chronic leukemias, and nonmalignant causes of leukocytosis.

2. Know the diagnostic criteria and staging system for CLL.

3. Be familiar with the complications of CLL.

Considerations

In a patient presenting with marked leukocytosis, the first consideration is to try to distinguish between malignant and nonmalignant (usually infectious) causes of the elevated white blood cell count. This man is afebrile without any symptoms of infection, so infectious causes are unlikely. Since he is essentially asymptomatic and does not have anemia or thrombocytopenia, acute leukemia is also unlikely. The most common type of chronic leukemia is CLL. The next steps would be to confirm the diagnosis of CLL with peripheral blood flow cytometry to demonstrate that the lymphocytosis is due to monoclonal proliferation, and then to stage the disease such as with imaging test, so he can be advised regarding treatment options.

APPROACH TO:

Lymphocytosis

DEFINITIONS

CHRONIC LYMPHOCYTIC LEUKEMIA: Increased number of circulating mature lymphocytes (usually >10,000/μL) that are *monoclonal* B-cells expressing the CD5 antigen.

SMALL LYMPHOCYTIC LYMPHOMA (SLL): Malignancy of mature B-lymphocytes that are *monoclonal* in origin. Synonymous with CLL, considered the same disease at different stages. If the clinical presentation is lymphadenopathy without peripheral lymphocytosis (<5000/μL), it is termed SLL.

LEUKEMOID REACTION: Leukocytosis with neutrophilia, and WBC count >30,000-50,000/μL, with immature neutrophils (myelocytes, metamyelocytes, promyelocytes) that are not monoclonal.

CLINICAL APPROACH

In patients who are found to have a significantly elevated WBC count, a common clinical problem is to differentiate a hematologic malignancy from a reactive leukocytosis as a response to infection or inflammation.

If the elevated WBCs are predominantly myeloid cells, the differential diagnosis is usually between a **leukemoid reaction** and **chronic myelogenous leukemia (CML)**. In patients with a leukemoid reaction, the peripheral smear may show myelocytes, metamyelocytes, promyelocytes, and sometimes myeloblasts. **Leukocyte alkaline phosphatase (LAP)** is **elevated in leukemoid reaction**, but is low in CML cells. Leukemoid reactions are not dangerous in and of themselves, but they typically represent a response to a significant underlying disease state.

Patients with **CML** typically present with elevated WBC count, with increased mature and immature granulocytes, basophilia, and may also have a mild normocytic anemia and elevated platelet count. Patients with significant anemia or thrombocytopenia should be evaluated for an alternative diagnosis. At diagnosis, many patients with CML are asymptomatic, or may have mild nonspecific symptoms such as fatigue, or might report some abdominal discomfort or early satiety due to splenomegaly. If CML is suspected, the diagnostic test of choice is an assay for the presence of the **Philadelphia chromosome t(9;22)**, using either cytogenetics or fluorescence in situ hybridization (FISH), or *polymerase chain reaction* (PCR) for the **BCR-ABL fusion gene**, which is a constitutively active tyrosine kinase. This dysregulation of tyrosine kinase activity is part of the pathogenesis of CML. Initial treatment of patients in the chronic stable phase is usually with one of the targeted agents imatinib, dasatinib, or nilotinib, **tyrosine kinase inhibitors (TKIs)** that blocks BCR-ABL-mediated signal transduction, and induce apoptosis in cells expressing BCR-ABL.

In contrast to the asymptomatic or subacute presentation of patients with CML, patients with **acute leukemia** present with **marked leukocytosis but with anemia and thrombocytopenia**, or with **pancytopenia**. Symptoms may include weakness, easy fatigability and dyspnea due to anemia, infections due to neutropenia, or bleeding symptoms such as gingival bleeding, epistaxis, or menorrhagia. Occasionally, patients present with an extramedullary tumor mass due to accumulation of blast cells. Patients with **hyperleukocytosis** (WBC >50,000-100,000/μL) may develop **leukostasis**, which is the symptomatic state caused by microvascular ischemia due to white cell plugs, typically produces respiratory or neurologic distress, and is a medical emergency. The diagnosis of **acute myeloid leukemia (AML)** or **acute lymphoid leukemia (ALL)** is established by **bone marrow biopsy** using morphologic, cytogenetic, and molecular analysis. Initial management is stabilization and

Table 57–1 • CAUSES OF LYMPHOCYTOSIS	
Viral	Infectious mononucleosis (Epstein-Barr virus) Mononucleosis syndrome (cytomegalovirus, adenovirus type 12, herpes virus 6) HIV-1 Mumps, varicella, influenza, hepatitis, rubella, roseola Enteroviruses including poliovirus
Bacterial	Pertussis Tuberculosis, brucellosis, syphilis
Protozoal	Toxoplasmosis
Parasitic	Babesiosis
Immune mediated	Drug-induced Serum sickness Rheumatoid arthritis Thymoma
Endocrine	Hyperthyroidism

supportive care for acutely ill patients, and treatment with **induction chemotherapy** to try to achieve complete remission (CR).

Lymphocytosis

The most common clinical scenario involving elevated WBC count is a patient presenting with **lymphocytosis**. To determine if a lymphocytosis is present, one must calculate the absolute lymphocyte count (ALC), which is equal to the product of the total WBC and the fraction of lymphocytes on the WBC differential: ALC = Total WBC (cells/μL) × % lymphocytes ÷ 100. **Lymphocytosis is present if the ALC >4000/μL.**

Causes of lymphocytosis are listed in Table 57–1.

Lymphocytosis is most frequently found in **viral infections** and only rarely in bacterial infection except **pertussis. Pertussis** (whooping cough) may be associated with ALC of 20,000-30,000/μL. The lymphocytes are small and mature appearing on peripheral smear. Other infections that can cause lymphocytosis are toxoplasmosis, brucellosis, and sometimes syphilis. The most common viral infection associated with lymphocytosis is **Epstein-Barr virus (EBV)**. The clinical syndrome of infectious mononucleosis caused by EBV or other viral infections that are listed is characterized by fever and lymphadenopathy, and may produce larger, reactive lymphocytes **(atypical lymphocytosis)**.

Chronic Lymphocytic Leukemia

CLL/SLL is an indolent disorder characterized by the monoclonal proliferation of **mature B-lymphocytes** that express the CD5 antigen. It may present either as a leukemia or a lymphoma, depending on whether lymphocytosis or lymphadenopathy is the predominant finding. Patients with CLL or SLL are often asymptomatic, and present with incidental discovery of lymphocytosis or painless adenopathy, respectively. On the peripheral blood smear of patients with CLL, there is an increased number of small, well-differentiated lymphocytes, which are fragile and are often seen

Table 57–2 • RAI STAGING OF CLL			
Risk	**Stage**	**Clinical Features**	**Median Survival**
Low	0	Lymphocytosis in blood or bone marrow	>10 y
Intermediate	I	Lymphocytosis + lymphadenopathy	7 y
	II	Lymphocytosis + splenomegaly + hepatomegaly	
High	III	Lymphocytosis + anemia	1.5 y
	IV	Lymphocytosis + thrombocytopenia	

as broken or **"smudge" cells.** Diagnosis of CLL is confirmed by peripheral blood **flow cytometry demonstrating a monoclonal B-cell population that shows aberrant expression of a T-cell antigen (CD5).**

CLL is a generally indolent disease but prognosis is extremely variable, with survival times from initial diagnosis that range from 2 to 12 years. The prognosis depends on the stage of disease, and a commonly used staging system is the Rai system based on the concept that there is a gradual and progressive increase in the body burden of leukemic lymphocytes, starting in the blood and bone marrow (lymphocytosis), progressively involving lymph nodes (lymphadenopathy), then spleen and liver (organomegaly), with eventual compromise of bone marrow function (anemia and thrombocytopenia). Median survival time ranges from 12 years at stage 0, 6 to 8 years at stage I/II, and 2 years at stage III/IV (Table 57–2).

Patients with CLL have an imbalance of lymphocyte subsets and may develop altered immune responses including **autoimmune hemolytic anemia (AIHA) and autoimmune thrombocytopenia**, as well as recurrent viral and bacterial infections. In a small percentage of cases, CLL may **transform into an aggressive large cell lymphoma (Richter syndrome)** characterized by constitutional symptoms (fever, night sweats), progressive lymphadenopathy, and often extranodal (eg, liver) involvement.

CLL is considered an incurable disease, but many patients do not require treatment initially. Treatment is usually indicated if the patient develops any of the following symptoms: pancytopenia, autoimmune hemolytic anemia or thrombocytopenia, symptomatic bulky adenopathy or splenomegaly, or Richter syndrome.

Emerging Concepts

Chromosomal testing and prognostic markers can be used for prognosis. Patients with deletion of the short arm of chromosome 17 (17p), long arm of chromosome 11 (llq), or nonmutation in the immunoglobulin variable heavy chain (IgVH) gene have a poorer prognosis. Monoclonal antibodies are being developed and may be useful for treatment in these circumstances.

CASE CORRELATION

- See also Case 54 (Iron Deficiency Anemia), Case 56 (ITP), and Case 58 (Sickle Cell Anemia).

COMPREHENSION QUESTIONS

57.1 A 25-year-old man presents with a 2-week history of low-grade fever, slight cough, malaise, and myalgias, and is noted on physical examination to have enlarged posterior cervical lymph nodes and significant splenomegaly. His CBC shows a lymphocytosis with ALC 10,000/µL, normal hemoglobin level, and normal platelet count. The peripheral smear shows large atypical lymphocytes. What is the most likely diagnosis?

A. ALL

B. CLL

C. Acute HIV infection

D. EBV infection

E. Pertussis

57.2 Which of the following statements regarding CML is true?

A. Peripheral smear shows elevated WBC count with mature and immature granulocytes, toxic granulation, and high LAP score.

B. Usually presents initially with splenomegaly, anemia, and thrombocytopenia.

C. Chromosomal translocations, most often t(9;22), are found in 90% to 95% of patients.

D. Is an indolent disease, and should be monitored without treatment until patients enter accelerated or blast phase.

57.3 A 75-year-old woman, diagnosed with stage 0 CLL 1 year ago and being monitored without treatment, now complains of fatigue and dyspnea. She has no palpable adenopathy or splenomegaly, no rashes or arthritis, and her CBC shows ALC 11,000/µL, with hemoglobin 6.8 mg/dL, and platelet count 127,000/µL. What is the most appropriate diagnostic test?

A. Direct antiglobulin (Coombs) test

B. Antinuclear antibody

C. Bone marrow biopsy

D. Test for Lewis alloantibody

ANSWERS

57.1 **D.** The clinical presentation of fever, malaise, adenopathy, and splenomegaly is consistent with infectious mononucleosis, which is most often associated with EBV, but can also be due to CMV or other viral infections. The absence of cytopenias makes ALL unlikely. The lymphocytosis in CLL and pertussis consist of mature small lymphocytes. Acute HIV infection can present similarly to mononucleosis, but does not typically cause massive splenomegaly.

57.2 **C.** Definitive diagnosis of CML is established by demonstrating the presence of the Philadelphia chromosome or the underlying t(9;22) translocation, the BCR-ABL1 fusion gene or mRNA fusion product, which is found in nearly all patients. Toxic granulation and high LAP score are features of leukemoid reaction. Splenomegaly is common in CML, but significant cytopenias are not seen. Before imatinib and other TKIs, median survival in CML was 4 years with progression to blast (acute leukemic) phase and death. Imatinib or other TKIs are indicated as initial treatment for patients in chronic phase, with the goals of achieving remission and preventing progression of disease.

57.3 **A.** The most likely diagnosis is AIHA (autoimmne hemolytic anemia), which can be confirmed by detection of antibody and/or complement components on the surface of the red blood cell (RBC), usually by the direct antiglobulin (Coombs) test. AIHA is a common complication of CLL. Antinuclear antibody (ANA) to screen for systemic lupus erythematosus (SLE) has a low probability in a woman of this age, without other clinical features of SLE. Bone marrow biopsy to evaluate for bone marrow failure due to CLL could be considered, but rapid progression to stage III/IV would be unlikely. Lewis alloantibodies have no clinical significance.

CLINICAL PEARLS

▶ Low leukocyte alkaline phosphatase (LAP) and presence of basophilia are seen in CML, and help distinguish it from leukemoid reaction (high LAP).

▶ The BCR-ABL fusion gene found in the Philadelphia chromosome t(9;22) produces a deregulated tyrosine kinase that is implicated in the pathogenesis of CML, and is the target of therapy.

▶ Acute leukemias present with symptoms due to symptomatic anemia, bleeding due to thrombocytopenia, infection due to neutropenia, or with hyperleukocytosis and symptoms of central nervous system (CNS) or pulmonary microvascular ischemia.

▶ CLL/SLL is an indolent disease characterized by the monoclonal proliferation of mature B-lymphocytes expressing the CD5 antigen, and typically presents as asymptomatic lymphocytosis or painless lymphadenopathy.

▶ Complications of CLL include autoimmune hemolytic anemia or thrombocytopenia, recurrent infections due to immune dysfunction, or transformation to a more aggressive large cell lymphoma.

REFERENCES

Longo DL. Malignancies of lymphoid cells. In: Kasper DL, Fauci AS, Hauser SL, et al., eds. *Harrison's Principles of Internal Medicine*. 19th ed. New York, NY: McGraw-Hill; 2015:695-710.

Tsimberidou AM, Wen S, O'Brien S, et al. Assessment of chronic lymphocytic leukemia and small lymphocytic lymphoma by absolute lymphocyte counts in 2,126 patients: 20 years of experience at the University of Texas M.D. Anderson Cancer Center. *J Clin Oncol*. 2007;25(29):4648.

Wetzler M, Marcucci G, Bloomfield CD. Acute and chronic myeloid leukemia. In: Longo DL, Fauci AS, Kasper DL, et al., eds. *Harrison's Principles of Internal Medicine*. 18th ed. New York, NY: McGraw-Hill; 2012:905-918.

A 25-year-old African-American man is admitted to your service with the diagnosis of a sickle cell pain episode. He was admitted to the hospital six times last year with the same diagnosis, and he was last discharged 2 months ago. This time, he presented to the emergency department complaining of abdominal and bilateral lower extremity pain, his usual sites of pain. When you examine him, you note he is febrile to 101°F, with respiratory rate 25 bpm, normal blood pressure, and slight tachycardia of 100 bpm. Lung examination reveals bronchial breath sounds and egophony in the right lung base. His oxygen saturation on 2 L/min nasal cannula is 92%. Besides the usual abdominal and leg pain, he is now complaining of chest pain, which is worse on inspiration. Although he is tender on palpation of his extremities, the remainder of his examination is normal. His laboratory examinations reveal elevated white blood cell and reticulocyte counts, and a hemoglobin and hematocrit that are slightly lower than baseline. Sickle and target cells are seen on the peripheral smear.

▶ What is the most likely diagnosis?
▶ What is your next step?
▶ What are the potential complications of this condition?
▶ What is the best treatment for the probable condition?

ANSWERS TO CASE 58:

Sickle Cell Crisis

Summary: A 25-year-old African-American man with a history of numerous pain crises is admitted for abdominal and bilateral lower extremity pain. He is febrile to 101°F, with respiratory rate 25 bpm, and slight tachycardia of 100 bpm. Lung examination reveals bronchial breath sounds and egophony in the right lung base. His oxygen saturation on 2 L/min nasal cannula is 92%. He is now complaining of chest pain, which is worse on inspiration. He has a leukocytosis, an elevated reticulocyte count, and a hemoglobin and hematocrit that are slightly lower than baseline. Sickle and target cells are seen on the peripheral smear.

- **Most likely diagnosis:** Acute chest syndrome.

- **Next step:** Chest radiograph and empiric antibiotic therapy.

- **Potential complications:** Respiratory failure, possible death.

- **Best treatment:** Aside from empiric antibiotic therapy (and possibly antiviral therapy such as for influenza), oxygen, pain control, incentive spirometry, and transfusion (simple if mild symptoms, or exchange transfusion if severe).

ANALYSIS

Objectives

1. Understand the pathophysiology of sickle cell anemia and acute painful episodes.

2. Learn the acute and chronic complications of sickle cell anemia.

3. Become familiar with treatment options available for the complications of sickle cell anemia.

Considerations

The patient in this case, a 25-year-old man with known sickle cell disease with a history of numerous pain crises is admitted with abdominal pain and bilateral leg pain. He also **has the acute onset of chest pain, cough, fever, and abnormal findings on the pulmonary auscultation.** His **oxygen saturation is 92% on room air,** which is concerning, and should be followed up with an arterial blood gas. Pulmonary embolism, pneumonia, and **acute chest syndrome** should be considered as possible diagnoses. **Acute chest syndrome** is a constellation of symptoms that includes chest pain and tachypnea. It can result from infection, or noninfectious causes such as pulmonary infarction or fat embolism. It usually presents with some combination of **chest pain, fever, hypoxia, and a new pulmonary infiltrate on chest radiography.** Often, acute chest syndrome and pneumonia cannot be distinguished initially. Therefore, it is prudent to treat these patients with antibiotics, obtain a Gram stain and culture of the sputum, and admit them to the hospital. The treatment for acute chest syndrome is supportive and includes oxygen, intravenous fluid hydration, broad-spectrum antibiotics, and analgesia, and transfusion. With significant disease, an exchange transfusion may be necessary. These patients should be carefully evaluated, because significant morbidity or mortality can result.

APPROACH TO:
Sickle Cell Anemia

DEFINITIONS

SICKLE CELL ANEMIA: A congenital defect in hemoglobin formation such that both genes code for hemoglobin S, leading to hemolysis and an abnormal shape of the red blood cell. Affected individuals have numerous complications including pain crises.

ACUTE CHEST SYNDROME: A condition found in individuals with sickle cell disease characterized by **fever, tachycardia, chest pain, leukocytosis, and pulmonary infiltrates.**

CLINICAL APPROACH

Pathophysiology

The molecular structure of a normal hemoglobin molecule consists of two alpha-globin chains and two beta-globin chains. Sickle cell anemia is an autosomal recessive disorder resulting from a substitution of valine for glutamine in the sixth amino acid position of the beta-globin chain. This substitution results in an alteration of the quaternary structure of the hemoglobin molecule. Individuals in whom only half of their beta chains are affected are heterozygous, a state referred to as *sickle cell trait*. When both beta chains are affected, the patient is homozygous and has sickle cell anemia. In patients with sickle cell disease, the altered quaternary structure of the hemoglobin molecule causes polymerization of the molecules under conditions of deoxygenation. These rigid polymers distort the red blood cell into a sickle shape, which is characteristic of the disease. **Sickling** is promoted by **hypoxia, acidosis, dehydration, or variations in body temperature.**

Epidemiology

Sickle cell anemia is the most common autosomal recessive disorder, and the most common cause of hemolytic anemia in African Americans. Approximately 8% of African Americans carry the gene (ie, sickle cell trait), with one in 625 affected by the disease.

Complications of Sickle Cell Disease

Acute painful episodes, also known as *pain crises*, are a consequence of microvascular occlusion of bones by sickled cells. The most common sites are the long bones of the arms and legs, the vertebral column, and the sternum. Acute painful episodes are precipitated by infection, hypoxia (for instance, at high altitude), cold exposure, dehydration, venous stasis, or acidosis. They usually last 2 to 7 days.

Infections are another complication. Patients with sickle cell disease are at greater risk for infections, especially with encapsulated bacterial organisms. **Auto-infarction of the spleen** occurs during early childhood secondary to microvascular obstruction by sickled red blood cells. The spleen gradually regresses in size and by age 4 is no longer palpable. As a consequence of infarction and fibrosis, the immunologic capacity of the spleen is diminished. Patients with sickle cell disease are at greater risk for pneumonia, sepsis, and meningitis by encapsulated organisms such as *Streptococcus pneumoniae* and *Haemophilus influenzae*. For the same reason, patients with sickle cell disease are at greater risk for osteomyelitis with *Salmonella* spp.

Acute chest syndrome is a vaso-occlusive crisis within the lungs and may be associated with infection or pulmonary infarction. It is characterized by the presence of the following signs and symptoms: **new pulmonary infiltrate, chest pain, fever, and respiratory symptoms such as tachypnea, wheezing, or cough.** These episodes may be precipitated by pneumonia causing sickling in the infected lung segments, or, in the absence of infection, intrapulmonary sickling can occur as a primary event. It is virtually impossible to clinically distinguish whether or not infection is present; thus, empiric antibiotic therapy is used.

Aplastic crisis occurs secondary to viral suppression of red blood cell precursors, most often by parvovirus B19. It occurs because of the very short half-life of sickled red blood cells and consequent need for brisk erythropoiesis. If red blood cell production is inhibited, even for a short time, profound anemia may result. The process is acute and usually reversible, with spontaneous recovery.

Other complications of sickle cell disease include hemorrhagic or ischemic stroke as a result of thrombosis, pigmented gallstones, papillary necrosis of the kidney, priapism, pulmonary hypertension, and congestive heart failure.

Treatment

The mainstay of treatment of pain crisis is hydration and pain control with nonsteroidal anti-inflammatory agents and narcotics. It is important to also provide adequate oxygenation to reduce sickling. One must search diligently for any underlying infection, and antibiotics are often used empirically when infection is suspected. **Acute chest syndrome** is treated with **oxygen, analgesia, and antibiotics.** Sometimes exchange transfusions are necessary.

In general, blood transfusions may be required for aplastic crisis, for severe hypoxia in acute chest syndrome, or to decrease viscosity and cerebral thrombosis in patients with stroke. Transfusion does not shorten the duration of pain crisis. To protect against encapsulated organisms, all patients with sickle cell disease should receive **penicillin prophylaxis** and a **vaccination against pneumococcus. Hydroxyurea** is often used to reduce the occurrence of painful crisis by stimulating hemoglobin F production and thus decreasing hemoglobin S concentration, and should be considered in patients who have repeated episodes of acute chest syndrome or frequent severe pain crises. The antineoplastic agent 5-deoxyazacytidine (**decitabine**) may also elevate levels of hemoglobin F without excessive side effects.

Other Agents

Phosphodiesterase type 5 (PDE5) inhibitors such as sildenafil promotes smooth muscle relaxation in the lungs and can treat pulmonary hypertension and also priapism. Endothelin receptor agonists such as bosentan can improve pulmonary hypertension caused by sickle cell disease. The mechanism of this agent is competitive binding to ET-1 receptors endothelin A and endothelin B in the pulmonary vascular endothelium. Because of the numerous transfusions, sometimes iron chelators are needed to prevent iron overload (which may lead to heart or liver failure).

Emerging Concepts

Research is being concentrated on allogeneic hematopoietic stem cell transplantation, which can be curative. In children with severe disease, myeloablative stem cell transplantation has been effective with approximately 10% side effects if there is sufficient matched donor such as a sibling; however, adults have more complications and there is ongoing studies to find an optimal stem cell transplantation process. Gene therapy is only in its initial stages of research but holds promise.

CASE CORRELATION

- See also Case 54 (Iron Deficiency Anemia), Case 55 (Transfusion Medicine), Case 56 (ITP), and Case 57 (Lymphocytosis).

COMPREHENSION QUESTIONS

58.1 Which of the following therapies would most likely decrease the number of sickle cell crises?

    A. Hydroxyurea

    B. Folate supplementation

    C. Prophylactic penicillin

    D. Pneumococcal vaccination

For the following questions (58.2-58.4) choose the finding (A-E) that best matches with the syndrome to which it is commonly associated in persons with sickle cell anemia.

    A. *Salmonella* spp

    B. *S pneumoniae*

    C. Parvovirus B19

    D. Fat embolus

    E. Hematuria

58.2 Aplastic crisis

58.3 Osteomyelitis

58.4 Pneumonia

ANSWERS

58.1 **A.** Hydroxyurea and decitabine may decrease the incidence of sickle cell crises by increasing levels of hemoglobin F.

58.2 **C.** Parvovirus B19 is associated with aplastic crisis, especially in individuals with sickle cell disease.

58.3 **A.** Patients with sickle cell disease are at risk for *Salmonella* osteomyelitis.

58.4 **B.** *S pneumoniae* is the most common causative agent for pneumonia.

CLINICAL PEARLS

▶ Treatment of an acute painful episode in sickle cell disease includes hydration, narcotic analgesia, adequate oxygenation, and search for underlying infection.

▶ Acute chest syndrome is characterized by chest pain, fever, new radiographic pulmonary infiltrate, and respiratory symptoms; it can be caused by pneumonia, vaso-occlusion, or pulmonary embolism.

▶ Blood transfusion may be required for aplastic crisis, for severe hypoxemia in acute chest syndrome, or to decrease viscosity and cerebral thrombosis in patients with stroke.

▶ Hydroxyurea and decitabine increase hemoglobin F production (decreasing hemoglobin S concentration) and thus reduce the frequency of pain crises and other complications.

REFERENCES

Benz EJ. Disorders of hemoglobin. In: Kasper DL, Fauci AS, Hauser SL, et al., eds. *Harrison's Principles of Internal Medicine.* 19th ed. New York, NY: McGraw-Hill; 2015:631-639.

Centre for Clinical Practice at NICE (UK). Guidelines for the management of the acute painful crisis in sickle cell disease. *Br J Haematol.* 2012;120(5):744-752.

Steinberg MH. Management of sickle cell disease. *N Engl J Med.* 1999;340:1021-1030.

Vichinsky E. New therapies in sickle cell disease. *Lancet.* 2002;360:629-631.

Vichinsky EP, Styles LA, Colangelo LH, Wright EC, Castro O, Nickerson B. Acute chest syndrome in sickle cell disease: clinical presentation and course. Cooperative Study of Sickle Cell Disease. *Blood.* 1997;89:1787-1792.

A 57-year-old man was admitted to the hospital 2 days ago following a motor vehicle accident. He suffered multiple contusions and a femur fracture that was surgically repaired 24 hours ago. He also had a laceration on his forehead; a computed tomography (CT) scan of his head on admission that showed no intracranial bleeding. His hospital course has been uncomplicated, and the only medications he currently is taking are morphine as needed for pain, and sub-cutaneous enoxaparin for prophylaxis of deep venous thrombosis. This evening he has been agitated and combative, having pulled out his intravenous (IV) line. He is cursing at the nurses and is trying to get out of bed to leave the hospital. When you see him, he is febrile with a temperature of 100.8°F, heart rate of 122 bpm, blood pressure of 168/110 mm Hg, respiratory rate of 28 bpm, and oxygen saturations of 98% on room air. He is awake and fidgety, staring around the room nervously. He is disoriented to place and time; he seems to be having auditory hallucinations and is brushing off unseen objects from his arms. On examination, his forehead wound is bandaged, his pupils are dilated but reactive, and he is mildly diaphoretic. His lung sounds are clear to auscultation, his heart rhythm is tachycardic but regular, his abdomen is benign, and he is tremulous. You are able to contact family members by phone. They confirm that prior to his car accident, the patient had no medical problems, had no dementia or psychiatric illness, and was employed as an attorney. They report that he took no medications at home, did not smoke or use illicit drugs, and drank at least three to four mixed drinks every day after work, sometimes more on the weekends.

▶ What is your most likely diagnosis?
▶ What should be your next step?

ANSWERS TO CASE 59:

Delirium/Alcohol Withdrawal

Summary: A 57-year-old man has been hospitalized for 2 days for multiple contusions and surgery performed 24 hours ago for a femur fracture sustained in a motor vehicle accident. CT scan of his head is normal. His only medications are morphine and subcutaneous enoxaparin. This evening he is agitated and combative, and he is trying to leave the hospital. His temperature is 100.8°F, heart rate is 122 bpm, blood pressure is 168/110 mm Hg, respiratory rate is 28 bpm, and oxygen saturation is 98% on room air. He is awake, fidgety, and disoriented, and he seems to be having auditory and tactile hallucinations. His pupils are dilated, and he is mildly diaphoretic and tremulous. Family members confirm that the patient had no medical problems and no dementia or psychiatric illness. He took no medications, did not smoke or use illicit drugs, and drank three to four mixed drinks every day after work.

- **Most likely diagnosis:** Delirium as a result of an acute medical illness or possibly alcohol withdrawal.

- **Next step:** Look for serious or reversible underlying medical causes for the delirium. If no other medical problems are identified, based on the patient's daily alcohol use, a possible diagnosis is alcohol withdrawal syndrome.

ANALYSIS

Objectives

1. Be able to recognize delirium in a hospitalized patient.

2. Know the most common causes of delirium.

3. Understand the management of an agitated, delirious patient.

4. Know the special considerations applicable to an elderly demented patient with delirium.

5. Learn the stages, treatment, and complications of alcohol withdrawal syndrome.

Considerations

This 57-year-old man had been in a normal physical and mental state prior to hospitalization. He then developed an acute change in mental status, with fluctuating consciousness and orientation, the hallmark of delirium. There are many possible causes for his delirium: hypoxia, pulmonary embolism, acute electrolyte disturbances, hypoglycemia, occult infection, central nervous system (CNS) hemorrhage or infection, or drug intoxication or withdrawal. These conditions require investigation before ascribing the symptoms to alcohol withdrawal, because they are potentially very serious or even fatal. In addition, further investigation to quantify his alcohol intake is necessary. Rapid diagnosis and treatment is vital since this patient has findings of significant autonomic instability based on the hyperthermia, tachycardia and high blood pressure, and mortality if untreated can approach 20%. The use of a benzodiazepine such as lorazepam is a fundamental part of the treatment regimen.

APPROACH TO:
Delirium

DEFINITIONS

DELIRIUM: An acute confusional state that is one of the most common mental disorders encountered in hospitalized or otherwise medically ill patients.

DEMENTIA: Significant loss of intellectual abilities, such as memory capacity, severe enough to interfere with social or occupational functioning, usually over a long period of time.

CLINICAL APPROACH

Incidence and Mechanism

It is estimated that 5% to 10% of the population has alcoholism, and a fair proportion will have withdrawal symptoms upon cessation. Many Americans are also habituated to benzodiazepines, and the withdrawal syndrome is similar to alcohol withdrawal. The withdrawal findings of alcohol or benzodiazepine cessation are complex, and can be explained largely due to the interaction of ethanol to the postsynaptic gamma-aminobutyric acid (GABA)-A receptors, which are inhibitory neurons. Long-term alcohol use leads to downregulation of the GABA-A receptors; the brain compensates for this chronic loss of excitatory neurotransmission by increasing excitatory neurotransmitters such as norepinephrine, serotonin, and dopamine. Thus, with the sudden cessation of alcohol, these excitatory neurotransmitters are unopposed, leading to profound effects.

Diagnosis

The *Diagnostic and Statistical Manual of Mental Disorders, Fifth Edition (DSM-V)* defines delirium as a clinical diagnosis, and having the following features:

- Disturbance in attention (ie, reduced ability to direct, focus, sustain, and shift attention) and awareness

- Change in cognition (eg, memory deficit, disorientation, language disturbance, perceptual disturbance) that is not better accounted for by a preexisting, established, or evolving dementia.

- The disturbance develops over a short period (usually hours to days) and tends to fluctuate during the course of the day.

- Evidence that the above features are caused by a medical condition, medications, or intoxicants

One of the earliest signs of a disturbance of consciousness is an inability to focus or sustain attention, which may be evident as distractibility in conversation. Usually there also is disturbance of the sleep-wake cycle. In alcohol withdrawal, signs of autonomic hyperactivity predominate, and patients may become hypervigilant and agitated. As symptoms progress, patients may become lethargic or even stuporous (arousable only to painful stimuli).

Regarding changes in cognition or perception, patients may have difficulty with memory, orientation, or speech. It is important to ascertain from family members whether these impairments were chronic, as in dementia, or developed acutely. Delirious patients may have hallucinations or vague delusions of harm, but hallucinations are not a mandatory feature of the condition. **Delirium** is an acute process, with **symptoms developing over a period of hours to days.** Additionally, the patient's mental status fluctuates, with symptoms often becoming most severe in the evening and at night. Not uncommonly, hospitalized patients appear relatively lucid on morning rounds, especially if mental status is only superficially assessed, but then the night staff reports severe confusion and agitation.

Finally, **delirium is a manifestation of an underlying medical disorder.** Sometimes, the underlying condition is apparent. At other times, especially in elderly demented patients, delirium may be the first or the only sign of an acute illness, or it may be a serious decompensation or complication of a stable medical condition. Table 59–1 lists conditions that should be considered as causes of delirium. Of these conditions, the most common are drug toxicity (especially anticholinergics, sedatives, or narcotics in elderly patients), infection, electrolyte disturbances (most commonly hyponatremia or hypoglycemia), and withdrawal from alcohol or other sedatives.

Regardless of etiology, delirium produces a profound disturbance of brain function, and all etiologies are serious and potentially fatal illnesses. **Delirium must be approached as an acute medical emergency.** A detailed history, aggressively pursued, is mandatory, and because the responses from these patients cannot be relied upon,

Table 59-1 • MEDICAL CAUSES OF DELIRIUM
Discrete CNS lesion present
Head injury: stroke or intracranial bleed
Infection: meningitis, meningoencephalitis, brain abscess
Mass lesion: hematoma, tumor
Seizure, postictal
No discrete CNS lesion
Metabolic encephalopathy
• Anoxia: any cause, heart or respiratory failure, pulmonary embolus, sleep apnea, etc
• Hepatic encephalopathy
• Uremic encephalopathy
• Hypo-, hyperglycemia
• Hyponatremia/hypercalcemia
• Hypo-, hyperthermia
Toxic encephalopathy
• Drug withdrawal, especially alcohol and benzodiazepines, SSRIs
• Drug toxicity, eg, Dilantin
• Substance abuse
• Infections, especially pneumonia, urinary tract infections, intra-abdominal infection, bacteremia; all more frequent in the elderly

CNS, central nervous system; SSRI, selective serotonin reuptake inhibitor.

information from family, friends, or other caregivers is essential. A thorough physical examination with emphasis on neurologic status, clarity of speech, level of awareness, attention span, facial droop, and weakness of an extremity must be established because such changes must be carefully and frequently assessed. Basic laboratory studies should focus on chemical abnormalities (glucose, creatinine, bilirubin, serum sodium levels), drug intoxication, and evidence of hypoxia. The two threatening and potentially easily reversible conditions—**hypoxia and hypoglycemia**—should be immediately investigated and treated.

Delirium in the geriatric population can be the presenting manifestation of any acute illness, with an incidence of up to 10% on admission and up to 30% during an acute hospitalization. Causes of delirium in the elderly include pneumonia, urinary tract infection, myocardial infarction, gastrointestinal hemorrhage, traumatic injury, or virtually anything else that precipitates an acute hospitalization. This is even more of a problem after major surgery; nearly half of individuals (usually elderly) who suffer hip fractures develop delirium postoperatively.

Persons at any stage of dementia may develop delirium during an acute illness or injury or with additional pharmaceutical agent(s). Additionally, an acute delirium may "unmask" an early underlying, undetected dementia. The confused and disoriented geriatric patient cannot be dismissed as having one or the other, and the history on which this differential diagnosis is dependent should concentrate on any changes in the behavioral status of the patient since the acute event.

Management

The management of delirium is first and foremost the identification and treatment of the acute underlying illness. Adequate hydration, oxygenation, good nursing care, and round the clock careful supervision are always the initial measures. Management of agitation and disruptive behavior is the most challenging aspect of care of the delirious patient. If no specific treatable problem is identified, physical restraint should be used as a last resort. Frequent reassurance and orientation from familiar persons or constant supervision from a nurse or hospital aide are preferable. **Agitation with psychotic symptoms (hallucinations and delusions) can be treated with a neuroleptic such as low-dose haloperidol.** Older patients are more likely to experience extrapyramidal side effects, however, so newer atypical antipsychotics such as **risperidone** may be used. **Benzodiazepines** have a rapid onset of action but may worsen confusion and sedation.

Alcohol Withdrawal

Alcohol withdrawal manifests as a spectrum of symptoms, ranging from minor tremulousness and insomnia to the most severe form, **delirium tremens (DT)**, characterized by delirium, tremor, and autonomic hyperactivity. The severity of withdrawal can be assessed using a validated assessment tool, the Clinical Institute Withdrawal Assessment (CIWA) scale. Risk factors for the development of **delirium tremens** include a history of sustained drinking, prior withdrawal symptoms, age older than 30, and a concurrent medical illness. Withdrawal can coexist with or mimic other conditions, such as infection, intracranial bleeding, hepatic failure, gastrointestinal bleeding, or other drug overdose. DT is a diagnosis of exclusion;

Table 59–2 • ALCOHOL WITHDRAWAL SYMPTOMS	
Stage	**Symptoms**
Tremulousness	Earliest symptom occurring within 6 h of abstinence, caused by CNS and sympathetic hyperactivity, often referred to as the "shakes" or "jitters," and can occur even when patients still have a significant blood alcohol level. In addition to the typical 6- to 8-Hz tremor, which can be violent or subtle, insomnia, anxiety, gastrointestinal upset, diaphoresis, and palpitations can occur. Tremor typically diminishes over 48-72 h, but anxiety, easy startling can persist for 2 wk.
Withdrawal seizures	Also called "rum fits": Typically generalized tonic-clonic seizures, often occurring in clusters of two to six episodes, and almost always within 6-48 h of abstinence. Seen in patients with a long history of chronic alcoholism.
Alcoholic hallucinosis	Typically develops within 12 h of abstinence and resolves within 48 h. Hallucinations are most often visual (eg, bugs, pink elephants) but can be auditory or tactile. When auditory, they are often maligning or reproachful human voices. Despite the hallucinations, patients maintain a relatively intact sensorium.
Delirium tremens (DT)	Most dramatic and serious form of alcohol withdrawal, but occurs in only 5% of patients with withdrawal symptoms. DT typically begins within 48-72 h after the last drink and can last several days, often with a resolution as abrupt as its onset. Characterized by hallucinations, agitation, tremor, and sleeplessness, as well as signs of sympathetic hyperactivity: dilated pupils, low-grade fever, tachycardia, hypertension, diaphoresis, and hyperventilation. Delirium tremens is a serious condition with an in-hospital mortality of 5%-10%, usually from arrhythmias or infection, which is often unsuspected.

other serious diagnoses must be excluded before the patient's mental status and autonomic signs are attributed to withdrawal (see Table 59–1).

It is important to understand the temporal course of the spectrum of alcohol withdrawal syndromes (Table 59–2).

In contrast to other causes of delirium, **benzodiazepines are the drugs of choice in alcohol withdrawal.** They can be given on a fixed schedule in high-risk patients (previous history of DT or withdrawal seizures) to prevent withdrawal symptoms. If symptoms have already developed, benzodiazepines can be given according to one of two strategies. **Long-acting benzodiazepines such as diazepam or chlordiazepoxide** can be given in high doses until withdrawal symptoms cease and then the slow clearance of the drug is allowed to prevent further withdrawal symptoms. Alternatively, shorter-acting agents such as **lorazepam** can be **given as needed**, only when the patient has symptoms. Both strategies are effective. In either case, the key to successful management is initially aggressive upward titration of dosage until the patient is heavily sedated but responsive, followed by rapid downward titration as agitation decreases, usually over 48 to 72 hours. Supportive measures are also important, such as adequate hydration, replacement of electrolytes such as magnesium, and supplementation with **thiamine** and other B vitamins in malnourished, chronic alcoholics to prevent the development of Wernicke encephalopathy.

> ## CASE CORRELATION
> • See also Case 53 (Thyrotoxicosis) and Case 60 (Alcohol Ketoacidosis).

COMPREHENSION QUESTIONS

59.1 Which of the following agents most closely resembles the action of alcohol in the brain?

    A. Amphetamines

    B. Marijuana

    C. Cocaine

    D. Benzodiazepine

    E. Acetaminophen

59.2 Compared with dementia, which of the following is a characteristic of delirium?

    A. A fluctuating level of consciousness

    B. Slow onset

    C. Can be due to deficiencies of thiamine or cyanocobalamin

    D. Decreased memory ability

59.3 A 34-year-old man is brought to the emergency room for extreme tremors and auditory hallucinations. Which of the following statements is most likely to be correct?

    A. Auditory hallucinations are unique to alcohol withdrawal and cannot be caused by a brain tumor.

    B. If the serum blood alcohol level is higher than the legal limits of intoxication, these symptoms cannot be alcohol withdrawal.

    C. This patient should receive glucose intravenously for possible hypoglycemia.

    D. If the patient also has hypertension, fever, and tachycardia, he has a 5% to 10% chance of mortality.

ANSWERS

59.1 **D.** Alcohol and benzodiazepines both interact with the GABA system; thus, benzodiazepines are the drugs of choice for treatment of acute alcohol withdrawal. Cocaine and amphetamines both act as stimulants in the brain, increasing levels of dopamine.

59.2 **A.** Fluctuating levels of alertness and consciousness are typical of delirium. Remember that delirium is usually acute in onset and fluctuates, whereas dementia (the other answers) is slower and more gradual in onset, and consistent in alteration of cognition.

59.3 **D.** DT with autonomic instability and sympathetic overactivity is associated with a 5% to 10% mortality. Auditory hallucinations can occur from a number of illicit agents or even brain tumors. The fall in serum blood alcohol level and not the absolute level may induce symptoms of withdrawal. An individual who abuses alcohol should first be given thiamine, before glucose is administered, to prevent acute Wernicke encephalopathy.

CLINICAL PEARLS

▶ Delirium is characterized by acute onset of impaired attention and cognition, and fluctuating levels of consciousness, often with psychomotor and autonomic hyperactivity.

▶ Delirium requires urgent investigation to search for serious underlying systemic or metabolic causes.

▶ Frequent reassurance and orientation and constant observation are useful in managing the agitated delirious patient. Low-dose haloperidol can be used to control agitation or psychotic symptoms. Physical restraint is used as a last resort.

▶ Delirium tremens is the most severe and dramatic form of alcohol withdrawal, with abrupt onset from 2 to 4 days after cessation of drinking and sudden resolution several days later, and is associated with a mortality rate of 5% to 10%.

▶ Therapy for alcohol withdrawal syndromes includes benzodiazepines, hydration, electrolyte replacement, and B vitamins to prevent Wernicke encephalopathy.

▶ The mechanism of alcohol withdrawal is due to excitatory neurotransmitters due to sudden cessation of alcohol, which binds to GABA-A (inhibitory) receptors.

REFERENCES

Inouye SK. Delirium in older persons. *N Engl J Med*. 2006;354:1157-1165.

Cassidy EM, O'Sullivan I, Bradshaw P, Islam T, Onovo C. Symptom-triggered benzodiazepine therapy for alcohol withdrawal syndrome in the emergency department: a comparison with the standard fixed dose benzodiazepine regimen. *Emerg Med J*. 2012;29(10):802-804.

Goodson CM, Clark BJ, Douglas IS. Predictors of severe alcohol withdrawal syndrome: a systematic review and meta-analysis. *Alcohol Clin Exp Res*. 2014;38(10):2664-2677.

Josephson SA, Miller BL. Confusion and delirium. In: Kasper DL, Fauci AS, Hauser SL, Longo DL, Jameson JL, Loscalzo J, eds. *Harrison's Principles of Internal Medicine*. 19th ed. New York, NY: McGraw-Hill; 2015:196-201.

Shuckit MA. Alcohol and alcoholism. In: Kasper DL, Fauci AS, Hauser SL, Longo DL, Jameson JL, Loscalzo J, eds. *Harrison's Principles of Internal Medicine*. 19th ed. New York, NY: McGraw-Hill; 2015:3546-3556.

A 45-year-old man with a history of alcohol abuse is brought to the emergency department complaining of nausea and vomiting and mild abdominal pain. He had been on a 5-day drinking binge until the onset of these symptoms. He has no other medical history and was taking no other drugs and no medications.

On examination, he is sleeping on the stretcher but is easily arousable. He is afebrile with a pulse rate of 115 bpm, blood pressure of 122/72 mm Hg, and respiratory rate of 18 bpm. His breath has a strong odor of alcohol. His eyes are bloodshot but anicteric, his chest is clear to auscultation, and his heart is tachycardic but regular in rhythm, and no murmurs are appreciated. His abdominal examination is significant for mild epigastric tenderness with hypoactive bowel sounds, but no guarding or tenderness is noted. He has peripheral edema, and no focal neurologic deficits.

Initial laboratories show sodium 145 mEq/L, potassium 5 mEq/L, chloride 105 mEq/L, and bicarbonate 14 mEq/L, with blood urea nitrogen (BUN) 20 mg/dL, and creatinine 1.5 mg/dL. Serum glucose is 142 mg/dL. A serum Acetest is weakly positive for ketones. Urinalysis shows ketonuria but no glycosuria and no cells, casts, or crystals. Urine drug screen is negative, and abdominal x-rays show a normal bowel gas pattern with no signs of obstruction.

▶ What is the most likely diagnosis?
▶ What is the best initial treatment?

ANSWERS TO CASE 60:

Alcoholic Ketoacidosis

Summary: A 45-year-old man with a history of alcohol abuse is brought to the emergency room with nausea and vomiting after a prolonged drinking binge. His physical examination is significant only for tachycardia and mild epigastric tenderness. His laboratory studies are most significant for a low serum bicarbonate level, suggestive of an acidotic state. The Acetest is weakly positive for ketones, but his serum glucose is not elevated.

- **Most likely diagnosis:** Alcoholic ketoacidosis.

- **Best initial treatment:** Infusion of 5% dextrose with 0.9% saline.

ANALYSIS

Objectives

1. Understand how to diagnose and classify simple acid-base disorders.

2. Know how to calculate the anion gap (AG), and how to manage the causes of high AG acidosis.

3. Understand the two causes of nongap acidosis (bicarbonate losses from the gastrointestinal [GI] tract and renal tubular acidosis).

4. Understand how to distinguish between saline-responsive and saline-resistant metabolic alkalosis.

Considerations

This 45 year old man presents with nausea and vomiting after an alcohol binge. The most significant finding in this case is an apparent acidosis with an elevated anion gap. In this patient with a history of alcoholism and an alcohol binge, alcoholic ketoacidosis is most likely, but one must also consider the possibility of other ingestions (methanol, ethylene glycol), either accidental or intentional, that would also present with similar laboratory findings, but may be more serious or even fatal. Alcoholic ketoacidosis (AKA) is characterized by metabolic acidosis with an elevated anion gap, elevated serum ketones, and a normal or low serum glucose level. Sometimes, due to persistent vomiting, there is a coexisting metabolic alkalosis due to volume depletion.

APPROACH TO:

Alcoholic Ketoacidosis

DEFINITIONS

ANION GAP = $[Na^+] - [Cl^- + HCO_3^-]$. An estimation of unmeasured anions in the plasma (phosphate, sulfate, organic acids), with normal being 10 to 12 mmol/L.

OSMOLAL GAP: The difference between the measured and calculated serum osmolality. If elevated (eg, >10 mOsm), then suggestive of the presence of significant serum concentration of an additional osmotically active solute such as methanol or ethylene glycol.

URINE ANION GAP (UAG) = urine $[Na^+ + K^+]$ − urine $[Cl^-]$. An estimation of urinary ammonium ion (NH_4^+) excretion.

CLINICAL APPROACH

In normal physiology, systemic pH is maintained between 7.35 and 7.45. The main homeostatic mechanisms are respiratory and renal. Under normal conditions, body CO_2 production is relatively stable, and CO_2 excretion by the respiratory system keeps the arterial CO_2 tension around 40 mm Hg. The main renal mechanisms for maintaining normal pH are the reabsorption of filtered HCO_3^- in the proximal tubule, and excretion of NH_4^+ in the distal tubule. Disturbances in one of these systems cause a compensatory change in the other system. For instance, the development of a metabolic acidosis would stimulate the respiratory system to increase the ventilation and lower the $PaCO_2$, which affects the HCO_3^- to $PaCO_2$ ratio and thus the pH would move toward but not quite to normal. Simple acid-base disorders can be classified and understood using the pH, the $PaCO_2$, and the HCO_3^- (Table 60–1).

Metabolic Acidosis

If metabolic acidosis is evident, the first step in evaluating the cause is to calculate the **AG.** The AG represents unmeasured anions in the plasma including phosphates, sulfates, organic anions, as well as anionic proteins such as albumin. **The normal AG is usually 10 to 12 mmol/L.** When evaluating the AG, one should remember the role of charged proteins. The calculated AG will be lowered if patients are hypoalbuminemic as in nephrotic syndrome (decreased anionic albumin), or if there are high levels of immunoglobulins as in multiple myeloma (increased cationic paraproteins). The causes of high AG metabolic acidosis are listed in Table 60–2.

Lactic acidosis most commonly occurs in the setting of an **acute illness with poor tissue perfusion** such as septic shock, heart failure, severe anemia, or poisoning affecting tissue oxygen delivery or cellular respiration (carbon monoxide, cyanide). Treatment is aimed at correcting the underlying condition. Sodium bicarbonate may be used in severe acidemia (pH <7.1), sufficient to correct to a pH of 7.2. Acute bicarbonate use has been associated with increased mortality, heart failure, and volume overload. (See also Case 52 DKA for discussion).

Table 60–1 • SIMPLE ACID-BASE DISORDERS

Disorder	pH	$PaCO_2$	HCO_3^-
Metabolic acidosis	Low	Low	Low
Metabolic alkalosis	High	High	High
Respiratory acidosis	Low	High	High
Respiratory alkalosis	High	Low	Low

Table 60–2 • CAUSES OF ANION GAP METABOLIC ACIDOSIS[a]
1. Lactic acidosis
2. Ketoacidosis
a. Diabetic
b. Alcoholic
c. Starvation
3. Toxins
a. Ethylene glycol
b. Methanol
c. Salicylates
d. Propylene glycol
4. Renal failure (acute and chronic)

[a]Mneumonic: MUDPILES- Methanol, Uremia, DKA, Propylene glycol, Isoniazid, Lactic acid, Ethylene glycol, Starvation/ Salicylates.

Diabetic ketoacidosis (DKA) is caused by insulin deficiency with increased lipolysis and fatty acid metabolism, with accumulation of the ketoacids acetoacetate and beta-hydroxybutyrate. Diagnosis and treatment of DKA is discussed in Case 52.

In **alcoholic ketoacidosis**, decreased carbohydrate intake reduces insulin secretion, and alcohol-induced inhibition of gluconeogenesis leads to stimulation of lipolysis and contributes to increased ketoacid formation, predominantly beta-hydroxybutyrate. The nitroprusside reaction test to detect serum ketones (Acetest) can detect acetoacetate, but not beta-hydroxybutyrate, so the nitroprusside reaction may only be weakly positive, and can lead one to underestimate the degree of ketosis. With treatment, as the patient improves, the formation of acetoacetate is favored, so the degree of measured ketosis may appear to paradoxically worsen. In contrast to the markedly elevated glucose levels in DKA, the plasma glucose concentration in alcoholic ketoacidosis may be low, normal, or somewhat elevated. In alcoholic or fasting ketoacidosis, the primary treatment is administration of dextrose and saline solutions; the dextrose will increase insulin secretion and reduce lipolysis, along with saline to replenish fluid deficits. Electrolyte deficiencies such as hypophosphatemia, hypokalemia, or hypomagnesemia are also common, and should be corrected. **In alcoholics, thiamine 100 mg IV should be administered prior to any glucose-containing solution to decrease the risk of precipitating Wernicke encephalopathy or Korsakoff syndrome.**

In a patient with an elevated AG acidosis and a suggestive social history, one must also consider the possibility of other ingestions, such as methanol or ethylene glycol. Methanol and ethylene glycol are frequently found in high concentration in automotive antifreeze and deicing solutions, windshield wiper fluid, and other solvents. They may be ingested as a substitute for ethanol, by accident, or intentionally, for example, in a suicide attempt. **Methanol** is metabolized via the alcohol dehydrogenase (ADH) enzyme to formaldehyde and formic acid, causing **optic nerve and CNS injury. Ethylene glycol** is metabolized by ADH to glycolate, glyoxylate, and oxalate and can cause acute renal failure due to glycolate-induced damage to tubules, and tubular obstruction from precipitated oxalate crystals. If either of these ingestions is suspected, direct laboratory assays of the substances are not usually available, so their presence may be inferred by an elevated **osmolal gap.**

Serum osmolality is primarily determined by solutes that can be directly measured: sodium, glucose, and urea. Other unmeasured solutes, especially low-molecular-weight substances such as methanol will also affect osmolality. Serum osmolality can be calculated using the following formula:

$$SmOsm = (2 \times [Na]) + [glucose, in\ mg/dL]/18 + [BUN, in\ mg/dL]/2.8.$$

If the difference between the directly measured serum osmolality and the calculated serum osmolality is greater than 10, then the presence of another solute is suspected. Ethanol itself can be directly measured in most laboratories, so a patient with a suspicious ingestion with a high AG acidosis, elevated osmolar gap, and low or absent blood alcohol level may be suspected to have methanol or ethylene glycol ingestion. If ethylene glycol is suspected, one may also examine the urine for oxalate crystals. For either methanol or ethylene glycol ingestion, therapy includes the administration of **fomepizole**, an ADH inhibitor that reduces the formation of the toxic metabolites.

Non-AG metabolic acidosis: Causes of non-AG metabolic acidosis are listed in Table 60–3. With bicarbonate losses from the GI tract or kidney, there is a rise in chloride concentration that approximates the fall in bicarbonate concentration (hyperchloremic metabolic acidosis), so the AG remains normal. Most GI causes can be elicited by the clinical history (diarrhea, external pancreatic, biliary, or small bowel drainage). In patients with diarrhea and hypokalemia, renal synthesis and secretion of ammonia are stimulated, causing a buffering of the urine with a pH greater than 5.5 (higher than expected in acidosis). Acidosis with high urine pH

Table 60–3 • CAUSES OF NON-ANION GAP ACIDOSIS

Gastrointestinal bicarbonate loss
- Diarrhea
- External pancreatic or small bowel drainage
- Ureterosigmoidostomy, jejunal loop, ileal loop

Renal acidosis
A. Hypokalemia
  - Proximal RTA (type 2)
  - Distal (classic) RTA (type 1)
B. Hyperkalemia
  1. Generalized distal nephron dysfunction (type 4 RTA)
    - Mineralocorticoid deficiency
    - Mineralocorticoid resistance

Drug-induced hyperkalemia (with renal insufficiency)
- Potassium-sparing diuretics (amiloride, triamterene, spironolactone)
- Trimethoprim
- ACE inhibitors and ARBs
- NSAIDs

Other causes
- Acid loads (ammonium chloride, hyperalimentation)
- Expansion acidosis (rapid saline administration)

(*Data from Longo*. Harrison's Principles of Internal Medicine. *18th ed. New York: McGraw-Hill, 2012. Table 47-5.*)

due to GI losses (has high urinary NH_4^+) can be differentiated from renal tubular acidosis (RTA) (has low urinary NH_4^+) by assessing urinary NH_4^+ excretion. Urine NH_4^+ cannot be directly measured, but it can be estimated with the UAG.

When **[Na + K] – [Cl] is negative** (usually –20 to –50 mEq/L), then urinary NH_4^+ is appropriately increased, suggesting a **GI or extrarenal cause of acidosis.**

When the **UAG is positive**, it suggests **impaired NH_4^+ excretion.** Causes include **distal (type 1) RTA**, hypoaldosteronism, or **type 4 RTA.** In patients with advanced chronic kidney disease, decline in functional renal mass also causes a proportional reduction in renal NH_4^+ excretion.

Distal or type 1 RTA in adults is most commonly caused by autoimmune diseases such as **Sjögren syndrome** or rheumatoid arthritis. Patients have a high urine pH, and often have **hypokalemia.** Most patients have hypocitraturia and hypercalciuria, so **kidney stones** and nephrocalcinosis commonly occur. Treatment usually involves alkalinization and citrate supplementation with sodium or potassium citrate to normalize pH and prevent stone formation.

Type 4 RTA is due to generalized distal nephron dysfunction, and is commonly seen in patients with **diabetic nephropathy.** Low plasma renin activity is common in diabetic patients, leading to hyporeninemic hypoaldosteronism. Patients typically present with **hyperkalemia** and a mild hyperchloremic metabolic acidosis. The hyperkalemia is usually managed with a low potassium diet and use of loop or thiazide diuretics.

Respiratory Acidosis

Respiratory acidosis can occur acutely or chronically. The pathophysiology is reduction in minute ventilation leading to rising $PaCO_2$ and falling pH. Renal adaptation occurs but requires several days, with increased reabsorption of HCO_3^-. **In a chronic compensated state, the HCO_3^- increases 4 mmol/L for every 10 mm Hg increase in $PaCO_2$. (This is also called the "4 for 10 rule" for chronic respiratory acidosis).** The most common cause of acute respiratory acidosis in hospitalized patients is drug-induced respiratory depression with hypoventilation, due to narcotics, sedatives, or anesthesia. The most common cause of chronic respiratory acidosis is chronic obstructive pulmonary disease (COPD). Many of these patients live with chronic elevations of $PaCO_2$ of 50 mm Hg or higher.

Respiratory Alkalosis

This condition most often occurs acutely, with increased respiratory rate and tidal volume, leading to an acute fall in $PaCO_2$ and rise in pH. After several days, the **HCO_3^- decreases 5 mmol/L for every 10 mm Hg decrease in $PaCO_2$. (This is also called the "5 for 10 rule" for chronic respiratory alkalosis).** It can be a response to any disease that causes hypoxia, such as a pulmonary embolism, but is also often seen as a manifestation of an anxiety disorder with hyperventilation. Hypocapnia causes decreased cerebral blood flow, so symptoms manifest as light-headedness or dizziness. With acute alkalosis, there is increased affinity between albumin and calcium, so more calcium becomes protein bound. Patients may then experience symptoms of hypocalcemia (perioral numbness, paresthesias).

Metabolic Alkalosis

Metabolic alkalosis most often occurs when there is loss of acid or excess endogenous production of HCO_3^- by the kidney. Under normal physiologic circumstances, the kidney can excrete very high quantities of HCO_3^-, so for a metabolic alkalosis to be maintained, there must be some impairment in their normal ability to excrete excess alkali. The kidneys will retain rather than excrete excess HCO_3^- under the following common conditions:

1. Hyperaldosteronism causes increased tubular reabsorption of Na^+ and HCO_3^-, and excessive loss of Cl^- in the urine (**urine chloride >20 mEq/L**). **These disorders require** correction of the metabolic alkalosis which requires treatment of the underlying condition (eg, primary aldosteronism, renal artery stenosis, Cushing syndrome). This alkalosis is termed "**chloride resistant**" or "saline resistant," meaning that it cannot be corrected by the administration of sodium chloride solution.

2. Extracellular fluid (ECF) volume contraction and hypokalemia due to various causes (vomiting, nasogastric suction, diuretics), causing augmented distal H^+ secretion (**urine chloride <10 mEq/L**).

Correction of hypokalemia and administration of saline solution to restore ECF volume are usually sufficient to reverse the alkalosis. This alkalosis is termed "**chloride responsive**" or "saline responsive." A patient with persistent emesis such as due to gastroenteritis may develop saline responsive metabolic alkalosis.

COMPREHENSION QUESTIONS

60.1 A 34-year-old woman presents to your office for a checkup. Her only medical history is recurrent kidney stones. She is currently asymptomatic. Her laboratories show Na 136, K 3.0, Cl 110, HCO_3 16, creatinine 1, and glucose 110. Her urine pH is 6.5. Which of the following is the most likely diagnosis?

   A. Bulimia with chronic hypokalemia

   B. Ethylene glycol ingestion with calcium oxalate stones

   C. Type 1 distal RTA

   D. Type 4 RTA due to diabetic kidney disease

60.2 Which of the following urine electrolytes is most useful in estimating the ECF volume status of a patient with metabolic alkalosis?

   A. Urine Na

   B. Urine Cl

   C. Urine urea

   D. Urine anion gap

60.3 A 59-year-old man is brought to the emergency room obtunded and unable to give a history. He is afebrile and normotensive. He has edema of the optic disc, and his neurologic examination does not reveal any focal neurologic deficits. His laboratories include pH 7.25, $PaCO_2$ 23, Na 145, K 5.3, Cl 105, HCO_3 10, BUN 25, creatinine 1.3, and glucose 80. His measured serum osmolality is 335 mOsm, and his blood alcohol level is 0. Urinalysis shows no crystals. What is the most likely cause of his mental status and acidemia?

A. Ethanol intoxication

B. Acute stroke with hypoventilation

C. Methanol intoxication

D. Ethylene glycol intoxication

ANSWERS

60.1 **C.** She has a non-AG acidosis with alkaline urine, suggestive of RTA. Patients with type 1 RTA tend toward hypokalemia, whereas type 4 RTA has hyperkalemia. With alkaline urine and hypercalciuria, patients are predisposed to recurrent calcium phosphate stones. Vomiting from bulimia might cause metabolic alkalosis. Ethylene glycol would cause AG acidosis.

60.2 **B.** Urine chloride is useful for judging the volume status of patients with metabolic alkalosis, and is used to classify them as either volume depleted (low urine Cl) or volume repleted (high urine Cl). If low urine chloride, they are considered chloride responsive, and the alkalosis can be corrected with the infusion of saline. Urine Na is not a good indicator of volume status, since urinary HCO_3 losses will force a certain amount of Na with it.

60.3 **C.** The patient has a high AG metabolic acidosis. He has a high osmolal gap, but his ethanol level is undetectable. The most likely intoxication is methanol, which is metabolized to formic acid. This toxic metabolite causes mental status depression, papilledema, optic neuritis, and metabolic acidosis. Hypoventilation would cause respiratory acidosis. Ethylene glycol may cause the formation of calcium oxalate crystals in the urine.

CLINICAL PEARLS

▶ Causes of AG metabolic acidosis include lactic acidosis, ketoacidosis, toxic ingestion, and renal failure.

▶ In AG acidosis, a large osmolal gap (>10) can be caused by ingestion of methanol or ethylene glycol.

▶ In non-AG acidosis, positive urine anion gap is suggestive of RTA, and negative urine anion gap is consistent with extrarenal (GI) cause of acidosis.

▶ Patients with respiratory alkalosis may experience symptoms of cerebral vasoconstriction (dizziness) and transient hypocalcemia (perioral numbness and paresthesias).

▶ In metabolic alkalosis, low urine chloride can determine that the alkalosis can be corrected by saline infusion (chloride responsive).

▶ The 5 for 10 rule for chronic respiratory alkalosis means the bicarbonate level is expected to decrease **5 mmol/L for every 10 mm Hg decrease in $PaCO_2$** below 40 mm Hg.

▶ The 4 for 10 rule for chronic respiratory acidosis means that the bicarbonate level is expected to rise **4 mmol/L for every 10 mm Hg increase in $PaCO_2$** above 40 mm Hg.

REFERENCES

Beck LH, Salant DJ. Tubulointerstitial diseases and the kidney. In: Kasper DL, Fauci AS, Hauser SL, Longo DL, Jameson JL, Loscalzo J, eds. *Harrison's Principles of Internal Medicine.* 19th ed. New York, NY: McGraw-Hill; 2015:2367-2374.

DuBose TD. Acidosis and alkalosis. In: Kasper DL, Fauci AS, Hauser SL, Longo DL, Jameson JL, Loscalzo J, eds. *Harrison's Principles of Internal Medicine.* 19th ed. New York, NY: McGraw-Hill; 2015:363-373.

Rose BD, Post TW. *Clinical Physiology of Acid-Base and Electrolyte Disorders.* 5th ed. New York, NY: McGraw-Hill; 2001:328-347.

Review Questions

REVIEW QUESTIONS

R1.   A 55-year-old white man with a history of end-stage renal disease (ESRD) secondary to chronic uncontrolled hypertension (HTN) presents to the emergency department (ED) after sustaining a fall in his bathroom on to his right hip. He complains of pain with passive motion of the hip and on physical examination the hip has limited range of motion upon internal rotation. An x-ray of the right hip shows a fracture. Which of the below series of serum laboratory values are consistent with the underlying condition predisposing to this patient's fracture?

	Serum Ca	Serum PO3	Serum PTH
A.	Increased	Decreased	Increased
B.	Increased	Decreased	Decreased
C.	Increased	Increased	Decreased
D.	Decreased	Increased	Increased
E.	Decreased	Increased	Decreased
F.	Decreased	Decreased	Decreased

R2.   A 24-year old African-American man comes into clinic from a referral after having significant bleeding following a wisdom tooth extraction 1 week ago. He has no significant medical history and took aspirin 1 week ago for a headache. However, he reports getting nosebleeds lasting over 10 minutes as a child. He reports no family history of diagnosed bleeding disorders but endorses his mother easily bruises and has heavy menstrual bleeding. Laboratory values include a normal platelet count, increased bleeding time, a normal prothrombin time (PT), and an increased partial prothrombin time (PTT). What is the most likely diagnosis?

A. Aspirin overdose

B. Bernard-Soulier syndrome

C. Hemophilia A

D. Vitamin K deficiency

E. von Willebrand disease

R3.   A 40-year-old woman with known HIV presents to clinic with complaints of difficulty and pain with swallowing. She has been experiencing substernal burning chest pain for the past 2 weeks. Her most recent CD4+ count was 80 cells/mm^3 and her medications include trimethoprim/sulfamethoxazole (TMP-SMX) and highly active antiretroviral therapy (HAART). On physical examination there are white plaques visible in the oral cavity and posterior pharynx that are easily removed with a tongue blade. No vesicular lesions are visible in the posterior pharynx. An endoscopy is performed that demonstrates additional white plaques in the proximal esophagus. Biopsies are significant for pseudohyphae. What is the best pharmacotherapy for this patient's condition?

A. Acyclovir

B. Azithromycin

C. Fluconazole

D. Ganciclovir

E. Sulfadiazine-pyrimethamine

R4. A 55-year-old man with known alcoholic cirrhosis presents to the ED with confusion and diffuse abdominal pain. Blood pressure is 98/68 mm Hg, temperature is 100.4°F, and pulse is 102 bpm. The abdomen is distended and a fluid wave present on physical examination. In the past, his ascites was controlled with furosemide and spironolactone. Paracentesis is performed and found to have an absolute polymorphonuclear (PMN) count of 280 cells/mm^3, albumin of 1 mg/dL, and cultures are pending. Serum albumin is 2.6 g/dL. Which of the following is the best next step?

A. Administer oral lactulose.

B. Empiric IV ceftriaxone.

C. Empiric IV octreotide.

D. Liver transplantation.

E. Protein-restricted diet.

R5. A 30-year-old woman is admitted to the shock trauma intensive care unit (ICU) after sustaining a motor vehicle collision. She has required multiple major surgeries as well as mechanical ventilation for the past week. Vital signs have been stable during this time and her chest x-rays have been clear. On hospital day 8 she develops a temperature of 102.2°F, blood pressure is 110/70 mm Hg, heart rate is 104 bpm, SpO$_2$ is 92%, and new purulent secretions from the endotracheal tube are sent for Gram stain and culture. A chest x-ray is found to have a new infiltrate in the right lower lobe. Initial antibiotic coverage should include coverage for what organism?

A. *Chlamydia pneumoniae*

B. *Haemophilus influenzae*

C. *Legionella pneumophila*

D. *Pseudomonas aeruginosa*

E. Methicillin-sensitive *Staphylococcus aureus*

R6. A 60-year-old man with a history of hyperlipidemia controlled on simvastatin and well-controlled hypertension complains of nonbloody, watery diarrhea for over 1 year. He complains of episodes of wheezing and increased redness and heat in his face, neck, and upper chest that last up to 5 minutes. On physical examination there is hepatomegaly and a 2/6 holosystolic murmur is auscultated on the left lower sternal boarder that is accentuated with inspiration. Blood pressure is 135/85 mm Hg, heart rate is 85 bpm, and respiratory rate is 16 breaths per minute. What is the next best diagnostic test?

    A. 24-Hour urine 5-hydroxyindoleacetic acid

    B. 24-Hour urine metanephrines

    C. Endoscopy with colonoscopy

    D. Methacholine challenge

    E. Secretin injection test

R7. A 37-year-old woman with a history of intravenous (IV) drug use and prostitution presents with complaints of fatigue and increased swelling around her eyes, hands, and feet. She has also noticed increased abdominal girth. She is on no medications. Physical examination shows temperature 98.9°F, blood pressure 125/80 mm Hg, heart rate 76 bpm, respiratory rate 14 breaths per minute, periorbital edema, and shifting dullness on abdominal examination. Laboratory values include serum albumin 2.4 g/dL, negative rapid plasma reagin (RPR), positive hepatitis B surface antigen (HBsAg), positive HBeAg, and negative Anti-HIV antibody. Urinalysis is negative for red blood cells (RBCs) and positive for waxy casts. 24-Hour urine protein excretion is 3.7 g/d. What is the most likely diagnosis?

    A. Diabetic nephropathy

    B. Focal segmental glomerulosclerosis

    C. IgA nephropathy

    D. Membranous nephropathy

    E. Minimal change disease

R8. The patient in Question R7 suddenly develops redness, swelling, and pain in her left calf. On physical examination there is pain with dorsiflexion of the foot. What is the most likely pathophysiology of her current condition?

    A. Increase in clotting factor VIII

    B. Decrease in antithrombin III

    C. Decrease in protein C

    D. Decrease in protein S

    E. A mutation in clotting factor V

R9. A 61-year-old man presents to the hospital complaining of substernal chest pain and malaise. He was previously hospitalized 3 weeks ago for a myocardial infarction (MI). He reports increased pain when taking deep breaths but denies shortness of breath or palpitations. His chest pain improves when he is leaning forward. Electrocardiogram (ECG) is performed and shows diffuse ST elevation and his erythrocyte sedimentation rate (ESR) is elevated at 35 mm/h. What is the best treatment for this patient's condition?

    A. Nitroglycerin and metoprolol

    B. Morphine and supplemental oxygen

    C. High-dose aspirin and nonsteroidal anti-inflammatory drugs (NSAIDs)

D. IV heparin and clopidogrel

E. IV vancomycin and ceftriaxone

R10. A 45-year-old man with history of seizure disorder and alcohol abuse is hospitalized after a 30-minute tonic-clonic seizure. 24 hours after the seizure he is found on physical examination to have a blood pressure of 157/90 mm Hg, heart rate is 110 bpm, and temperature is 98.6°F. Urine draining from the Foley catheter is dark and sent for analysis. Laboratory values include the following:

Serum sodium 143, serum potassium 5.1, serum bicarbonate 19, serum Cr 3 mg/dL, and blood urea nitrogen (BUN) 32 mg/dL. Urinalysis reveals negative protein, negative leukocytes, negative nitrites, 4+ blood with microscopy 2 to 5 RBCs, 0 to 1 white blood cells (WBCs).

What is the most likely underlying pathophysiology to this patient's condition?

A. Vascular inflammation

B. Outflow tract obstruction

C. Poor renal perfusion

D. Toxic injury to glomerulus

R11. A 65-year-old man with a 30-year history of smoking 2 packs per day complains of increased swelling in both of his legs, increased dyspnea, and fatigue on exertion. He denies having to use extra pillows at night to help him breathe. He also notes an increase in number of times he urinates during the night. On physical examination there is distention of the right jugular vein when firm pressure is applied over the liver, presence of a parasternal heave, and there are diffuse expiratory wheezes heard on auscultation of the lungs. What is most likely to be found on chest x-ray?

A. Bilateral pulmonary infiltrates

B. Depressed diaphragm with prominent pulmonary artery

C. Unilateral lobar consolidation

D. Widened mediastinum

E. Multiple pulmonary nodules

R12. A 40-year-old woman comes into clinic complaining of a 15-lb weight gain over the past 6 months despite a decrease in appetite. She states she is more bothered by cold temperatures, her hair is thinner, and recently has more difficulty passing bowel movements. She states that 8 months ago she was experiencing diarrhea, felt like her heart was beating quickly, and was always hot. Today her blood pressure is 125/85 mm Hg, heart rate is 70 bpm, and she is afebrile. On physical examination there is no exophthalmos, thyroid is nontender and diffusely enlarged with a rubbery texture without any isolated nodules, and her skin is dry to the touch. Laboratory values include elevated thyroid-stimulating hormone (TSH), decreased free T_3 and T_4, and positive antithyroid peroxidase (anti-TPO) antibodies. This patient is now at risk for which of the following complications?

A. Anaplastic carcinoma of the thyroid

B. Follicular carcinoma of the thyroid

C. Lymphoma of the thyroid

D. Medullary carcinoma of the thyroid

E. Papillary carcinoma of the thyroid

ANSWERS

R1. **D. This patient suffered a hip fracture with minimal trauma.** ESRD patients can be at risk for bone fractures due to a decrease in bone mineral density described as osteitis fibrosa cystica. Those with ESRD are unable to activate vitamin D in the kidney; this creating hypovitaminosis D, which impairs the absorption of calcium from the gastrointestinal tract. Decreased serum calcium then impairs regulation of parathyroid hormone (PTH) production, causing a secondary hyperparathyroidism. Furthermore, decreased kidney function impairs the excretion of phosphate, causing serum levels to become elevated, sometimes requiring treatment with phosphate binders. Choice A (increased Ca, decreased PO_3, increased PTH) is consistent with osteitis fibrosa cystica due to a primary hyperparathyroidism where an increased PTH causes an increase in calcium from the bone as well as an increased excretion of phosphate in the kidney. Choice C (increased Ca, increased PO_3, decreased PTH) is consistent with hypervitaminosis D caused by excessive supplementation or granulomatous disease such as sarcoidosis. In sarcoidosis immune cells in the granulomas outside of the kidney increases the active form of vitamin D. Hip fractures secondary to osteoporosis are unlikely to demonstrate abnormal laboratory values where those caused secondary to Paget disease will show an elevated alkaline phosphatase (See Case 35 [Osteoporosis] and Case 50 [Hypercalcemia]).

R2. **E. This man has both platelet and clotting factor dysfunction inherited in an autosomal dominant fashion.** Von Willebrand disease (vWD) is caused by a deficiency of von Willebrand factor (vWF). vWF plays a role in primary (platelet driven) and secondary (clotting factors) hemostasis. In primary hemostasis vWF is released by damaged endothelium which is where the platelet glycoprotein Ib (GpIb) receptor initially binds. If vWF is decreased or absent, platelets are unable to bind to the damaged endothelium, which causes clinical manifestations of platelet dysfunction (increased bleeding time) such as petechiae, epistaxis, and increased bruising without affecting the number of platelets. vWF is also responsible for protecting clotting factor VIII from rapid breakdown in the blood; therefore, a deficiency of vWF can cause a deficiency of factor VIII, elevating the PTT without affecting the PT. Choice A (aspirin overdose) causes platelet dysfunction without decreasing the number of platelets by irreversibly inhibiting thromboxane

A2 (TXA2), making platelet aggregation ineffective in primary hemostasis; however, aspirin does not affect secondary hemostasis laboratory values (PT/PTT). Choice B (Bernard-Soulier syndrome) is also an isolated dysfunction of platelets whereby there is a deficiency of the receptor GpIb preventing platelets to bind to the vWF expressed by the damaged epithelium. This produces the same effect as vWD in primary hemostasis; however, there is no dysfunction of clotting factors and no elevation in PT or PTT. Choice C (hemophilia A) is an X-linked inherited disorder characterized by a deficiency in factor VIII that causes dysfunction in secondary hemostasis alone which is clinically manifested by an elevated PTT, normal bleeding time and PT, and increased deep bleeding such as hemarthrosis (bleeding into joints). Choice D (vitamin K deficiency) would manifest as an elevated PT, mildly increased PTT, and no effect on bleeding time or platelet number from the inability to activate clotting factors II, VII, IX, and X through gamma-carboxylation (see Case 56 [Immune Thrombocytopenia Purpura]).

R3.   **C. This patient needs an antifungal treatment for *Candida esophagitis*.** When the CD4 counts fall below 100 cells/mm³, patients infected with HIV are at risk for developing esophagitis. Esophagitis presents with primary complaints of odynophagia (painful swallowing), dysphagia, and a substernal burning chest pain. White plaques that are easily removed with a tongue blade are consistent with oral thrush caused by the opportunistic fungus—*Candida* that can cause esophagitis when it extends beyond the oral cavity to the proximal esophagus. *Candida esophagitis* is the most likely diagnosis in patients presenting with oral thrush. Endoscopy and biopsy are not necessary before initiating treatment with oral fluconazole. However, if patients show no improvement and have no signs of oral thrush, endoscopy with biopsy is warranted. Choice A (acyclovir) would be appropriate treatment for herpes simplex virus (HSV) esophagitis that would present with multiple, small vesicles and round/ovoid ulcers on endoscopy. Cells on biopsy would contain eosinophilic intranuclear inclusions. Choice D (ganciclovir) is appropriate for treating cytomegalovirus (CMV) esophagitis that demonstrates large linear ulcerations likely in the distal esophagus. Biopsy would be positive for intranuclear and intracytoplasmic inclusions. Choice B (azithromycin) is appropriate for *Mycobacterium avium* complex (MAC) prophylaxis when the CD4 count is <100. Choice E (sulfadiazine/pyrimethamine) is appropriate treatment for toxoplasmosis that usually presents as ring-enhancing lesions in the brain when the CD4 count is <100 cells/mm³ (see Case 46 [HIV Infection]).

R4.   **B. This patient is suffering from spontaneous bacterial peritonitis.** This patient is likely in end-stage liver failure due to known alcoholic cirrhosis. One of the many complications of cirrhosis is spontaneous bacterial peritonitis, an infection of the ascitic fluid most often caused by flora of the gastrointestinal (GI) tract such as *Escherichia coli* or *Klebsiella*. It is associated with a high mortality rate (20%-30%) and is likely to reoccur. Clinical presentation is subtle and there should be a high index of suspicion in order to initiate treatment as soon as possible. Common symptoms include fever, diffuse abdominal pain, and altered mental status in a patient with known cirrhosis. Diagnosis is confirmed with a diagnostic paracentesis evaluating fluid for WBCs, in particular PMNs, Gram stain, and culture. There will be a serum ascites-albumin gradient (SAAG) ≥1.1 g/dL and fluid will have a PMN count ≥250 cells/uL and a positive culture. However, empiric treatment should be initiated with a third-generation cephalosporin (ceftriaxone, cefotaxime) while awaiting culture results given the most common cause is gram-negative organisms. Choice A (oral lactulose) would be the appropriate treatment for hepatic encephalopathy to prevent reabsorption of the toxic metabolite ammonia. Clinical presentation would include an altered mental status; however, this diagnosis is less likely given the patient's fever and diffuse abdominal pain. Choice C (empiric IV octreotide) would be appropriate during the treatment of bleeding esophageal varices that usually present as a patient in liver failure with massive hematemesis. It acts as a vasoconstrictor to the splanchnic vessels and helps reduce portal pressure. Choice D (liver transplant) and choice E (protein restricted diet) would not be appropriate initial treatment for this patient (see Case 24 [Cirrhosis]).

R5.   **D. This patient has developed a ventilator-associated pneumonia (VAP) and empiric antibiotics should include antipseudomonal coverage.** VAP is a pneumonia that occurs after 2 days in the intubated patient. It should be suspected when there is an acute change in the intubated patient including a new fever, decrease in oxygen saturation, and new purulent secretions. A chest x-ray should be obtained, and VAP should be suspected if there is an acute change in previously clear chest x-rays showing new infiltrates. A lower respiratory tract endotracheal sample should be sampled and cultured. Pending cultures, empiric antibiotics should include gram-positive coverage, anti-*Pseudomonas* and gram-negative coverage, and coverage for methicillin-**resistant** *Staphylococcus aureus* (MRSA) should be considered. Once sensitivities come back, coverage can be narrowed to the specific organism. Choice A (*C pneumoniae*) is a cause of community-acquired atypical pneumonia where the patient presents with an insidious onset of various symptoms such as headache and fatigue with dry cough and fever—"walking pneumonia." Chest x-ray will most likely demonstrate interstitial infiltrates. Choice B (*H influenzae*) is the organism associated with pneumonias found in patients with other comorbidities such as chronic obstructive pulmonary disease (COPD), diabetes, or alcoholism. Clinical presentation will be similar to patients with community-acquired pneumonia such as fever, cough, and shortness of breath. Choice C (*L pneumophila*) is the causal organism associated with pneumonia named "Legionnaires' disease" usually in patients who are heavy smokers and have been exposed to a contaminated water source. A urine antigen test can confirm this diagnosis. Choice D would be incorrect because in a hospitalized patient, MRSA would be a more likely cause of ventilator-associated pneumonia. (See Case 19 [Community-Acquired Pneumonia] and Case 42 [Neutropenic Fever].)

R6. **A. This patient has carcinoid syndrome caused by metastasis of a neuroendocrine serotonin secreting tumor.** Carcinoid tumors are neuroendocrine tumors usually arising in the appendix that secrete serotonin. The serotonin excretion is usually asymptomatic when the tumor arises in the GI tract due to the liver detoxifying the serotonin into inactive metabolites. However, when there are metastases to the liver serotonin excretion becomes symptomatic. Clinical manifestations often include profuse watery diarrhea, episodes of flushing and bronchospasm, and valvular lesions affecting the right side of the heart, such as tricuspid regurgitation. Niacin deficiency is a potential complication due to increased conversion of tryptophan to serotonin, manifesting as dermatitis, diarrhea, and dementia. The next best test would be 24-hour urine 5-hydroxyindoleacetic acid levels which would be increased with someone suffering from carcinoid syndrome. Choice B (24-hour urine metanephrines) would be a screening test for pheochromocytoma that would present as a patient suffering from persistently high blood pressure and episodes of severe HTN and severe headache. Choice C (endoscopy with colonoscopy) would be the next appropriate test to diagnose Crohn disease, an irritable bowel disease that presents with chronic nonbloody diarrhea, weight loss, possible anemia from diseased ileum and other manifestations such as uveitis, arthritis, and skin lesions. Choice D (methacholine challenge) is the appropriate diagnostic test to evaluate for asthma which is characterized by bronchospasm and wheezing though it is usually diagnosed as a child and without long-standing diarrhea. Choice E (secretin injection test) is the diagnostic test of choice to evaluate for Zollinger-Ellison syndrome (ZES), a gastrinoma that is a pancreatic islet cell tumor. Clinical manifestations include side effects related to excessive gastrin production such as gastric ulcers, abdominal pain, and diarrhea. Secretin usually suppresses gastrin; however, patients with ZES would demonstrate high gastrin levels after the secretin injection test (see Case 47 [Syndrome of Inappropriate Secretion of Antidiuretic Hormone]).

R7. **D. This patient has a nephrotic syndrome secondary to hepatitis B.** Nephrotic syndrome is defined as an abnormal glomerular permeability secondary to many causes. It results in urine protein excretion >3.5 g/24 h, hypoalbuminemia, hyperlipidemia, edema, hypercoagulable state, and an increased risk for infection. Membranous nephropathy is the most common cause of primary nephrotic syndrome in Caucasian adults, and the most common secondary cause is hepatitis B. Histologic examination will demonstrate diffuse capillary and glomerular basement membrane thickening. Choice A (diabetic nephropathy) presents as a nephrotic syndrome from nonenzymatic glycosylation of the basement membrane in a patient with long-standing uncontrolled diabetes that on histologic examination will demonstrate mesangial expansion, eosinophilic nodular glomerulosclerosis also known as Kimmelstiel-Wilson lesions. Choice B (focal segmental glomerulosclerosis) is a nephrotic syndrome associated with African Americans and Hispanics and can be secondary to conditions such as HIV and sickle cell disease. Choice C (IgA nephropathy) usually presents as a nephritic syndrome characterized by HTN, azotemia, oliguria, and hematuria following a upper respiratory infection or gastroenteritis. Choice E (minimal change disease) is the most common cause of nephrotic syndrome in children that is caused by T-cell dysfunction (see Case 24 [Cirrhosis] and Case 29 [Nephrotic Syndrome]).

R8. **B. This patient is suffering a deep venous thrombosis (DVT) secondary to a hypercoagulable state.** Those with nephrotic syndrome are in a hypercoagulable state primarily due to a loss of antithrombin III in the urine (see Case 29 [Nephrotic Syndrome]).

R9. **C. This patient is suffering from Dressler syndrome, which is an autoimmune reaction occurring 2 to 10 weeks after a myocardial infarction.** Dressler syndrome is caused by an autoimmune reaction to the pericardium several weeks after a MI that results in fibrinous pericarditis. Appropriate treatment is NSAIDs and high-dose aspirin. Clinical presentation is usually weeks to months after a myocardial infarction that presents with fever, malaise, and pericarditis (chest pain with a friction rub that improves when leaning forward). Choices A (nitroglycerin and metoprolol) and B (morphine and supplemental oxygen) are appropriate treatments during the acute phase of a MI, and only nitroglycerin and metoprolol should be initiated as maintenance therapy after the MI. Choice D (IV heparin and clopidogrel) are appropriate treatments for anticoagulation during another MI or for a left ventricular mural thrombus. Choice E (IV vancomycin and ceftriaxone) is appropriate treatment for bacterial endocarditis that would most likely present with fever and a new murmur (see Case 3 [Acute Myocardial Infarction]).

R10. **D. A urine dipstick that is positive for blood and a urinalysis with few microscopic RBCs is highly suggestive of myoglobinuria.** Rhabdomyolysis is caused by excessive rapid muscle breakdown as a result of crush injury, trauma, seizures (in this patient), prolonged immobility, or snake bites. As muscle breaks down, myoglobin is released into the blood stream and filtered by the kidneys. Myoglobin is toxic to the glomerulus and can cause an acute kidney injury via acute tubular necrosis. Typically, the creatinine kinase levels are markedly elevated. Given the injury to the kidney is intrinsic and impairs renal function, BUN:Cr ratio will be <20 and the kidney will be unable to conserve sodium and concentrate the urine. Choice A (vascular inflammation) is more consistent with the pathophysiology of nephritic syndrome that is characterized by HTN, azotemia, oliguria, and hematuria. Choice B (outflow obstruction) is more consistent with a postrenal kidney injury secondary to obstruction of the ureter, bladder, or urethra. Diagnosis would be made by physical examination, ultrasounds, and catheterization, noting renal failure is present when kidneys are obstructed bilaterally and when the obstruction is removed, renal function is restored. Choice C (poor renal perfusion) is the pathophysiology behind prerenal failure usually secondary to decreased cardiac output, hypotension, or volume loss/sequestration. Laboratory values will include a BUN:Cr of

>20 and a preserved function of the kidney to concentrate urine and reabsorb sodium (see Case 30 [Acute Renal Failure]).

R11.   **B. This patient is suffering from cor pulmonale, right-sided heart failure secondary to a chronic lung disease.** Clinical signs suggestive of cor pulmonale in this patient include jugular venous distention, hepatojugular reflex and no crackles on lung auscultation. Differentiating between left and right heart failure can be difficult especially when left ventricular failure can often lead to right ventricular dysfunction. However, given this patient's long-standing smoking history and no evidence of left ventricular dysfunction such as orthopnea or pulmonary edema, the cause of his heart failure is most likely due to right ventricular dysfunction (as evidenced by the parasternal heave) due to long-standing pulmonary disease. On chest x-ray the lungs would be clear and there would be evidence of hyperinflation with depression of the diaphragm. The pulmonary artery will also be prominent from increased pulmonary pressures over time. Choice A (bilateral pulmonary infiltrates) is more consistent with pulmonary edema and the transduction of fluid into the lungs from increased pulmonary venous pressure via left ventricular dysfunction. Choice C (unilateral lobar consolidation) is consistent with a lobar pneumonia that presents as a patient with fever, cough, and shortness of breath with or without secretions and crackles on auscultation of the lobe with consolidation. Choice D (widened mediastinum) is consistent with an aortic dissection that usually presents as a patient with tearing chest pain radiating to the back that has long-standing hypertension or collagen-vascular disease such as Marfan syndrome. Choice E (multiple pulmonary nodules) would be consistent with pulmonary cancer (see Case 4 [Congestive Heart Failure]).

R12.   **C. There is an increased risk for lymphoma of the thyroid for patients diagnosed with Hashimoto thyroiditis.** Hashimoto thyroiditis is an autoimmune condition common in middle-aged females characterized by antibodies toward components of the thyroid gland. Initially patients may present with a transient period of hyperthyroidism due to release of thyroid hormone from follicle rupture. Eventually patients will present with symptoms of hypothyroidism such as weight gain, fatigue, cold intolerance, constipation, dry cool skin, and thin, brittle hair. Diagnosis of Hashimoto thyroiditis is made clinically by physical examination of diffusely enlarged thyroid with possibly rubbery texture, symptoms of hypothyroidism and elevated TSH with positive antithyroid peroxidase antibodies or histologically from thyroid fine-needle aspiration. These patients are at an increased risk for lymphoma of the thyroid. Other neoplasms of the thyroid are associated with different disease processes. Choice A (anaplastic carcinoma of the thyroid) is associated with older patient population with history of long-standing follicular or papillary carcinoma and is highly malignant. Choice B (follicular carcinoma of the thyroid) may be associated with iodine deficiency and more malignant than papillary cancer. Biopsy would be the only way to differentiate follicular carcinoma from a benign adenoma, by assessing whether there is extension into surrounding vasculature or through the capsule. Choice D (medullary carcinoma of the thyroid is associated multiple endocrine neoplasia type 2A (MEN2A) and MEN2B syndromes arising from the parafollicular cells (C cells) that produce calcitonin. Choice E (papillary carcinoma of the thyroid) is associated with a history of radiation of the head and neck during childhood and histologic examination would demonstrate empty-appearing nuclei with central clearing (see Case 53 [Thyrotoxicosis]).

INDEX

Page numbers followed by f or t indicate figures or tables, respectively.

A

AAA. *See* abdominal aortic aneurysm
abatacept, 319
ABCD^2 score, 334t
abdominal aortic aneurysm (AAA),
    60–61, 63–65, 284
ABGs. *See* arterial blood gases
ABI. *See* ankle-brachial index
abnormal bleeding, 509–515
ABO blood types, 502
abruptio placentae, 511
abscess
    in diverticulitis, 209t, 211
    pancreatic, 236, 239
acarbose, 467t
ACAS. *See* Asymptomatic Carotid Artery
    Stenosis trial
accelerated idioventricular rhythm, 44
ACE inhibitors. *See* angiotensin-converting
    enzyme inhibitors
acetaminophen, 97, 137, 241, 242, 514
    for low back pain, 301
    nomogram for, 243f, 246, 248
    for osteoarthritis, 288, 290, 292
acetaminophen hepatitis, 246–248
acetaminophen hepatotoxicity, 242
Acetest, 539, 540, 542
acetylcholinesterase inhibitors, 340
N-acetylcysteine, 247
acid-base disorders, 541t
acid-fast bacillus (AFB) culture, 397
acidosis. *See also* diabetic ketoacidosis;
    metabolic acidosis
    lactic, 541
    nonanion gap, 478, 479
    renal tubular, 540, 544, 546
    respiratory, 541t, 544, 547
ACIP. *See* Advisory Committee on
    Immunization Practices
acoustic neuromas, 359, 361t, 362,
    363

acquired immunodeficiency syndrome
    (AIDS), 183, 417, 418, 422, 423
    acetaminophen hepatitis and, 246
    adrenal involvement in, 447
    meningitis in, 391
ACTH. *See* adrenocorticotropic hormone
ACTH stimulation test, 446–447, 448, 450
acute adrenal insufficiency, 447
acute angle-closure glaucoma, 350t
acute arterial occlusion, 133, 136
acute chest syndrome, 526, 527, 528, 530
acute cholecystitis, 237, 238
acute coronary syndrome, 38, 50
acute cough, 156
acute cystitis, 375, 380
acute diarrhea, 215–216, 221
acute diverticulitis, 207, 211
acute endocarditis, 123
acute glomerulonephritis, 260–261, 264f
acute heart failure, 52
acute hemolytic reaction, 501, 502
acute hepatic failure, 248
acute hepatitis, 243
acute hepatocellular necrosis, 254t
acute HIV syndrome, 418
acute kidney injury (AKI), 262, 278, 279
    causes of intrinsic, 281t
    causes of prerenal, 280t
    dialysis indications in, 282
acute leukemia, 386, 513, 514
acute lymphoblastic leukemia (ALL), 381
acute lymphoid leukemia (ALL), 519
acute myeloid leukemia (AML), 519
acute myocardial infarction, 38–47, 48,
    50, 108
    acute pericarditis *versus*, 109t
    cardiac biomarkers and, 41–42
    complications, 44–45
    diagnostic criteria, 39–42
    electrocardiogram for, 40–41, 41f
    history and, 39

563